The **EYE** and **NUTRITION**

www.slackbooks.com

ISBN: 978-1-55642-964-4

Graphic design and page layout for the Italian edition:
I.N.C. Innovation-News-Communication s.r.l.

Published by: SLACK Incorporated
6900 Grove Road
Thorofare, NJ 08086 USA
Telephone: 856-848-1000
Fax: 856-848-6091
www.slackbooks.com

Library of Congress Cataloging-in-Publication Data

Buratto, Lucio.
[Occhio e nutrizione. English]
The eye and nutrition / Lucio Buratto ; with invaluable assistance from Eugenio Del Toma ... [et al.] ; presented by Umberto Veronesi.
p. cm.
Includes bibliographical references and index.
ISBN 978-1-55642-964-4 (pbk. : alk. paper) 1. Eye--Diseases--Nutritional aspects. 2. Cookery. I. Del Toma, Eugenio. II. Title.
RE48.B8713 2010
641.5'63--dc22
2010001126

Bianca... I hope that joy, happiness and love will always surround you and guide you throughout your life... Your Lucio

Printed in the United States of America.

Last digit is print number: 10 9 8 7 6 5 4 3 2 1

The **EYE** and **NUTRITION**

Lucio Buratto, MD

With invaluable assistance from

Eugenio Del Toma and Nazareno Marabottini

and

Mauro Febbrari Defendente, Natalya Ushakova,
Riccardo De Prà, Stefania Agrigento

Foreword by

Umberto Veronesi

SLACK
INCORPORATED

Authors

LUCIO BURATTO, MD
Specialist in Ophthalmology
Centro Ambrosiano di Microchirurgia Oculare
Milan, Italy

NAZARENO MARABOTTINI
Chief Consultant for the U.O.C. Ophthalmology I Department
Health Trust S. Giovanni Addolorata
Rome, Italy

EUGENIO DEL TOMA
Emeritus Chief Consultant in Dietology and Diabetology
Health Trust San Camillo-Forlanini
Rome, Italy
Honorary President of the Italian Association of Dietetics and Clinical Nutrition

MAURO FEBBRARI DEFENDENTE
Endocrinologist, Diabetologist, and Nutritionist
Bergamo, Italy

RICCARDO DE PRA'
Chef
Hotel-Restaurant "Dolada"
Plois d'Alpego
Belluno, Italy

NATALYA USHAKOVA
Graduate in Economics and Commerce
University "Luigi Bocconi"
Milan, Italy

STEFANIA AGRIGENTO
Biologist Specializing in Nutrition
Freelance
Rome, Italy

Contents

Good Food Recipes Contents

Good Food Recipes Contents

Good Food Recipes Contents

Good Food Recipes Contents

ABOUT THE AUTHOR

Dr. Lucio Buratto graduated with degrees in medicine and surgery from the University of Milan where he also specialized in clinical ophthalmology.

As an eye surgeon, Dr. Buratto specializes in the surgical treatment of cataract; he also specializes in refractive surgery (correction of myopia, astigmatism, and hyperopia); for his work in both sectors, he has earned international acclaim.

The principal milestones of his professional career follow:

- *He was one of the first surgeons in Europe to perform Kelman's phacoemulsification, a technique for cataract extraction that is still considered to be the most sophisticated surgical method today.*
- *In parallel, he started using artificial lenses for insertion in the posterior chamber following phacoemulsification.*
- *Subsequently, he performed sutureless cataract surgery and began implanting foldable artificial lenses.*
- *He published the first book on modern cataract surgery that, for many years, was considered to be the Italian "bible" for this type of surgery; in the years that followed, he published a number of other books dealing with the same topic.*
- *He was the first surgeon worldwide to suggest and use the excimer laser inside the cornea for the treatment of severe myopia (a technique now known as LASIK). Subsequently, he began treating mild myopia with surface techniques (PRK).*
- *He then invented and was the first surgeon worldwide to use the new LASIK down-up technique, a major improvement to the original LASIK procedure for the correction of myopia. He holds the US patent for this technique.*
- *He was appointed by the US FDA to monitor studies involving some new artificial lenses.*
- *Due to his groundbreaking innovations in the field of eye surgery, he was nominated "Maestro dell'Oftalmologia Italiana" by the Italian Ophthalmology Society.*
- *He was presented with the highest international award for a refractive surgeon—the "Barraquer" award—for his research and innovative developments to laser refractive surgery.*
- *In 2002, he published* Phacoemulsification: Principles and Techniques *in English and Spanish, a book that proved to be an international bestseller.*
- *He received the Award Certificate issued by the American Academy of Ophthalmology.*
- *In 2006, he was the first surgeon in Europe to transplant a cornea using the Intralase femtosecond laser.*
- *Each year in Milan, he organizes the most important Italian conference on cataract surgery with the participation of the most renowned international surgeons.*
- *He has participated in 370 Italian and international conferences as speaker and lecturer and has organized 54 teaching courses specific for cataract surgery.*
- *He has been included in the Italian Who's Who listing since 1984.*
- *He has performed many thousands of cataract and refractive surgeries.*

He is a member of 12 Societies of Ophthalmology, including American Academy of Ophthalmology (AAO), International Society of Refractive Surgery (ISRS), American Society of Cataract and Refractive Surgery (ASCRS), European Society of Cataract and Refractive Surgery (ESCRS), and The International Intra-Ocular Implant Club (IIIC).

He is a past President of the Associazione Italiana di Chirurgia della Cataratta e Chirurgia Refrattiva (Italian Association of Cataract and Refractive Surgery).

He is the current honorary president of AISO, Accademia Italiana di Scienze Oftalmologiche (Italian Academy of Ophthalmology Sciences).

FOREWORD

I have known Lucio Buratto for many years. I harbor deep admiration for him on both a professional and cultural level. We have a common passion for scientific research, and though we travel along different medical paths, the roads we take often lead us to common goals. One of these is prevention, which we both consider to be essential in safeguarding our health.

Prevention is something that drives us to change a number of factors that are sometimes beyond our control. They do not depend on us; we can transform them into factors that we can influence and change into something better. The core component of prevention is personal behavior (which is approximately 40% responsible for our health according to some American studies). Don't smoke, eat a healthy diet, and exercise daily. These are just some of the activities that we, and only we, can control. These are the cornerstones of prevention. However, prevention must be supported by valid, good quality information, which is exactly what can be found in the pages of this book.

Buratto is a top expert in his scientific field, and with this latest book, he takes an in-depth look at a topic that many may take for granted: diet and the preventive value of correct nutrition. It is a well-known fact that a well-balanced diet plays an extremely important role not only in maintaining the body in good health, but in supplying the body with all the nutrients it requires for correct performance. In this book, Buratto focuses his attention on the eye, the organ at the core of his work as a surgeon and the object of all his research. He does this in a way that is captivating, curious, and rich with valuable information (wonderful recipes!), and I admit that I read it with great interest.

In brief, Buratto describes the eye as an organ of extreme importance and in order to work to the best of its ability, like every other structure in the body, and possibly more than any other, it must be given the right nutrients at the right doses. But that's not all. A good diet specifically for the eye can reduce the incidence of two sight-threatening conditions—the onset of cataract and age-related macular degeneration. Numerous epidemiological studies and clinical observations have underlined the protective role of some antioxidants; vitamins A, B, and E; and the macular pigments (luteine, which is found in many types of vegetables, and zeaxathine).

Buratto emphasizes that the role of the ophthalmologist or eye specialist lies not only in the identification of pathologies of the eye, the prescription of the right drugs to treat the problems, or good surgical procedures, he or she must also be able to give advice regarding the prevention of the illnesses and even suggest a correct diet. A healthy lifestyle is the theme of the book, where readers can understand the importance of the quality of the food and the quantity, which must never be excessive. I am a vegetarian and have always recommended that my patients eat frequent small meals. Once again, my dear friend Lucio Buratto and I agree wholeheartedly on this philosophy.

Umberto Veronesi

INTRODUCTION

A proper diet means loving oneself

For millions of years, the photoreceptors in the human eye have been working under relatively constant conditions; the light sources were natural (the sun), the physical properties of the light were stable, the amount of illumination corresponded to the length of the day, the workload for the eye was relatively limited, and the diet was simple and based on unprocessed produce from nature.

Down through the millennia, the histological organization and the functional state of the eye has evolved on the basis of the above-mentioned conditions, with minor variations based on the earth's different latitudes.

However, during the past century, this has all changed: the eye operates with a range of illumination types for 12 to 16 hours every day, and the amount of work the eye performs from the moment it opens in the morning to the final blink before the regenerating night's sleep is enormous; the commitment asked of the eye every day is quite incredible, but it is unlikely to stop here. On the contrary, it is destined to increase with the future evolution of the human race.

The eye should be assisted and supported as much as possible; but this is not necessarily the case because, during the past century in particular, diet has changed drastically, with a huge shift toward carbohydrates and fats. As a result, there is not just an increase in the number of people affected by dyslipidemia, the amount of fruit and vegetables included in the diet has decreased, and with it the quantity of antioxidants, which are protective agents for the eye. Moreover, the alteration in the ozone layer has greatly increased the amount of radiation in the blue band that generates a greater quantity of free radicals particularly in the eye. This can lead to a state of precocious aging of the structures, and this in conjunction with smoking and other toxic factors, psychophysical stress and atmospheric and environmental pollution means that drastic measures need to be taken to protect the eye.

For several decades, the eye's requirement for antioxidants has increased and continues to increase. Consequently, we must increase the quantities through food consumption. A normal diet does not supply a sufficient amount of antioxidants; in fact, the daily requirement for luteine in our latitudes is much higher than the amount normally supplied by food.

However, is it really necessary to increase the quantity of antioxidants introduced with food? The answer is yes and not only where the eye is concerned but for the human body as a whole. This is because the protective effect of antioxidants has been demonstrated in numerous trials. Among them, luteine is possibly the most important antioxidant agent because it impounds free electrons and reduces the formation of radicals.
Man must pay more attention to the everyday diet, and if necessary, use carefully selected integrators.
A correct diet is something that everyone should follow if they wish to enjoy good health and maintain an optimal body weight.
In the first place, a correct diet means the right amount of food consumed, selected on the basis of the calorie intake on the one hand and the energy requirements of the individual on the other. It also means an intake of all the necessary ingredients, consumed in a well-balanced and suitably proportioned diet.
Second, people should eat large quantities of raw and cooked fruit and vegetables as these products are rich in minerals, vitamins, fibers, and particularly antioxidants.
Third, food should be consumed in smaller quantities throughout the day as opposed to concentrating the whole daily intake into 2 or 3 meals.
Keeping in mind these simple rules, which will be presented in more detail in this book, we can give our body all its daily requirements without overloading it with extra work, and we can create the matrix for the excellent performance of all its functions. And our eyes, these precious organs of sight, which are so important for our daily lives, will enjoy considerable benefit from the right diet, or at least be less susceptible to eye pathologies that can negatively influence our everyday visual activities.

Lucio Buratto

Part I

Eugenio Del Toma

Dietary Prevention

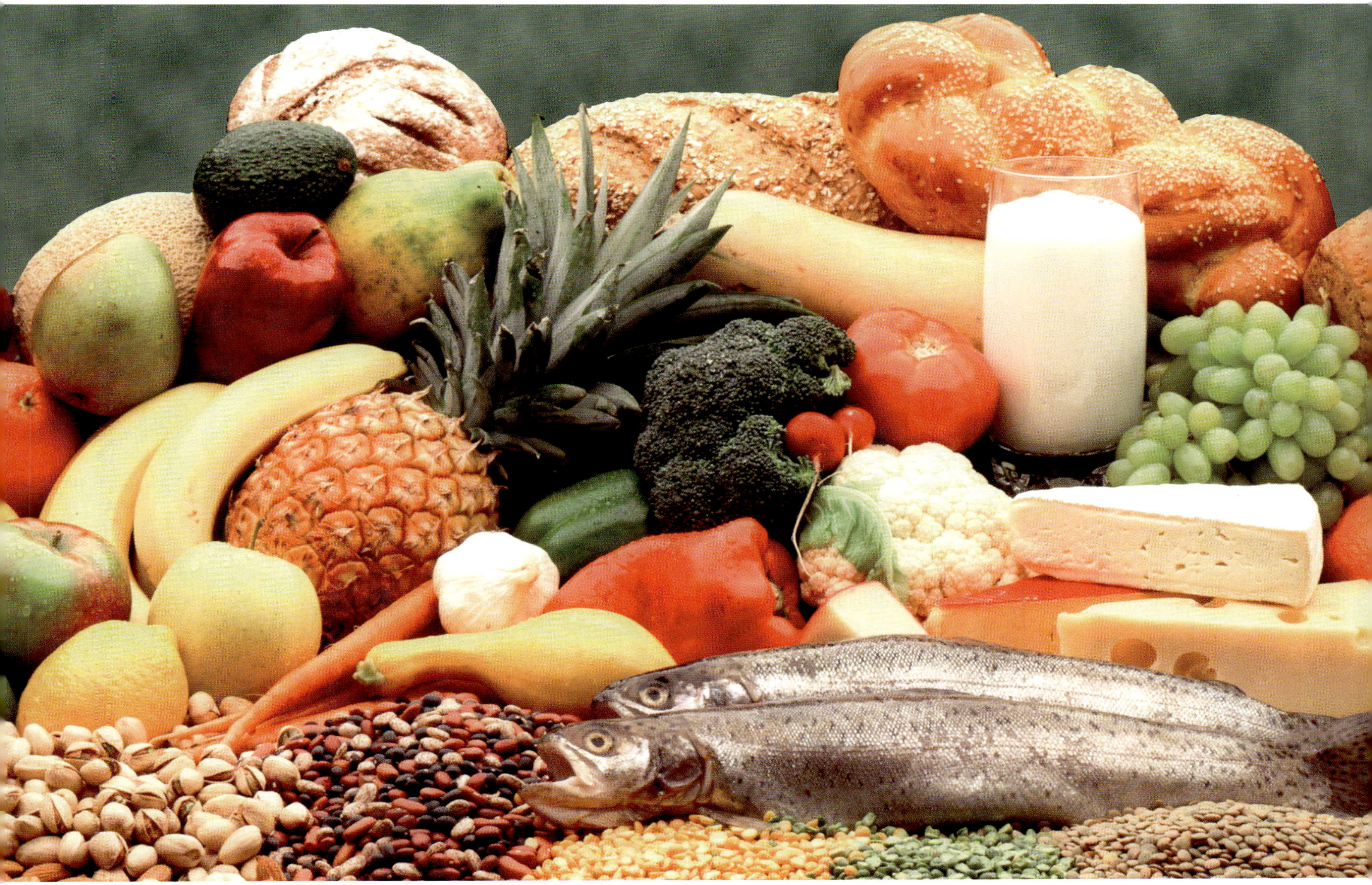

Guidelines, food pyramids, and other advice

For some years, the health officials of the more developed countries have used the mass media to broadcast the more important rules for human nutrition. Nevertheless, it is not easy, even for the experts, to translate into a handful of phrases a summary of a complex subject such as food science, based on the principles of physiology and biochemistry, which occasionally upset the ancient and empirical old wives' tales regarding the nutritional value of each food.

First, we need to mediate between the complexity of the subject and the need to supply, in simplified terms, the practical conclusions that can prevent or delay the appearance of pathologies caused or encouraged by the persistence of dietary errors. If the widespread availability of food has eliminated, at least in Italy, the phenomenon of malnutrition, contributing to increasing life expectancy, it is also true that the excess and the disorder of the choices encourage obesity and the appearance of a series of chronic degenerative pathologies such as arteriosclerosis, diabetes, macular degeneration, and even some tumors.

Excess and disorder in the choice of food will encourage obesity and the appearance of chronic degenerative pathologies, such as arteriosclerosis, diabetes, macular degeneration, and even tumors.

Food pyramids

Americans, who are more attentive to simplicity and efficacy of the message when compared to the Europeans, have adopted the symbol of the pyramid, which provides a visual representation of the concept of the frequency and recommended amount of consumption of the food at the base of the pyramid, with respect to those on the upper levels *(Figure 1.1)*.

The transposition of the American pyramid in Italy, without the appropriate adaptations to our great tradition of gastronomic history, gave rise to many complaints. The Guidelines for a Healthy Italian Diet was better accepted. It was processed by the National Research Institute for Food and Diet (INRAN) and will be summarized in this book.

In fact, the American food pyramid and the excessive number of variants that derived from it, without any precise references to the portions and the frequency of consumption *(Table 1.1)*, could have suggested that only the foods at the base were truly essential. This is not the case because all the foods can and must make their individual contribution to the total and to the variety of the diet, in very different quantitative limits.

For greater clarity, we can state that in the gasoline used by some types of car engines, there must be a quantity of oil, possibly only 2% but this does not mean that the oil is less important than the gas with which it is mixed. In actual fact, both ingredients are essential for the good performance

Each food can and must provide their individual contribution to the total and the variety in a well-balanced diet, though in greatly differing quantities.

of the engine, even though the percentages and quantities differ greatly. The same applies to the vitamins, minerals, or certain molecules that the body is not able to synthesize such as some amino acids or certain fatty acids defined as essential because of the dependency of our body's metabolism on the external intake.

Figure 1.1

Food Pyramid, proposed by USDA (1992) and then updated to promote a well-balanced healthy diet, thanks to the number of servings (see Table 1.1)

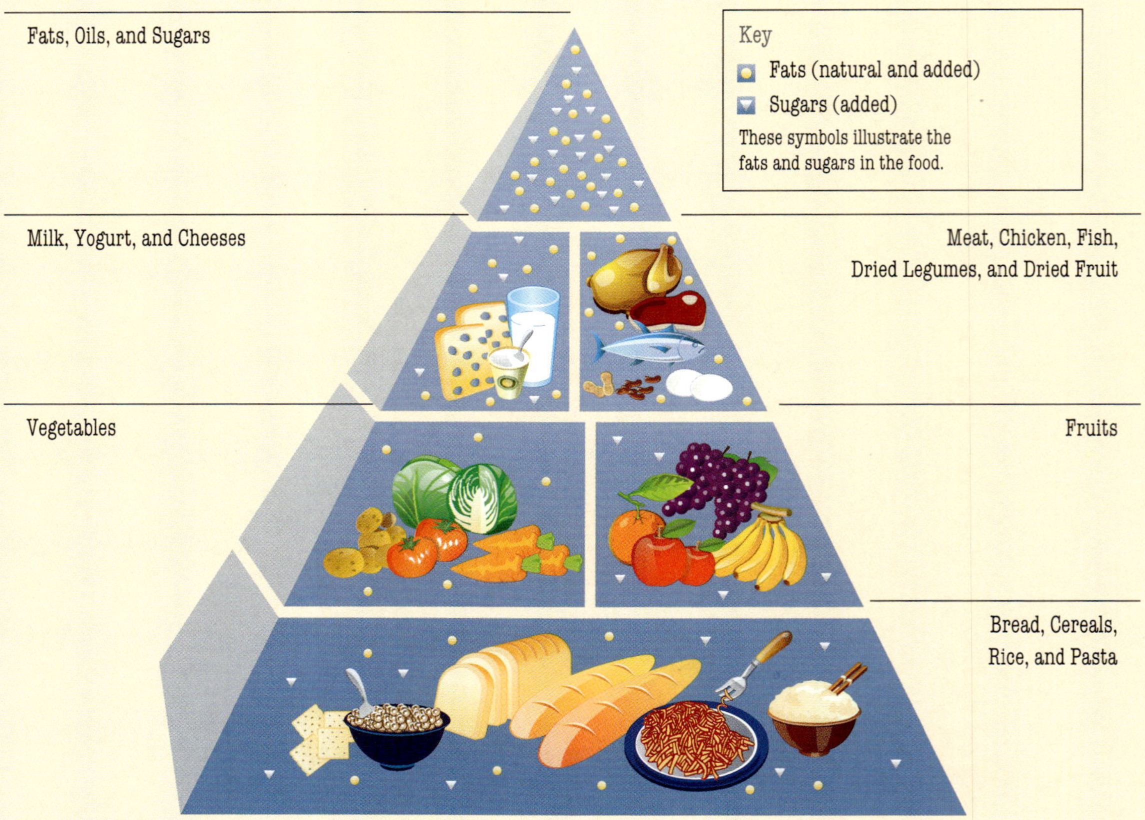

Table 1.1

Servings of the main food in the various groups and the number of servings needed to create a daily food intake of approximately 2000 kCal.

FOOD GROUPS	FOOD	Serving	NUMBER OF ServingS/DAY
MILK AND DAIRY	Milk	½ cup (1 glass)	2
	Yogurt	½ cup (1 tub)	2
	Mature cheese	1.8 oz	0 to 1
	Fresh cheese	3.5 oz	0 to 1
MEAT, FISH, EGGS	Fresh meat	3.5 oz	1
	Cured meats	1.8 oz	1
	Fish	5.3 oz	1
	Eggs	one (approx 50 g)	0 to 1
LEGUMES	Fresh beans	3.5 oz	0 to 1
	Dried beans	1 oz	0 to 1
CEREALS AND POTATOES	Potatoes	7 oz	0 to 1
	Bread	1.8 oz	3 to 4
	Baked products	1.8 oz	0 to 1
	Pasta or rice (*)	2.8 oz	1
	Fresh egg pasta (*)	4.2 oz	1
	Fresh filled pasta (*)	6.3 oz	1
FRUITS AND VEGETABLES	Lettuce	1.8 oz	2 to 4
	Vegetables	1 cup	2 to 4
	Fruits or juices	5.3 oz	2 to 4
FATS FOR SEASONING	Oil	2 tsp	3
	Butter	2 tsp	0 to 1
	Margarine	2 tsp	0 to 1

(*) In soups, the amount should be halved.

Bread should be eaten every day in the recommended amount. Baked goods must be eaten at breakfast or between meals. For the main courses, over a week, the following frequency of consumption is recommended: 3 to 4 servings of meat, 2 to 3 servings of fish, 2 to 3 servings of cheese, 2 to 3 servings of egg, and 1 to 2 servings of cured meat. Once or twice a week, the main course should be replaced with a single dish based on pasta or rice with beans, in the servings indicated for each of the 2 foods. Milk and/or yogurt should be consumed every day (2 servings). A bowl of milk is equivalent to 2 glasses. The servings of vegetables (2 to 4 per day) can include a serving of minestrone or creamed vegetable soup; alternately, a serving can be used to season pasta or rice (zucchini, eggplant, mushrooms, fresh tomatoes, artichokes, asparagus, etc). The servings of fresh or dried fruit can be consumed between meals. Olive oil is the recommended fat for seasoning; butter or margarine is occasionally permitted.

RDA and Guidelines published by the National Research Institute for Food and Diet are the official sources of information that assemble scientific recommendations, traditions and legitimate gastronomic satisfaction.

The 10 guidelines and RDAs

Given that the pyramid can lend itself to blatant advertising, it would be a good idea to examine the 10 golden rules that have been reviewed and reproposed by INRAN in 2003, in harmony with the dietary goals set by the American experts *(Table 1.2)*.

Each guideline should also be examined in relation to the recommended daily allowance (RDA), presented by INRAN in collaboration with the experts of the major Italian Scientific Societies, jointly interested in the dietary problems of research, clinical application and prevention.

The latest edition of RDAs is a scientific document intended for experts, unlike the Guidelines.

With the guidelines of these technical elements, originating from official sources, we can summarize the behavior of the consumer who wishes to combine his or her love of food and dietary traditions with respect for the nutritional rules.

The objective is difficult only in appearance; it can be reached with fewer sacrifices than would generally be imagined as long as within the quantitative and qualitative selection of food; that is, the energy intake is associated with the attention for the energy consumption, which the excessively sedentary lifestyle has reduced in recent decades beyond every possible physiological compensation.

Control weight and keep active.

On the other hand, this concept is a priority even as part of the INRAN Guidelines where the #1 rule is *"Control weight and keep active."*

Table 1.2

The 10 golden rules/guidelines established by INRAN for a healthy Italian diet

1. Control weight and keep active.
2. Eat more cereals, legumes, fruits, and vegetables.
3. Fats: choose the quality, restrict the quantity.
4. Sugars, sweets, and sugary drinks: in the appropriate amounts.
5. Drink plenty of water every day.
6. Salt: use small amounts.
7. Alcoholic drinks: if consumed, only in moderation.
8. Frequently vary your diet.
9. Special advice for special people.
10. The guarantee of safety in the food depends exclusively on you.

Cereals, beans, fruits, and vegetables: the antioxidants

The second piece of advice proposed by the Guidelines is: "*Eat more cereals, legumes, fruits, and vegetables*." This vegetarian orientation recommends eating more fruits and vegetables every day and is more suitable for people who have reduced their physical activity to a minimum, with respect to the increased availability of food, which exceeds the recommended daily requirements of proteins and fats.

The rules of physiology teach that in a well-balanced diet, at least 50% to 60% of the food intake must originate from carbohydrates *(Table 2.1)*. By way of clarification, we should remember that there are complex carbohydrates (found in cereals and legumes) that are absorbed slowly by the intestine, and there are simple carbohydrates (sucrose, glucose, fructose) that consist of just one or two molecules and are easier to digest and rapidly absorbed.

It should be emphasized that the carbohydrates in the food intake for the most part (at least 75%) must originate from complex carbohydrates. No more than 25% can be derived from simple carbohydrates, for example sucrose, common table sugar from cane, or beetroot used as a sweetener. This is because an excessively rapid introduction of glucose (the simplex sugar molecule that along with fructose is the final form of carbohydrate utilization) leads to excessive insulin stimulation with hormonal problems and metabolic overload.

The rules of physiology teach that in a well-balanced diet, at least 50% to 60% of the food intake must originate from carbohydrates.

It should be emphasized that the carbohydrates in the food intake for the most part (at least 75%) must originate from complex carbohydrates.

Table 2.1

Optimal proportions for the nutrients in the daily portions for an energy input of 2000 kCal

ENERGY 2000 kCal					
Protein 75 g (15% of the energy)	Carbohydrates 290 g (55% of the energy)		Lipids 65 g (30% of the energy)		
	Starch 220 g	Carbohydrates soluble	Saturated (7% energy)	Mono-unsaturated (18% energy)	Poly-unsaturated (4% energy)
Fiber 23 g		Cholesterol 255 mg			

Carbohydrates and the glycemic index

The most important feature of a carbohydrate is the simplicity of the molecule. Following digestion and absorption, it does not produce any waste that has to be eliminated (as happens for the nitrogen that characterizes the protein molecules), and it does not overload digestion and metabolism (as happens with fats).

Carbohydrates are a source of energy that is more congenial to cellular requirements, and if we compare them to the automobile, they are less "polluting" for the metabolism.

It should be mentioned at this point that everyone who "invents" his or her own diet for weight loss, without medical supervision, eliminating bread, pasta, and legumes, will be introducing fewer calories into his or her body but will also be changing the proportion of the nutrients in the food that form the basis of good metabolic performance.

When carbohydrate intake is excessively low, in order to satisfy the constant demand for glucose by the brain and other vital organs, the body is forced to obtain glucose from the glycogenetic amino acids before fats, which destroys the precious protein-building material to produce energy and this increases the workload for the kidneys in expelling the excess of nitrogen. So, we need to be careful that we do not start using a "green gas" for the machine that is our body.

We should also remember that foods rich in complex carbohydrates such as legumes, bread, and whole grain pasta also contain a considerable quantity of soluble and insoluble fiber.

Dietary fiber is a material with little or no energetic importance for man. However, it is useful for creating the sensation of fullness, for modulating the absorption times, and for encouraging intestinal peristalsis.

Fiber contained in food is a material that has little or no energetic value for man; nevertheless, it is useful for avoiding the sense of fullness, for modulating the absorption time, and for encouraging intestinal peristalsis. All of this is lost in a diet that has a low quantity of fruits and vegetables. The same applies to diets that are poor in cereals and that contain an excessive quantity of refined carbohydrates free from every trace of bran (eg, white pasta, widespread use of plain flour).

Sugar and sweets are the prototypes of food that are high in calories and lacking fibers. These are always reduced or eliminated from the diets of the obese and diabetics because of a perverted short-circuit of insulin resistance (hyperinsulinemia), which leads to obesity and hyperglycemia.

The studies that were initiated in the 1980s by Woolever and Jenkins et al introduced the concept of a glycemic index from the various starch- and sugar-based foods. In other words, with an equal total content of carbohydrates, some foods (legumes and pasta) have a lower glycemic index (ie, they raise the glycemic levels to a lesser degree) than potatoes, bread and rice, and necessitate a minimum production of insulin.

Other factors intervene on this characteristic (an important factor for diabetics, the obese, and athletes) such as the technological treatments and method of cooking but above all the simultaneous presence of vegetable fiber in terms of quality and quantity.

At a later stage, Jenkins used bread instead of glucose as the reference; nevertheless, this choice was criticized because of the relative variability of the terms of comparison with respect to the standard value of glucose.

Different foods, calculated to contain a similar quantity of carbohydrates (50 g) when consumed separately, provoke different glycemic responses. This is due to a number of factors such as the nature of the carbohydrate (complex or simple), the prevalence of amylose or amylopectin, the physical structure of the food, the type of cooking procedure, the presence and the viscosity of the fiber, etc *(Table 2.2)*. It stands to reason that, in a complete meal, the glycemic index of the individual food loses a good part of its mean, in relation to the complexity of the mouthful and the interference of the speed of intestinal transit, the rates of digestion and absorption of the carbohydrates.

Table 2.2

Glycemic index (GI) of various foods compared to bread

FOOD	GLYCEMIC INDEX
Glucose	138
Potatoes	106
Bread	100
Sucrose	90
Polished rice	83
Bananas	80
Oranges	66
Parboiled rice	65
Grapes	62
Spaghetti	59
Apples	53
Chick peas, garden peas	50
Beans, lentils	42 to 40

(Mod. from «Dietetica e Nutrizione». G. Fatati, 2007. Il Pensiero Scientifico Editore)

How much fiber and which types?

An appropriate daily consumption is recommended and even essential for good health and for the prevention of pathologies that are constantly on the increase such as the onset of diverticulitis (intestinal extroflexion) or chronic constipation. However, an excessively high intake of fiber should be avoided in states of acute intestinal inflammation (diarrhea, ulcerous colitis, etc) because it can restrict the absorption of mineral salts and some medicinal products. The recommended daily dose of fiber is approximately 30 g. Without consulting complicated tables, we can confirm that the typical Mediterranean diet, which is rich in cereals, legumes, and particularly fruits and vegetables, supplies an appropriate amount of dietary fiber with no need for any pharmacological supplements.

Not just vitamins and minerals but also antioxidants

In addition to their invaluable vitamin, mineral, and fiber content, fruits and vegetables have the added benefit of reinforcing the body's defenses and supplying an antioxidant heritage. In other words, they combat the excessive formation of free radicals that current scientific research blames for aging and cell degeneration.

In addition to their invaluable vitamin, mineral, and fiber content, fruits and vegetables have the added benefit of reinforcing the body's defenses and supplying an antioxidant heritage. In other words, they combat the damage caused by the excessive formation of free radicals.

The international scientific societies active in the fields of cardiology, metabolism, and oncology agree that consumption of fruits and vegetables is essential to reduce the possible damage from the excessive use of fats and animal protein. In particular, the wealth of natural antioxidants in fruits and vegetables appears to contain to a large degree the formation of free radicals (ie, the residues of metabolic activity that contribute to precocious cell aging and the deterioration of organic defenses).

Further studies, derived from this statistical evidence, aimed at identifying in particular which specific elements in fruits and vegetables (β-carotene, polyphenols, etc) contribute to strengthening the organic defenses even with regard to anticarcinogenic properties. The results were not conclusive but nevertheless justify the recommendation of increasing the consumption of fruits and vegetables (2 portions of vegetables and 2 portions of fruit each day in the quantity routinely served in any restaurant would be the optimum).

However, we still need to define whether the advantages of protection and prevention are derived from the individual dietary components or from the predominantly vegetarian eating habits.

The recommendation to increase the daily consumption of fruits and vegetables applies to everyone, but in particular to children, as it is essential that they learn to enjoy and appreciate the benefits of fruits and vegetables from a very young age. Moreover, this message should also be intercepted by the people involved in the food industry to ensure that everyone has the option of choosing the right type of vegetables.

How much fat, **which type** of fat

One of the first recommendations listed in the Guidelines, "*Fat: choose the quality and restrict the quantity*," tackles the problem that has upset the dietary habits not just of the Italians but of all the people who, thanks to industrial progress, no longer burn the large number of calories provided by dietary fat through physical activity, compared to the similar quantities of protein or carbohydrates.

Fats: choose the quality and restrict the quantity.

In fact, contemporary man puts on weight not just because of the almost unlimited availability of high-calorie food but also because of the reduced energy requirements of his lifestyle, where muscle power has been replaced by every imaginable type of useful instrument.

Manual work and living in a cold climate without adequate protection requires a much greater expenditure of energy compared to sitting at a desk, sitting in front of a computer in an acclimatized room, wearing clothes that reduce the cost of maintaining body temperature to a minimum!

One gram of edible fat, irrespective of the quality and the hepatic overload, will always provide 9 calories, compared with 4 calories of protein or carbohydrate.

Only the unadvisable energy source provided by alcohol approaches the calorie value of fats, in terms of energy potential (7 calories per gram).

Nevertheless, the fatty seasoning and foods that contribute so generously to our daily supply of energy is not a danger in itself, as long as the caloric intake counterbalances those effectively consumed and the energetic mixture of the food respects the percentage ratio of fats, proteins, and carbohydrates considered by metabolic physiopathology to be optimal.

It is no coincidence that past books on food biochemistry and physiology stated that, "Fats are burned on the pyre of carbohydrates"; even now, it is no rare occurrence to see patients attending diet clinics who are in a state of ketone-acidosis, with an extremely negative nitrogen balance and ketone particles in the urine, because they have been following an absurdly hypoglycidic diet in order to achieve more rapid weight loss.

The generic phobia to fats has been emphasized by the prevention campaign for hypercholesterolemia and therefore cardiac infarction, arteriosclerosis, obesity, and other dysmetabolic conditions and has completely upset the nutritional role of fats, presenting these substances as nonessential and dangerous. In actual fact, it is the excessive quantity and the poor quality of fats that should be addressed, always with the awareness that fats, in the right proportions, are an essential nutrient for life.

Fats are also essential components of our diet as they carry special molecules that our bodies would otherwise not be able to provide.

Not just lipophobia and cholesterolphobia

Polyunsaturated fats, including oleic acid (monounsaturated) can reduce the levels of cholesterol in blood, but have different effects on the HDL and LDL fractions.

Cholesterol, the compound mentioned with apprehension as though it were some sort of poison, is a substance synthesized by the body and present in all human cells, where it has essential life functions. Unfortunately, some people have a genetic difficulty with disposing of cholesterol, aggravated by the excessive consumption of food of animal origin. In these cases, the amount of cholesterol circulating in the blood (in particular, the feared LDL fraction) can increase to levels that can actually damage the cardiovascular system. However, this often occurs in the presence of additional risk factors, such as smoking, obesity, a sedentary lifestyle, constant stress, inflammation, and, according to recent hypotheses, when our antioxidant systems do not sufficiently protect the LDL lipoproteins from oxidation.

On the basis of many statistical-clinical observations, it has been shown particularly that some medium-chained saturated fatty acids (lauric, myristic, palmitic) electively but not exclusively present in fats of animal origin are atherogenic.

On the contrary, polyunsaturated fats (particularly linoleic acid contained in seed oils) and oleic acid (a monounsaturated fatty acid found in olive oil) tend to lower the levels of cholesterol in the blood.

Scientific studies in recent years have demonstrated that in addition to reducing the levels of the LDL lipoproteins, oleic acid has the advantage of not altering and in some cases improving the percentage of the artery-cleaning HDL cholesterol, which has the job of removing the excess cholesterol from blood and from the deposits in the arteries.

The benefits of fish oils and omega-3 fats

These thoughts lead to the renewed and consolidated appreciation that nutritionists have for olive and for fish oils (oily fish—anchovies, sardines, and mackerel; the salmon family—which should be eaten at least 2 to 3 times a week). They have characteristics of encouraging a reduction in the triglycerides, with better blood flow and a lower risk of thrombosis, so the consumer should pay more attention to the quantity and also the quality of fat in the diet *(Table 3.1)*.

Regarding the quantity, it is generally accepted by all specialists that the total amount of fat in the diet (and not just for seasoning but also the structural fats and those deposited in some foods) must not exceed 30% of the total caloric intake (although cardiologists suggest a level of approximately 25%).

In a normal healthy diet, 30% is equivalent to a maximum of 600 kCal per day, in other words 65 g of fat, given that 1 g of fat provides approximately 9 calories.

As part of the total that has already been indicated, the optimal percentage split between the various types of fatty acids is reported in *Table 3.2*.

Table 3.1

Total fat content, saturated fat, and cholesterol in some foods

FOODS	g OF FAT IN 100 g OF FOOD[1]	WEIGHT OF ONE PORTION	CONTENT PER PORTION		
			FAT	SATURATED FATTY ACIDS	CHOLESTEROL
	g	g	g	g	mg
Olive oil	100.0	10 (1 dessert spoon)	10.0	1.6	0
Butter	83.4	10 (1 portion)	8.3	4.9	25
Dried walnuts	68.1	16[2] (4 nuts)	4.1	0.3	0
Dried hazelnuts	64.1	16[2] (8 hazelnuts)	4.5	0.3	0
Milk chocolate	36.3	4 (1 square)	1.5	0.9	0.4
Dark chocolate	33.6	4 (1 square)	1.3	0.8	0
Salami	31.1	50 (8 to 10 medium slices)	15.5	4.9	45
Gruyére cheese	29.0	50 (1 portion)	14.5	8.8	9*
Parmesan	28.1	10 (1 dessert spoon)	2.8	1.8	9
Mozzarella (cow's milk)	19.5	100 (1 portion)	19.5	10.0*	46
Parma ham	18.4	50 (3 to 4 medium slices)	9.2	3.1	36
Plain croissant	18.3	40 (1 piece)	7.3	4.1*	30
Beef (lean meat)	10.2	70 (1 small slice)	7.1	2.2	46
Pork steak	8.0	70 (1 small slice)	5.6	2.5	43
Egg	8.7	50 (1 egg)	4.3	1.6	186
Pizza with tomato sauce	6.6	150 (1 portion)	9.9	1.0*	0
Parma ham (free of visible fat)	3.9	50 (3 to 4 medium slices)	2.0	0.7*	36
Whole milk	3.6	125 (1 glass)	4.5	2.6	14
Beef (silverside)	2.8	70 (1 small slice)	1.9	0.6	42
Anchovies or sardines	2.6	100 (1 small portion)	2.6	1.3	61
Partially skimmed milk	1.5	125 (1 glass)	1.9	1.1	9
Bread	0.4	50 (1 medium slice)	0.2	0.02*	0
Cod or hake	0.3	100 (1 small portion)	0.3	0.1	50
Skim milk	0.2	125 (1 glass)	0.3	0.2	3

N.B.: The values in the table have been taken from the Table of Food Composition (INRAN-Update 2000). Those marked with (*) have been taken from the Databank of Food Composition for epidemiological studies in Italy, European Institute of Oncology, 1998.
[1]Edible part, void of any waste.
[2]Gross weight.

(Mod. from «Linee Guida per una sana alimentazione italiana». INRAN, 2003)

Table 3.2

Optimal split of the lipid component in the diet

Quota	→ For healthy subjects: up to 30% of the daily caloric intake
	→ For prevention of atherosclerosis: 20% to 25%
SPLIT OF THE VARIOUS FATTY ACIDS	
Saturated fatty acids	Not more than 7% to 10% of the total calories
Monounsaturated fatty acids	Up to 20% of the total calories
Polyunsaturated fatty acids	Approximately 7% of the total caloric intake
	Have a ratio of omega-6/omega-3 of around 6

It is recommended that fats (particularly when unsaturated) be used in their crude form to avoid any alteration of their structure and the production of free radicals.

The popularity of the polyunsaturated oils has waned to some degree because their ability to lower cholesterol, different to the action of oleic acid, also involves the protective fraction (HDL cholesterol). Polysaturated fats have the tendency to oxidize, which can cause damage.
On this subject, people use crude fats (particularly the unsaturated ones) to avoid any alteration and the production of free radicals due to the action of heat and oxygen from the air.
Contrary to what too many consumers still believe, it is preferable to use olive oil or peanut oil for frying, instead of seed oils, which are highly unsaturated (particularly when the oil has to be used several times, a practice that should be discouraged).
However, the suggestion to moderate the daily quota of saturated fats should not be interpreted by healthy and physically active people as a total avoidance of butter, cheese, and meat, but should be accepted as a warning to limit the weekly consumption with respect to other preferential choices such as olive oil, fish, cereal, and legumes.
For people who are seriously affected by high cholesterol, these restrictions must be even more severe, and prior to using drug therapies (of the invaluable statin group), they should switch to the "low-fat" versions of many foods, which have a lipid content that is considerably lower than those of the traditional "full-fat" options.
Finally, the benefits of the polyunsaturated fatty acids such as the omega-3 deserve mention. These are found typically in oily fish such as sardines, anchovies, mackerel, and fish of the salmon family. In particular, eicopentaenoic acid (EPA) and docosahexaenoic acid (DHA) have been acclaimed primarily by cardiologists for their recognized cardioprotective and blood-thinning properties.

The omega-3s also have many other properties that are generally favorable and associated with their presence in the membrane phospholipids and therefore at the core of a number of physiopathological processes. In particular, it should be remembered that DHA accounts for some 8% to 20% of all fatty acids in the retina; it follows that a reduction in the retinal DHA levels will be associated with altered performance of the retinal tissue.

Docosahexaenoic acid (DHA) represents approximately 8% to 20% of all the fatty acids in the retina. It follows that a reduction in retinal DHA will be associated with altered performance of the retinal tissue.

Chapter 4

Animal and **vegetable proteins**

Man does not require proteins, but the amino acids that form the protein structures. The animal proteins supply all of the 8 "essential amino acids."

Everyone is aware that proteins play a complex role not only in cell turnover but in a series of functions essential for life. Science has managed to resist the antidemocratic distinction between "noble" proteins, or complete proteins of animal origin, and the "incomplete" proteins of plant origin.

In reality, the situation is very different. Man does not require proteins but the amino acids, the protein building blocks. If by mistake, the intestinal mucosa permitted the protein molecules to enter the blood before they are denatured into amino acids, unpleasant allergic reactions would result. The human body requires approximately 20 amino acids, and only 8 of these cannot be assembled from the elementary materials available in the body and must be introduced with the diet.

Animal proteins provide all 8 amino acids, labeled as the "essential amino acids," along with other more or less essential amino acids, which can be sourced independently and are incorrectly labeled "nonessential."

Vegetarians are well aware that this problem can be resolved because the proteins found in cereals and legumes (pasta and beans to be precise!) compensate synergetically for the mutual lack of one or more "limiting" amino acids, guaranteeing the necessary final completeness.

In times of poverty and famine, animal proteins when ingested in small quantities have provided a safety net for protein synthesis. However, the current abundance of food in Western countries, particularly red meat (at one time much fattier than the so-called "white meats"), leads to the danger of excessive intake of saturated fats.

Now, the myth "meat is always good" has been changed. Red or white meat is now only a commercial distinction because all meats have a lower fat content through genetic selection or the feed choices made by the breeder.

Due to worries associated with health and hygiene issues (eg, mad cow disease) and epidemiological factors (saturated fat as a concomitant cause of atherosclerosis), the number of vegetarians is increasing, at least in more developed societies. There are no criticisms of the vegetarians who still eat eggs and consume dairy products. However, there are various perplexities when—for ideological motives or for disputable health reasons—the strictest vegetarians (vegans) even refuse to feed their adolescent children with any food of animal origin, preventing them from ingesting a series of useful collateral nutrients (the guarantee of the complete amino-acid range, the vitamin B complex, iron, zinc, creatine, etc). Moreover, the voluntary abolition of animal proteins cancels the evolutionary advantage in the variety of food sources that omnivorous man has shown to possess over other animal species that are less ductile in metabolic terms.

Nevertheless, it should not be ignored that the International Scientific Societies recommend a daily intake of 1 g of protein per kg body weight (in other words, between 12% and 20% of the daily caloric intake). The average consumption is considerably higher, even when we exclude the trends of high-protein slimming regimens and the routine abuse (by professional and amateur athletes of all ages) of the so-called "protein integrators" used in the gyms and in a number of sporting disciplines.
From epidemiological studies and the published scientific literature regarding the protein requirements, there is the "evidence-based" conclusion that a deficiency in amino acids is harmful (leading to protein-energy malnutrition); however, it is also true that the excessive administration (in excess of 2 g/kg body weight) is of no use to anyone (athletes included) but long term, it is likely to be detrimental due to the consequent overload on the kidneys and liver.

The International Scientific Societies agree that a daily intake of 1 g of protein for every kg of body weight is appropriate (in other words between 12% and 20% of the daily caloric intake).

Chapter 5

Sweets and **desserts**: **irresistible temptations** (**allowed** in **just** the **right amounts**)

Diet fanatics have firmly condemned table sugar contrary to the scientific reality.

Thanks to the persuasive ability of mass advertising and the loud protests by critics of sugar—a group that includes the manufacturers of artificial sweeteners—attempts have been made to force people to give up sugar in their coffee or prevent them from eating a pastry or ice cream.

It has never been demonstrated that sugar can cause illness (not even diabetes, which has complex genetic and environmental causes), with the exception of dental cavities in subjects with poor oral hygiene or people more likely to develop cavities because of their naturally lower salivary pH.

Not even obesity can be blamed simply on an excessive sweet-tooth. The majority of the severely obese prefer other types of food, those that have a greater fat content with 9 calories per gram and not just the 4 calories per gram found in sucrose or any other simple or complex carbohydrate.

Many sweets and desserts are overloaded with both sugar and fats. In this case, the dietary danger lies with the excessive total caloric intake and not specifically the sugar.

However, it is true that many sweets and desserts (containing sugars, a heterogeneous family of molecules all with a sweet taste but with an extremely varied bromatological composition) are overloaded with both sugar and fats. In this case, the high number of calories is the real danger and not sugar in particular.

The INRAN Guidelines that we mentioned earlier dedicated one of its titles to this debate: "*Sugars, sweets and sugary drinks, allowed in just the right amounts*."

It should be mentioned that table sugar used for sweetening (ie, sucrose, extracted from sugar cane or sugar beet, consisting of a molecule of glucose and one of fructose) is a completely natural product even when refined. In nutritional terms, its molecule is easily metabolized, similar to fruit sugar or honey.

The problem lies in the fact that the refining process allows us to consume an excessive quantity in a small volume, and as we have repeated several times, all the food of high-energy density are a risk for people who live an excessively sedentary lifestyle.

The real problem lies with the speed with which the simple carbohydrates, and consequently sugar, are digested and metabolized.

A standard apple, weighing between 150 to 170 g, contains no less than 15 to 18 g of simple carbohydrates; however, it also includes fiber, vitamins, and minerals and can create a sense of fullness that can certainly not be compared to the corresponding 3 teaspoonfuls of sucrose (15 g) that we would have used to sweeten a drink.

The real problem lies with the speed with which the simple carbohydrates and, therefore, sugars are digested and metabolized.

Glucose, in particular, provokes an immediate rise in the glycemic levels, which should correspond to an appropriate production of insulin, the pancreatic hormone that controls the entrance and the utilization of glucose inside our cells.

It is common knowledge that diabetics are unable to rapidly counterbalance the glycemic peak provoked by the sugar intake with a sufficient quantity of insulin, and must, therefore, strictly limit the ingestion of simple carbohydrates. Nevertheless, modern diabetology has documented that small quantities of simple sugars, with delayed intestinal absorption due to the simultaneous presence of fiber and other nutrients as presented in some baked products, and when used as an alternative and not in addition to other complex carbohydrates, can be consumed by well-controlled diabetics.

We have already stated that carbohydrates can and must form at least 50% of our diet, and as a result, we can include up to 10% simple sugars without causing any metabolic problems. It should be remembered that this proportion may already have been reached with fruit sugars, milk, industrially sweetened drinks, or other drinks that contain simple sugars (beer, fruit juices, sodas).

The conclusions recommend that a few spoonfuls of sugar, throughout the day, should not be demonized. People should pay more attention to the total quantity of simple sugars on the basis of the frequency of consumption of food and sweet drinks.

If the dietician will not agree to the patient consuming products with a high content of sucrose (candy, nougat, etc), he or she may be more indulgent toward traditional Italian baked confectionaries (cookies, simple sponge cakes, etc) where the sugar and fat contents are lower with respect to the complex carbohydrates of flour.

We should mention artificial sweeteners, such as aspartame or acesulfame, which are precious for diabetics who are unable to do without the sweet taste of coffee or other drinks, but they are almost totally useless in low-calorie diets. Eliminating a couple of spoonfuls of sugar is not the way of tackling a complex, chronic, or multifactorial problem such as the tendency to obesity. More complex protocols are required with changes to the dietary habits and lifestyle. First, behavioral and pharmacological countermeasures have little or nothing to do with a spoonful of sugar or a slice of cake, consumed as an alternative to the glycidic and caloric intake of bread, pasta, or other food based on complex carbohydrates.

Artificial sweeteners, such as aspartame or acesulfame, are of little or no use in low-calorie diets.

Chapter 6

Reduce salt intake: good advice for everyone

Epidemiological studies have demonstrated that where salt does not exceed 3 g per day, the average value of the population's blood pressure is lower.

The dietary recommendations of the experts agree on the good advice of reducing the daily consumption of salt (sodium chloride).

Modern man normally consumes a quantity of salt in excess of the daily requirements, and this excess, at least for certain ethnic groups or "sodium-sensitive" families, would appear to have latent danger.

Epidemiological studies have demonstrated that when the salt consumption does not exceed 3 g per day, the average value of the population's blood pressure is generally lower; for this and other reasons, the Guidelines state, "*Salt? Better not in excess.*"

It is undeniable that through the centuries, salt has been the predominant, but not only, substance used to preserve food, and this fact justified its use and contributed to our appreciation of the salty taste. Nevertheless, we are aware from physiology that the addition of salt, as it is done routinely in today's cuisine, is not justified and is certainly excessive.

An exaggerated consumption of salt, in addition to being damaging in concept, becomes a risk factor for cardiocirculatory disease and a predisposing cofactor in cancer of the stomach and the upper digestive pathways.

In practice, the content of sodium that is naturally present in food should be sufficient for the body's physiological needs with no additional quantity required.

Table 6.1 lists the foods that have a greater sodium content—cured meats, mature cheeses, stock cubes, ketchup, soy sauce, tinned food, bread, baked products, and water rich in sodium. When used on a regular basis, these foods can increase the daily intake of sodium *(Table 6.2)*.

Despite the fact that sodium plays an important role in the body, the recommended intake averages between 0.6 and 3.5 g per day with the exception of the manual workers and athletes who sweat a lot and who work in a warm, damp climate.

It should be specified that sodium accounts for approximately 40% of the weight of table salt. As a result, international consensus suggests that the daily salt consumption should not exceed 6 g, which is half the quantity the average person is estimated to consume.

Unfortunately, adding less salt to the food is not enough if people eat out a lot because prepared foods generally have a high sodium content.

Eating food without salt is not a pleasant experience, but it is recommended for patients with kidney problems, high blood pressure, or heart problems. However, it is also true that after a few weeks, the taste buds adapt to the lack of salt, and the palate will learn to appreciate the real taste of the food, which was previously suffocated by an excess of salt. Moreover, a whole range of seasonings, herbs, spices, and mild sauces can replace the flavor enhancement provided by salt.

Table 6.1

Preserved and processed foods that have a high salt content

FOOD	WEIGHT OF THE UNIT OF MEASUREMENT (g)	CONTENT PER UNIT OF MEASUREMENT	
		SODIUM (g)	SALT (g)
Processed table olives (5 olives)	35	0.46*	1.1
Vegetables in vinegar (3 tablespoons)	60	0.48*	1.2
Cured ham (mild) (3 to 4 medium slices)	50	1.29	3.2
Cooked ham (3 to 4 medium slices)	50	0.36	0.9
Salami Milano (8 to 10 medium slices)	50	0.75	1.9
Mozzarella (cow's milk) (3.5 oz)	100	0.20	0.5
Provolone cheese (1.8 oz)	50	0.34	0.9
Cheese spread (0.4 oz)	22	0.22*	0.6
Grated Parmesan cheese (1 tablespoon)	10	0.06	0.2
Tuna in oil (drained) (1 can)	52	0.16	0.4
Potato chips (small individual bag)	25	0.27	0.7
Ketchup (1 tablespoon)	14	0.15	0.4
Stock cube (one-quarter)	3	0.50	1.2

N.B.: The sodium values reported have been taken from the Table of Composition of Food (INRAN-2000 Update). The values relative to products marked with (*) have been taken from the information printed on the labels.

(Mod. from «Linee Guida per una sana alimentazione italiana». INRAN, 2003)

Table 6.2

"Hidden" sources of salt

FOOD	WEIGHT OF THE UNIT OF MEASUREMENT (G)	CONTENT PER UNIT OF MEASUREMENT	
		SODIUM (g)	SALT (g)
Bread (1 average slice)	50	0.15	0.4
Insipid bread (no salt) (1 average slice)	50	trace*	trace
Sweet cookies (2 to 4 cookies)	20	0.04	0.1
Simple croissant (1 unit)	40	0.16*	0.4
Sponge-like cake (1 serving)	35	0.12*	0.3
Breakfast cereals (4 tablespoons)	30	0.33*	0.8

N.B.: The sodium values reported have been taken from the Table of Composition of Food (INRAN—2000 Update).
The values relative to products marked with (*) have been taken from the information printed on the labels.
To facilitate the interpretation, the equivalent value of salt is reported, obtained by multiplying the value of the sodium content by 2.5.

(Mod. from «Linee Guida per una sana alimentazione italiana». INRAN, 2003)

The healthy population is not expected to eliminate salt completely but to use less salt when cooking pasta or vegetables and pay more attention to the choice of food. A rediscovery of seasonings and spices, pepper, and better still chili peppers can enhance the flavor of the food more than salt and without the danger.

Salt substitutes should not be used unless under medical supervision. It may help people with high blood pressure who find it difficult to reduce their salt intake, but this may actually be contraindicated for some nephropathic patients.

It should also be mentioned that the Italian health officials, like their European counterparts, recommend the use of iodized table salt to prevent the onset of gout and iodine deficiency.

Iodized salt is nothing more than salt with iodate added and should replace normal table salt in seasoning and cooking.

Salt substitutes should not be used unless under medical guidance; in fact, replacement of salt may actually be contraindicated in some nephropathic patients.

Chapter 7

Alcoholic beverages: a **problem** of **doses**

"It is the dose that is poisonous," according to Paracelso. This concept is absolutely fundamental in medicine and legitimizes one of the headings of one of the Guidelines: *"Alcoholic beverages: yes, but only in moderation."* Even LARN, despite hiding behind the saying "permitted quantities," encourages the moderate consumption of drinks with a low alcoholic content, such as wine and beer.

For healthy adults, the "acceptable" daily consumption is measured in alcohol units (AU) *(Figure 7.1)*.

Moderate alcohol consumption can be suggested within the limit of 2 to 3 AU per day for men (equivalent to approximately 2 to 3 glasses of wine) and 1 to 2 AU for women. This amount should be consumed at mealtimes and should be considered to be the maximum limit permitted. Above this amount, the negative effects will predominate any positive ones.

Unfortunately, the mass media have broadcast the positive findings from the scientific literature with excessive emphasis—namely the antioxidant and vasoprotective qualities of wine, particularly red wine, which is rich in resveratrol and other potentially useful polyphenols.

Moderate alcohol consumption can be suggested within the limit of 2 to 3 AU per day for men (equivalent to approximately 2 to 3 glasses of wine) and 1 to 2 AU for women.

Figure 7.1

Definition of alcohol unit (AU)

One AU corresponds to approximately 12 g of ethanol; this quantity is found in a small glass of wine (4 oz), of average strength; in a can of beer (12 oz); or in a standard measure of spirits ($1\frac{1}{3}$ oz).

One g of alcohol has the calorie equivalent of 7 kCal.

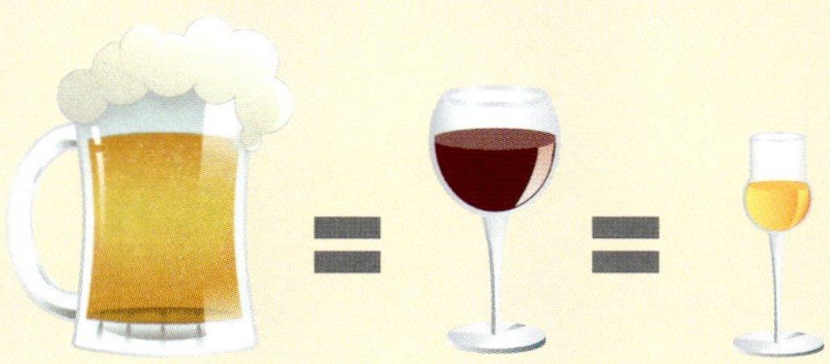

(Mod. from «Linee Guida per una sana alimentazione italiana». INRAN, 2003)

No food is good or bad; it all depends on the amount consumed and how it fits into the dietary context of the entire day.

We do not have the time needed to take a closer look at this topic or illustrate the certain benefits that counterbalance the notorious dangers associated with alcohol abuse.
It should be stressed that if the scientific investigations should confirm these minor benefits, it will never be possible to transform alcoholic beverages into a therapeutic drug, as it is not free from risks to the people who choose to abuse it.
The crux of the matter is that no food (and alcohol is also an energetic nutrient) is good or bad; it all depends on the amount consumed and how it fits into the dietary context of the entire day.
Drinking alcohol during meals has less obvious effects than when consumed on an empty stomach. However, it would be wise to consult *Table 7.1* for information regarding the time necessary to metabolize increasing quantities of ethanol in order to stay below the legal alcohol limits for drivers.
In a Mediterranean country, with the wonderful abundance of vines, olive trees, and a huge variety of fruits and vegetables, wine drinking is very much part of the country's history and traditions. However, it should be handled with care, so that the "acceptable" consumption is not transformed into abuse and dependency, as was tragically seen in the past with the tavern "winos."
Fortunately, the consumption of wine would appear to be substantially stationary, in contrast to the dangerous peaks just a few decades ago. It now seems that we have shifted our preference from quantity to quality!
For the people who are calorie counting *(Table 7.2)*, it should be mentioned that the alcohol strength printed on the label is expressed as a percentage volume and not in grams of alcohol (to obtain the quantity of alcohol in grams, it is sufficient to multiply the alcoholic strength by 0.79).
Drinking in moderation does not simply mean limiting the amount consumed, but it also means choosing the right moment (better to drink alcohol during mealtimes and not on an empty stomach), limiting the quantity (the total acceptable quantity should be spread over the entire day), and selecting low strengths (the nutritionist is unlikely to give his or her approval for spirits).
The social dangers associated with the excessive consumption of alcoholic drinks and in particular with respect to driving reflexes should also be taken into consideration. The figures reported in *Table 7.1* must act as warnings and reference values for the consumption of alcoholic beverages and the consequent dependency on alcohol.

Table 7.1

Indicative values of alcoholemia (g of alcohol per liter of blood) in function of the quantity of alcohol consumed (expressed in AU) and the period of time from consumption (under fasting conditions)

The values that exceed the legal values for driving are indicated in yellow.

	PERIOD OF TIME FROM CONSUMPTION (MEN)				
AU	1	2	3	4	5
1	0.13	0.01	0	0	0
2	0.38	0.26	0.14	0.02	0
3	0.63	0.51	0.39	0.27	0.15
4	0.88	0.76	0.64	0.52	0.40
5	1.13	1.01	0.89	0.77	0.65

	PERIOD OF TIME FROM CONSUMPTION (WOMEN)				
AU	1	2	3	4	5
1	0.23	0.10	0	0	0
2	0.57	0.45	0.33	0.21	0.09
3	0.92	0.79	0.67	0.56	0.44
4	1.26	1.14	1.02	0.91	0.78
5	1.61	1.49	1.37	1.25	1.1

The values reported have been calculated for a body weight of 154 lbs for men and 132 lbs for women.
Drinking during mealtimes reduces the level of alcohol in the blood by approximately 1 AU. To obtain the values achievable after mealtimes, the overall number of AU consumed must be reduced by one.
The formula applied takes into consideration the volume of alcohol introduced, the volume of body-water and the body's ability to eliminate alcohol.

(Mod. from «Linee Guida per una sana alimentazione italiana». INRAN, 2003)

Table 7.2

Quantity of alcohol and calorific value of some drinks

BEVERAGE	ALCOHOLIC STRENGTH	MEASUREMENT	QUANTITY (oz)	ALCOHOL (g)	TOTAL CALORIES
Table wine	11 to 13	1 average glass	5	13 to 15	90 to 110
Lager beer	4 to 5	1 can	12	11.7	112
Special brews	5.5 to 7.5	1 can	12	14.3 to 19.5	165 to 270
Aperitifs	19 to 22	1 shot glass	2½	11 to 13	90 to 140
Cognac, whisky	43	1 shot glass	1⅔	17	120

Chapter 8

The **benefits** of a **varied** and **well-balanced diet**

Food supplies the organism with calories and energy, but also has the job of introducing protective and plastic elements, essential for the repair and maintenance of this biological machine.

The problem of people being overweight has become such a priority, in terms of public health, that an incredible number of people have forgotten that food is not just something that replenishes the body with calories (ie, energy) but also has the job of introducing elements that are essential for the protection, repair, and maintenance of the biological machine.

A correct and well-balanced diet must contain an adequate amount of water, vitamins, and minerals (ie, elements with no energy value), in addition to the potential chemical energy of the food substances. Moreover, special nutrients that the body is unable to produce are also necessary. These must be ingested in preformed molecules, such as essential amino acids or essential fatty acids.

No food is able to satisfy all the organic requirements on its own. Not even milk, which is unquestionably closer to a theoretically complete nutritious substance, can satisfy the needs of the newborn child after the first few months of life. As a result, the simplest way to guarantee all the nutrients, and in particular the plastic and protective ones, where the needs including those considered essential are required in relatively modest quantities, is to vary the type of food, rotating the substances consumed.

"Frequently vary your diet" is also recommended by the Guidelines. Epidemiology has taught us that varying our diet in accordance with the changing seasons and, therefore, eating meals that are rich in fresh or frozen products will ensure the completion of the puzzle that forms the correct diet.

Moreover, varying the diet will avoid or reduce the danger of prolonged metabolic overload, which may occur if an excessive quantity of high protein, high fat, or high sugar foods are eaten in continuation. Varying the diet will also ensure a reduction in the risk of constant ingestion of foreign substances that are deliberately or casually present in foods that may be defined as "genuine," and compounds that are "antinutritional," which may occur naturally in some foods.

The diversification of food choices attenuates the potential risks of onset of certain tumor localizations, such as those of the intestinal tract; diversification also guarantees better protection of the state of health.

Dietary prevention of tumors is based on the dietary variation, a simple but useful means for reducing the risk of food; this may contribute to preventing the appearance of some tumors, for example of the intestinal tract, a localization that health statistics have shown to be in constant and considerable increase.

The diversification of the food choices attenuates these potential risks and guarantees better protection of our state of health. Diet studies in recent years have emphasized the protective importance of many natural elements, present particularly in fruits and vegetables, such as antioxidants, which are widely present in the plant kingdom. Without ideological reasoning, from the medical-scientific point of view, it is actually true that food for modern and highly sedentary man must shift more toward vegetarian choices with respect to the past overconsumption of meat and more generally food of animal origin.

For a more focused vision of the problem, we should remember that foods can be split into just a handful of categories; people should choose one or more of each according to taste.

Throughout the day, one or two substances from each food group *(Table 8.1)* must compete and combine to form the dietary ration. However, over 1 week, alternative choices should be selected from the 5 main groups.

For example, in the group of meat, fish, eggs, and dried legumes, fish should be selected at least twice a week; the same applies to eggs (even people with high cholesterol levels can still eat a couple of eggs each week); cold cuts should only be eaten 2 or 3 times a week, with a preference for those with a lower fat content (eg, Bresaola—cured beef, ham). Depending on the person's age and his or her individual taste, 2 to 4 rations of meat can be eaten each week. Once or twice each week, it would be a good idea to have a single dish based on legumes and cereals (a soup of pasta and chickpeas, rice and peas, etc) in perfect agreement with our internationally acclaimed Mediterranean diet.

INRAN has actually identified 7 (not 5) fundamental food categories that will allow us to diversify even more to include all the noncalorie-bearing nutrients such as vitamins and minerals, which are extremely important for a balanced diet. Nevertheless, in practical terms, 5 relatively homogeneous groups prevail *(see Table 8.1)*, ignoring the fruit and vegetable split, with the substances that are richer in vitamin C or precursors of vitamin A and including dried legumes in the group of protein sources.

For anyone who wishes to follow a varied and balanced diet, the first step is to select something from each nutrient group; however, it goes without saying that the rotation within the groups will make a further contribution to variations within the diet and lead to a balanced, well-rounded eating plan.

It is not right to choose meat alone and ignore fish. While the protein content can be considered to be

The food groups facilitate the equilibrium of the dietary choices.

Table 8.1

The five food categories
Milk, milk products, yogurt, cheese
Meat, fish, eggs, dried legumes
Cereals, their derivatives, potatoes
Animal and vegetable fats for seasoning
Vegetables (including fresh legumes) and fruit

A balanced and varied diet involves all 7 food groups, but also involves the frequent alteration of the individual foods within each group.

interchangeable, the same cannot be said for the different characteristics in the lipid fraction; meat fat is predominantly saturated, while fish consists largely of special polyunsaturated essential fatty acids, which also have a specific protective importance.
The same can be said for the different varieties of fruits and vegetables, those rich in vitamin C (oranges, lemons, broccoli, etc) or those rich in carotene and vitamin A (carrots, apricots, etc).

"Drink plenty of water every day"

Water is in a category of its own; water is an extremely precious commodity and without it, no form of life could survive. The Guidelines dedicated a specific chapter to this primary necessity: *"Drink plenty of water every day*."
Approximately 55% to 60% of human adult body weight consists of water, which accounts for 75% of the muscles and the internal organs.
If we consider that every organic system is influenced by water, it stands to reason that a correct balance between water intake and output is necessary to maintain a good state of health. As we are dealing with water balance, it is not possible to define the exact intake; the amount of fluid necessary will be different for an athlete who sweats a lot compared to the person who has a sedentary lifestyle, and possibly again in the vegetarian who regularly eats minestrones, which have a high fluid content.
Nevertheless, in general terms, the majority of the adult population should drink approximately 33 to 67 ounces of water each day.

The majority of the adult population should drink between 33 and 67 ounces of water each day.

Thirst is a clear sign of dehydration; however, it is a well-known fact that this invaluable and unavoidable signal is delayed in children and in the elderly. These 2 groups should be educated to drink plenty before they become aware of being thirsty.
This is particularly important in the warmer seasons because even an apparently modest loss of just 1% to 2% of our fluid will have negative repercussions on the entire body, as athletes will be fully aware. They know they must prevent dehydration to safeguard their efficiency and the resistance to the physical effort.

The **fresh versus engineered conflict**

People are very quick to criticize the modern diet and emotionally regret the past; however, those were the days when poverty and poor food hygiene had major responsibility in shortening man's lifespan, with deadly deficiencies (pellagra, beri-beri, malnutrition) or epidemics, poisoning and toxic food infections (typhus, paratyphus, brucellosis, bovine tuberculosis).

Most people quite rightly suspect the dangers of preservatives, chemical fertilizers, industrial animal feed, and the like; however, in practice, the age-old microbiological problems of food hygiene have been ranked first in the epidemiological listings for frequency and severity.

The old microbiological problems of food hygiene are still ranked first in the epidemiological listings, in terms of frequency and severity.

During the summer months, leaving a cream cake, minced meat, or hors d'oeuvres just a few hours at room temperature or handled by a number of different customers will lead to a microbial load enough to provoke intestinal problems and diarrhea. Germs also require nutrients, and they find them more readily in foods that are rich in proteins (meat, eggs, fish, and milk) and in foods that are processed in factories or workshops; microbial reproduction is highly likely at room temperature. Another myth to be dispelled is the value of "organic," regardless of whether or not it is true.

We are sorry to disappoint the large group of people who hope to rediscover organic food in the modern restyling of the farmhouse or the barn or chicken run of some unknown farmer. Unfortunately, there are not enough quality guarantees for the people who wish to drink fresh milk or eat raw fish, a freshly laid egg, or some homemade jam. Epidemiological studies have taught us that it is this type of product, all made by "traditional" means but not subjected to the technological controls, that is to blame for the majority of food-related health problems.

There is no doubt that homemade products are almost always tastier. The problem is upstream, in the hygiene controls of the animals or the food sources (mushrooms are the best example of dangerous organic products because of the excessive number of pseudoexperts who gather them from the fields) and especially with the various production phases. In view of this, the industry is "obliged" to give maximum guarantees to the consumer because any accident, even the simplest, such as a temporary interruption in the refrigerated chain, would provoke a destruction of the company's image, which would have a negative effect on the profits.

It would be impossible to even try to supply the large and medium-sized cities with "organic" and fresh products alone. Vegetables transported directly from the small-hold farm to the general markets in big cites, and successively to the local market to wait for a buyer who may cook it a couple of days later may have lost a greater quantity of vitamin C than the analogous product that was harvested at the right moment of ripeness and deep-frozen immediately by a modern industrial plant.

Scientific literature has stated quite clearly that frozen peas can be "nutritionally" fresher than those purchased in a market or store in a large city. However, for obvious reasons, this comparison does not apply to the produce that the farmer harvests from his or her fields and eats within a couple of hours.

We must accept technological progress that guarantees health, hygiene and freshness and reject the farming methods that use an excessive amount of chemical additives—from the indiscriminate use of the antiparasitic drugs to the chemical manipulation of colorants and preservatives, practices we feel should be abandoned.

We need to accept technological progress as it safeguards hygiene and freshness with no manipulation—as is the case with industrial "deep-freezing" techniques.

We hope that farming in the future will be able to maintain the balance. The biological battle (with the identification of species that will keep the main pests under control), the strategeic battle (monitoring the information from the field), and the "integrated" battle (attentive use of chemicals only as a support for what was activated in the previous phases) are a growing concept and reality.

With no pretext of completely resolving the problems of food pollution, this responsible orientation now warrants the attention of the consumers in the majority of cases and the greater cost of the products with truly guaranteed quality.

All the metropolitan consumer, who lives far from the production sites, can do is trust the brands of specific companies and hope that they responsibly control all the phases of the production, from the harvesting to the distribution. The experience that has already been matured in some sectors confirms that this will be the long-term success strategy for the consumer and the more attentive producers.

Modern living obliges us to delegate all the complex phases of the operations from production to end consumers exclusively to truly competent experts, educated and trained in all the delicate phases of the relationship between the "genuine" qualities and technological needs. The laws of competition and the commercial needs that do not betray the qualities guaranteed by the brand ensure that the producers must safeguard themselves; they must control that every phase of the production process is faultless and constantly controlled in-house, over and above the invaluable surveillance by the authorities (NAS—Nucleo antisofisticazione—Italian Antisophistication Squad).

Diet, ideal weight, and body composition

The press coverage given to the risks associated with being overweight and the myths, typical of our times, associated with efficiency, youthfulness, pleasure, and self-confidence has created a trend that isolates or marginalizes people who are obese and drives them to follow irrational diets.

If the dietetic quirks of the improvisers were not enough, there is also the temptation of drugs, possibly a Galenic cocktail where anorexants may be mixed with harmless plant extracts; this is not in accordance with Hippocratic Oath, which expects doctors to practice through science and conscience.

For people who wish to lose weight, the public health care structures, which also lack amenities for emergency medicine, do not offer suitable assistance; as always, in the official vacuum, the commercially inspired initiatives have become more consistent and more legitimate compared to initiatives of documented scientific validity.

The weight-loss business has produced every imaginable type of diet. These diets are rarely correct; they are often contradictory to the point of legitimizing the belief, formulated by an expert, "Diets lead to weight gain." This is true because they are difficult to follow, they are too restrictive, and they lead to the excessive loss of muscle mass that precludes the resulting yo-yo syndrome (weight cycle syndrome).

In any case, badly managed diets, oriented to immediate weight loss, are very rarely geared to dietary re-education and behavior. This is the only long-term method advised by people who correctly interpret their medical role and who worry about preventing the regular relapses of these unfortunate patients.

When should we consider ourselves to be overweight or obese?

Not everything can be defined with figures, not even our weight. Doctors are well aware that the quality of weight—in other words the "body composition" and, therefore, the ratio of muscle mass and fat mass—is more important than the overall weight.

Nevertheless, for practical reasons, the classification is based on the body mass index (BMI), which is calculated using the formula: Weight (in lbs)/Height (in inches) squared *(Table 10.1).*

When the BMI exceeds 37 to 40, the patient is considered to be morbidly obese and suitable for bariatric surgery. Sometimes, this is the only option, given the extreme difficulty of returning this patient to a stable acceptable condition long-term.

The ratio between the muscle mass and the fat mass is more important than the person's overall weight.

Drugs are not enough to address the "lifestyle" balance

The drugs available today cannot resolve the complex problem of obesity.

Unfortunately, obese people who would like to use drugs in order to lose weight because they are unmotivated or cannot make the effort (cases of obesity secondary to hormonal disorders are a minority) should be aware that the drugs available today cannot resolve the complex problem of obesity. If we exclude the amphetamine-based anorexants, which will be efficacious in the short term, there is little else available. These are not recommended as a long-term treatment because of the side effects and because of the certainty that when treatment is suspended, the patient's weight will increase as before.

Other products are available, but these are only the easily managed coadjuvant drugs such as sibutramine or orlistat. At the time of publication, a new, conceptually more active molecule (rimonabant) is currently being registered. Nevertheless, these drugs necessitate prescription by a specialist despite the fact that their action is not as stimulating as amphetamine (sibutramine prolongs but does not increase the secretion of serotonin) while the sense of fullness provided by many fiber-based preparations does not differ much from a placebo.

Other remedies are either not very efficacious (inhibitors of pancreatic lipase such as orlistat), almost totally useless (tisanes and other herbal products), or lack any scientific justification in that they eliminate large quantities of liquid or protein mass from the body rather than fat (thyroid extracts, ketogenic diets). Some contribute to creating a greater sense of fullness (eg, methylcellulose, bran, and various fibers) or they simply supply the exact amount of nutrient in "bars" or similar meal replacements, none of which will ever resolve the multiple reasons behind obesity.

Table 10.1

Body Mass Index (weight/height²)

< 18.5	Pathologically underweight
18.5 to 25	Normal
25 to 30	Overweight
> 30	Obese

Abdominal obesity is the worst kind

Many people will have attempted every method for weight loss in vain. However, it should be pointed out that not all forms of obesity have the same negative implications. Specialists now agree that obesity concentrated on the abdomen and the chest (ventral obesity, prevalent in males) as opposed to obesity concentrated on the hips and the thighs (peripheral obesity, prevalent in females) is certainly more dangerous. This is due to the association with high cholesterol levels, diabetes, and degenerative pathologies of the cardiovascular apparatus. The waist circumference should not exceed 34.5 in for women and 40 in for men. Ideally, the measurements should be at least 1.5 in less than this—33 and 38.5 in, respectively—for the 2 genders *(Table 10.2)*.

Obesity should be tackled, or better still, prevented; however, it is also true that not all overweight adults should be forced for the rest of their days to follow irrational and monotonous diets.

Not all forms of obesity have the same negative potential. Obesity that is concentrated in the abdomen and the chest is unquestionably more dangerous than fat deposits on the hips and thighs.

Table 10.2

Waist circumference: ventral and peripheral obesity

	MEN	WOMEN
Optimal circumference	< 38.5 in	< 33 in
Overweight	38.5 to 40 in	33 to 34.5 in
Obese	> 40 in	> 34.5 in

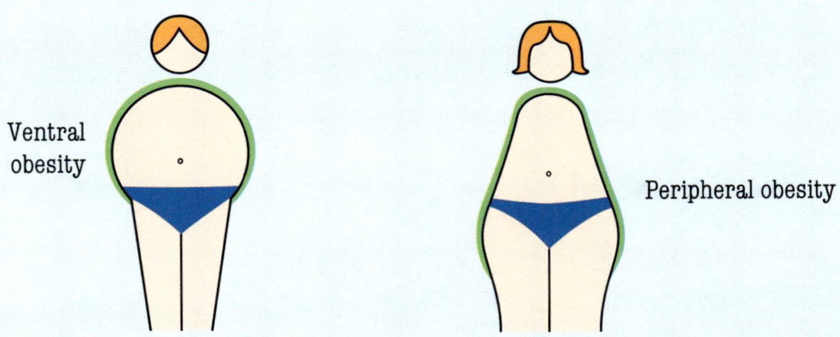

Faced with the difficulties and the failures in the treatment of obesity, the family doctor should tolerate a few pounds of fat in the gynoid areas. Unfortunately, life is limited, and for the adult—more so for the elderly—the price of continual sacrifices, essential for weight loss and to avoid returning to weight gain after just a few months, could exceed the presumed benefits.

Quality of life has an important value that every doctor must evaluate prior to asking the patient to overturn lifetime dietary habits.

Quality of life has a value that every doctor needs to evaluate before he or she presents the patient with a diet plan that will completely upset his or her eating habits. Unfortunately, dietary madness is not limited to the universe of the obese. The improvisers, the false prophets, and the diet gurus (and it should be said that the diet industry is not just part of the American reality), whether good or bad, have something for everyone and can broadcast lies that only serve to complicate the lives of the healthy, the ill, and their doctors, just like the fortune-tellers who publish the daily horoscopes.

It is time that the absurdity of certain dietary proposals is stopped and the information directed toward the idea of a well-balanced diet (possibly with a slightly lower content of protein) with reduced or even miniaturized portions.

The medieval restrictions of the food myths and prejudices no longer have a reason for existing in view of the modern scientific evidence.

nutrogenomic science and our diet

The idea that the way we nourish ourselves plays an essential role in our condition of health dates back to the ancient days of Hippocrates. However, the ideas were transformed into certainties and statistical facts thanks to the large-scale epidemiological studies of the last century. It was modern technology, the study of the role of DNA and the identification of the structure and sequence of the human genome, that confirmed and disproved the ancient doctrines.

With the advent of molecular biology, it was possible to investigate the direct influence of nutrients on gene expression and in 1999, Dean Della Penna drew up the basis of the nutritional gene science, coining the term ***nutrogenomic***, which was followed by other fairly unattractive yet technically appropriate "omic" terms—proteomic, transcriptomic, and metabolomic. Since then, there has been considerable progress yet the commercial intrusions have also made their mark, to the degree of legitimate titles such as "Hope and fraud at the dawn of Nutrogenomics!"

Without spending too much time on the little-known meanders of nutrogenomics, we can begin by giving it a simple definition: *"Science dedicated to the study of interactions between specific genes and nutrients."*

For too long, the dietary principles were studied simply as a source of energy or cofactors of cell metabolism and only once molecular biology entered the laboratories was it possible to identify, at least in part, the direct influence of the nutrients on gene expression.

Very briefly, the consequences of our lifestyle depend on our genetic profile, which is specific for each individual; however, the fate transcribed in the genes can, in turn, be delayed or anticipated by the way we eat.

There are racial, ethnic, and hereditary predispositions to the response to specific nutrients, and this is why the clinical responses, for example to phytoestrogens or to soya, differ considerably in Indian women compared to European women. Nutrogenomic science with the study of polymorphism (small but effective differences in the amino-acid sequences of the genes) provides plausible explanations regarding the differing clinical efficacy of the products legitimized by studies and numbers that are not coincidental.

Polymorphism of the gene for angiotensin may explain the different response of patients with high blood pressure to the diets rich in dietary fiber, or alternately other polymorphisms justify the fact that folic acid led to a reduction in the incidence of colon tumors in some studies conducted on ethnic groups with a long habit of substantially different food types but not in others.

These are just 2 examples of the well-known fact that some dietary precautions have proved useful in the prevention of tumors in some specific studies but not in others.

Nutrogenomics: "Science dedicated to the study of interactions between specific genes and nutrients."

The expression of what has been transcribed in the genes can be influenced, in turn, by a person's lifestyle.

We now know that the genes of an individual are involved in the beneficial or damaging response to a specific component of a food; however, the problem increases in complexity when concomitant interferences with other foods intervene. This could possibly be compared to the situation of the glycemic index of food tested in the laboratory and the real effect the same food has when ingested as part of a full meal where there is the superimposition and the interference of other foods and digestive variables!

Progress in the field of nutrogenomics will allow us to understand how a specific food, or more correctly, a diet, can interfere on a molecular level with the function of the body.

Progress in nutrogenomics will lead us to better understanding of a specific food or a special dietary style; it may actually interfere on the molecular functioning of the body. At the time of publication, this will still have its commercial and mystifying knock-off effects. Some companies are focusing on this business sector and have already produced nutrogenomic kits consisting of questionnaires and DNA analyses, which, for the moment, do not justify the dietary suppositions formulated in exchange for a few hundred dollars.

Gregory Kutz, director of the Special Investigations of the US Government Accountability Office, explained that for the meantime, *"These are just predictions with no medical or scientific value; they are extremely ambiguous in their formulation as in reality they do not supply any information to the consumer who will spend a lot of money basically for nothing*."

Josè M. Ordovas, the director of the Genomics Laboratory of Tufts University in Boston, probably made a valid comparison. He explained, *"In terms of development potential of our knowledge, today we are in the same situation we were in with computers in 1980. We played the very deliberate game of ping-pong on slow primitive computers, and look where we are today!*"

The forecast for a greater number of people being affected by ocular pathologies could lead to a different preventive use of vitamins; more correctly, the foods that naturally contain vitamins or have them artificially added—such as vitamin A to ß-carotene, to vitamin E, vitamin B2, vitamin C, the omega-3s, luteine, etc.

At the moment, nutrogenomics is a developing cultural fact for the future. However, clinical dieticians must not undervalue it but investigate it more closely and be ready to use it when the time is right. They should approach the new world of functional foods and custom diets with open minds that are free from conceptual preclusions.

The use of diets and nutraceutical food as an instrument for prevention and consequently for "wellness" or possibly an anti-aging strategy is certainly a very attractive proposition. Considering food as a daily necessity could create a sort of "continuative" therapy to be used for life, with no risks of toxicity or side effects that are conceptually intrinsic to the use of pharmaceutical products.

It is likely that the forecast of a greater incidence of ocular pathologies could authorize a different use of vitamins, or rather foods that contain them naturally or those with vitamins added (nutraceutical food), from vitamin A to β-carotene, vitamin E, vitamin B2, vitamin C, the omega-3s, luteine, etc.

The advent of dietary supplements

While waiting for diets that are increasingly oriented to the individuality of the genetic make-up and the lifestyle of each person, there has been an explosion of novel foods, functional foods, dietary foods in the pharmacies and even in the supermarkets (all for special diets) and "supplements" of every imaginable type.

The reason behind this commercial explosion lies in the population's increased awareness of the role of diet in the state of physical wellness, in the prevention of some pathologies, and in the delay of the chronic degenerative processes of aging.

Nevertheless, the majority of these products, with the exception of those for specific clinical conditions (celiac, diabetes, etc) are used by people who undertake normal physical activity. They should adopt a normal well-balanced diet or use hydrosaline supplements only when the physical or sporting activity results in excessive sweating.

Not by chance, in a specific directive on the role of supplements and the rules devised to govern their sales, the European Food Safety Authority stated, "*Under normal circumstances, an adequate and well-balanced diet will be sufficient to supply all the elements necessary for the normal development and maintenance of the body's state of health, in the proportions considered to be ideal and recommended by recognized scientific studies*."

The supplements should be used solely to redress the deficiencies of extremely low-calorie diets in the people who lead extremely sedentary lives, given that no diet containing less than 1200 to 1300 calories per day can guarantee the necessary amounts of vitamins and minerals.

Contrary to what one might think, the main—not to say the only—supplement for athletes, or better still, all healthy people involved in prolonged physical activity is fluid intake. It has been widely demonstrated that in physically demanding sports, practiced under the August sun or in the warm humid atmosphere of a sports center, rehydration can be so important as to necessitate a hydrosaline supplement.

Having said this, it is possible to ignore other supplements (energy sources, branched amino acids, creatine, etc) that are usually unnecessary for people who are involved in any sporting activity or amateur sport for just a few hours every week.

The functional foods are characterized by components that interact selectively on one or more physiological functions, with beneficial effects on the state of health and/or on prevention.

The hydro-saline supplements are particularly useful to redress the vitamin and mineral balance following excessive sweating.

Are supplements useful particularly for the people who eat little and badly?

In fact, it is generally amateur athletes who resort to the use of supplements (let's leave aside the major sporting professionals who are in a different world; eg, Formula 1 race cars cannot be compared to vehicles for the general public). They do this in the hope of replacing their training discontinuity or their modest physical progress with vitamin supplements or worse, with real medicines. The people who participate in even a small amount of physical exercise every day can and must consume a greater number of calories; as a result, given the fact that they are eating a much more varied diet, they should not be worried about taking vitamin-mineral supplements that have little or nothing to do with the high muscle mass objective set by the obsessive body builders.

People who perform limited amounts or sporadic weekly training sessions do not require any additional vitamin or mineral supplements.

Contrary to athletes who are always on the look-out for magical foods, physiologists believe that a slight increase in the vitamin and mineral intake in some distance and resistance sports may be useful or necessary. However, a varied and calorie-adequate diet should provide all the necessary elements. This statement will probably not please the numerous supplement producers but this is the scientific truth, save just a few exceptions.

The counteraction of the advocates of supplements was to encourage the individual to follow an incorrect food regime, not under the guidance of the sports doctors. The excuse given to the population as a whole, and the elderly in particular, was that the conservation, manipulation, and cooking processes of food may reduce the theoretical contents reported in the tables for the "ideal" foods rather than those purchased in the local markets.

All of this is partially true; however, in the majority of cases, it does not justify the continual use of these products, even when the diet is balanced and varied to include a good quantity of fresh seasonal products.

References

- Binetti P, Marcelli M, Baisi R. Manuale di Nutrizione clinica e scienze applicate. Società Editrice Universo, Roma, 2006.
- Capitano A, Dugo G, Restani P. Tossicologia degli alimenti. UTET, 1999.
- Del Toma E. Prevenzione e Terapia Dietetica. Il Pensiero Scientifico Editore, Roma, 2005.
- Del Toma E. Alimentazione: domande e risposte (2°ediz.). Il Pensiero Scientifico Editore, Roma 2006.
- Fatati G. Dietetica e Nutrizione. Il Pensiero Scientifico Editore, Roma, 2007
- INRAN Tabelle di consultazione degli alimenti. Edra, 2000.
- INRAN Linee Guida per una sana alimentazione italiana (rev. 2003).
- Shils ME, Olson JA, Shike M. ***Modern Nutrition in Health and Disease***. New York, NY: Lea and Febiger; 1994.

Part II

Nazareno Marabottini

Nutrition and Eye Disease

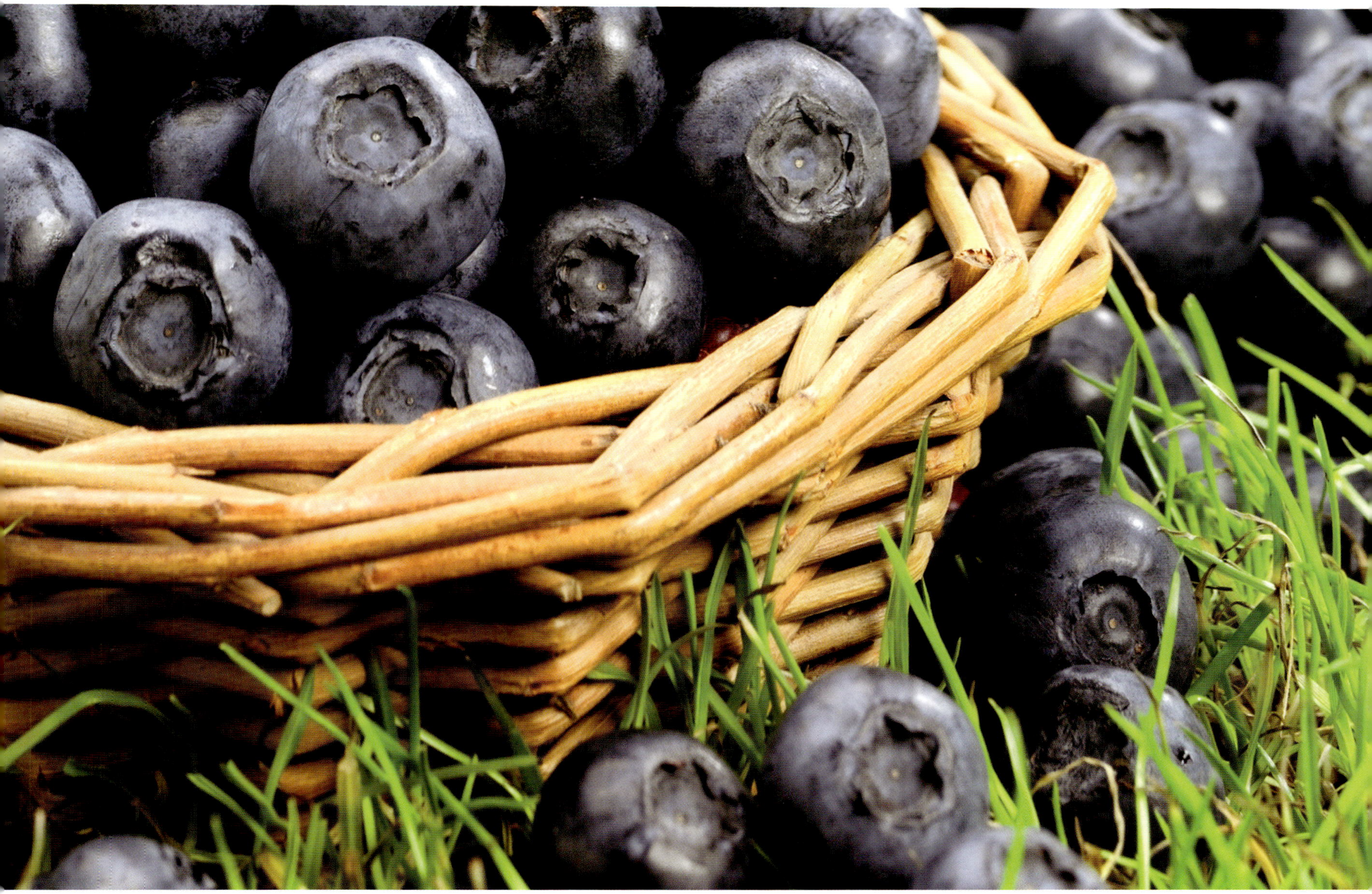

The **structures** of the **eyes**

Introduction

Our body is undergoing continual renewal. The molecules in the body's structures are always being replaced. For the molecules to work well, they must be new and free from damage. Our body expends a lot of energy to keep its systems efficient, to prevent them from being damaged, and to repair them. Despite this, any permanent damage will accumulate over time, giving rise to aging phenomena.
We will take a look at the eye from a different angle than the one to which we are accustomed. We will examine it as a collection of structures that, in order to have their shape and function, necessitate specific components. We will see how the normal metabolic activity and life events can modify and damage these components and we will see how the organism intervenes in order to maintain and defend itself. Lastly, we will see how we can supply our body with the weapons necessary to fight this war. All the structural components and energy that can contribute to defending our health is provided in the same way: nutrition.

Food contains substances that are useful for repairing and protecting our bodies.

The dioptric media

The cornea and the vitreous

The consistencies of the corneal stroma and the vitreous are unquestionably very different; however, they both contain the same structural molecules. They consist of a reticular structure of collagen with the interfibrillary spaces filled with glycosaminoglycans (GAG).
The stroma is the thickest of the 5 layers of the cornea, accounting for approximately 90%. It consists of water for the most part (78%). The remainder is collagen, intercellular substance, and a small number of fibroblasts,[1] called keratocytes.
The corneal collagen fibers are arranged parallel with the eye[2] at intervals of approximately 200 μm,[3] a distance that corresponds to approximately half the wavelength of visible light. This arrangement of the fibers permits the transparency of the structures. Sixty percent of corneal collagen is Type I, 10% is Type V, and 30% is Type VI.[4] The GAGs are largely sulforate proteoglycans, and these keep the collagen fibrils in their correct mutual positions.[5]
The vitreous is a gel that is 98% water. The structure consists of a network of thin collagen fibrils with the spaces filled with GAG, largely hyaluronic acid[6]: the collagen confers elasticity to the structure,

The cornea and the vitreous are formed by collagen and glycosaminoglycans.

while hyaluronate confers viscosity.[7] The GAGs are found in greater quantities at the center of the vitreous and to a lesser degree in the cortical portion.[8] The gel-like structure of the vitreous is maintained even when the hyaluronate is removed[9] because it depends on some specific proteins and other GAGs.[10,11] Collagen and GAGs are secreted by the hyalocytes, cells of macrophagic derivation.

The crystalline lens

The crystalline lens contains an extremely high concentration of protein, and also a high water content.

The crystalline lens contains a high concentration of protein but also a high water content of approximately 69%. The proteins are derived from the epithelial cells that lose their nuclei and organelles during differentiation.

The lens grows in concentric layers that overlap; there is no protein turnover nor diffusion between cells. As a result, the proteins that were synthesized during embryogenesis can still be found in the nucleus of the adult crystalline lens. For this reason, it is essential to have mechanisms that will maintain the transparency and the degree of hydration of the lens. These are based on maintenance of the osmotic equilibrium through NA,K-ATPases and the redox balance maintained by glutathione. These are mechanisms that consume energy; in the crystalline lens, energy is produced largely by anaerobic glycolysis and by means of the polyol pathway (sorbitol).[12] The sorbitol produced tends to spread into the aqueous humor but can accumulate in the lens in conditions of hyperglycemia, which can lead to the formation of cataract.[13] The hexose monophosphate pathway supplies NADH for glutathione reductase (GSH-red).

The crystalline lens is highly sensitive to oxidative damage because its proteins are not replaced.

Aging of the crystalline lens may lead to the appearance of cataract; this is encouraged by smoking, diabetes and exposure to UV light.[14] The oxidative stress on lipids and proteins plays an important role in this process.[15] Hydrogen peroxide is present in the aqueous humor, and this can damage the Na,K pump; this damage is associated with the onset of cataract.[16] In order to protect the eye against these events, the cellular antioxidant systems such as glutathione (the most important in the crystalline lens), catalase (CAT), superoxide dismutase (SOD), and the presence of some macro-nutrients (luteine) and micronutrients (Zn, Cu, Se) become essential.

The retina

The relationship between the photoreceptors and the retinal pigment epithelium

The production of electrical potential by the photoreceptors is the foundation of the sight and is guaranteed by the interaction between the photoreceptors and the retinal pigment epithelium (RPE). Both of these structures consist of cells that are not renewed; as a result, the replacement of the structural elements and the defense barriers against toxic agents becomes crucial.

RPE phagocytates the external segment of the photoreceptors.

The RPE is a structure of key importance: it facilitates the transition of nutritional elements directed to the photoreceptors and it phagocytates the external sector, allowing it to be renewed.

If the photoreceptor membrane contains peroxidated lipids (which are damaged), phagocytosis by the RPE is created.[17] Unfortunately, the peroxidated membranes are not completely digestible by the phagosomial enzymes[18]; as a result, we will witnesss the slow and progressive accumulation of undigested material in the phagosomes called lipofuscine, the quantity of which increases over time, proportional to the degree of peroxidative damage.[19] The cells of the RPE containing lipofuscine are more sensitive to damage induced by exposure to blue light.[20,21]

Lipofuscine accumulates in the RPE.

Material originating from the RPE cytoplasm is continually deposited on Bruch's membrane.[22] The accumulation of deposits leads to variations in the composition, because both of the increase in the percentage of lipids of photoreceptor origin and for the structural alterations of their proteins; the consequences of this are the calcification and the fragmentation of the membrane itself. Its permeability to water decreases with age, and this leads to a deterioration in the transport of soluble nutritional components.

The accumulation of residues of cell digestion on Bruch's membrane leads to the formation of drusen. The apoptosis of the RPE cells laden with lipofuscine leads to other waste products. The remaining cells will attempt to remove them by phagocytosis and will migrate to maintain contact between them, thinning the RPE layer and increasing the number of photoreceptors that each one is serving.[23] The absence of the RPE will result in the atrophy of choriocapillaris and the development of atrophic DMLE.[24]

Drusen and DMLE.

The cellular membrane of the photoreceptors

All the cell membranes contain amphipathic lipids, phospholipids, glycolipids, and cholesterol. When the fatty acids are long chain and polyunsaturated, they contribute to providing fluidity to the cell membranes; the opposite is true when the chains are short and the bonds saturated. The cell membranes of the photoreceptors are 80% to 90% phospholipids and 8% to 10%[25] cholesterol. The alcohols are usually choline, ethanolamine, serine, and inositol. DHA is the fatty acid with the largest concentration in the retina.

The membranes of the cones and rods are very smooth and contain DHA.

The external segment of the rods contains the highest concentration of polyunsaturated fatty acids compared to any other biologic membrane system. The concentration of DHA is high while the concentration of arachidonic acid is low. The reason why the membrane of the photoreceptors is structured in this way is unknown; it does not appear to depend on the selective incorporation of the fatty acids by specific membrane proteins but by a type of release controlled by RPE.[26-28] RPE possesses specific receptors for LDL, which contain phospholipids with DHA or free DHA; it controls the release into the inter-photoreceptor matrix[29] where some fatty acid-binding proteins (FABP) attach to the DHA and carry it inside the photoreceptors.

More detailed information

Collagen

Collagen is a fibrous protein, the most abundant found in the connective tissue where it has the role of matrix and support. Approximately 25% of all the protein in our body is collagen, and this is equivalent to approximately 6% of our body weight. It is synthesized by fibroblastic cells. To date, 28 different types of collagen have been identified. Type I collagen represents 90% of the total and is part of the corneal composition; Type II collagen is found in the vitreous body. Despite this wide variety, the structure is relatively simple.

The structural unit of collagen is tropocollagen, a protein with 3 polypeptide chains. The chains consist of a characteristic tripeptide unit with a glycine amino acid every 3 residues, while the other 2 are often proline and hydroxyproline, more infrequently lysine or hydrolysine. Some specific residues of proline and lysine are hydroxylate to hydroxyproline and hydroxylysine under the action of enzymes such as hydroxysilase, and the reaction requires vitamin C[30] as the essential cofactor.

The synthesis of the protein collagen requires vitamin C.

Collagen synthesis begins with the production of molecules of procollagen; it seems that the presence of vitamin C can affect the synthesis of RNA.[31] The chains are held together by S-S bonds and then twist to form a triple helix, which is then glycosylated and carried out of the cell through secretion vesicles.

At this point, some peptidases transform procollagen into tropocollagen, cutting off the ends. The molecules of tropocollagen are arranged in parallel rows, creating solid cross-linking–type bonds that give rise to the fibrils. Last, the fibrils can position themselves in undulated or parallel bands to form fibers, and the fibers then form fiber bundles *(Figure 1.1)*.

Collagen is endogenous but its precursors are consumed with the diet.

The collagen in our body is of endogenous origin. The dietary intake of the precursor amino acids (glycine, proline, and lysine) and vitamin C will influence the presence of collagen in the tissues. In bone tissue, the synthesis of collagen is predominantly associated with the diet; in muscles and tendons on the other hand, the synthesis is predominantly associated with physical exercise.[32]

The GAGs

The *glycoaminoglycans* (GAGs) or mucopolysaccharides are organic glucidic molecules consisting of long chains of disaccharide units. Several types exist, all with similar functions of support and protection in the majority of tissues.

Figure 1.1

Collagen synthesis

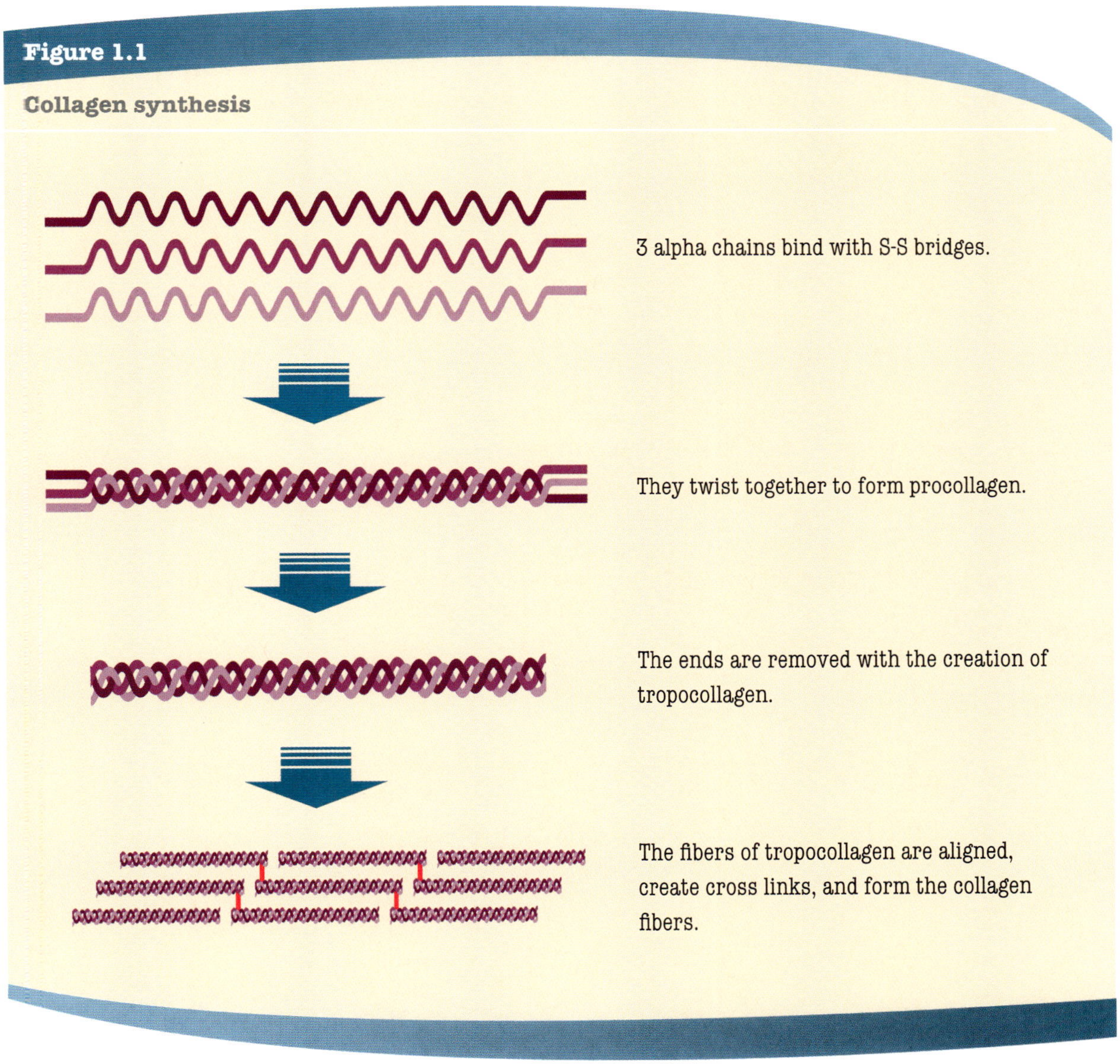

GAGs are highly hydrophyllic and easily form hydrated molecules that act as buffers that contribute to defending the body's structures from trauma caused by compressive forces. Moreover, they can permit the diffusion of hydrosoluble molecules inside their porous structure, and they can aggregate to each other and with some proteins, giving rise to glycoproteins and proteoglycans.

The GAGs are easily hydrated.

Hyaluronic acid is capable of creating reticular structures.

The glycoproteins are proteins bound to carbohydrates (ie, they are glycosylated proteins). Most of the proteins in nature are glycosylated. The percentage of the glucidic part with respect to the total molecule varies between 2% to 3%, as in the case of immunoglobulin, and 85%, as in the case of the glycoproteins that make up the blood groups.

The proteoglycans are macromolecules with a protein core that are covalently bonded to long chains of disaccharides or GAGs. There are 2 type of proteoglycans: the sulforates and the nonsulforates. The first group contains condroitin-sulfate, keratan-sulfate, heparan-sulfate and dermatan-sulfate; the second group contains hyaluronic acid and condroitin acid.

Hyaluronic acid is a GAG with an unbranched polysaccharide chain produced from the aggregation of thousands of disaccharide molecules consisting of glucuronic acid and N-acetylglucosamine *(Figure 1.2)*. In the amorphous matrix of the connective tissue, hyaluronic acid is the only GAG that may not be bonded to a protein core in order to form the proteoglycan. *In vivo*, all the carboxylic groups of hyaluronic acid are ionized, resulting in a highly polarized molecule that is highly soluble in water.

Figure 1.2

Hyaluronic acid

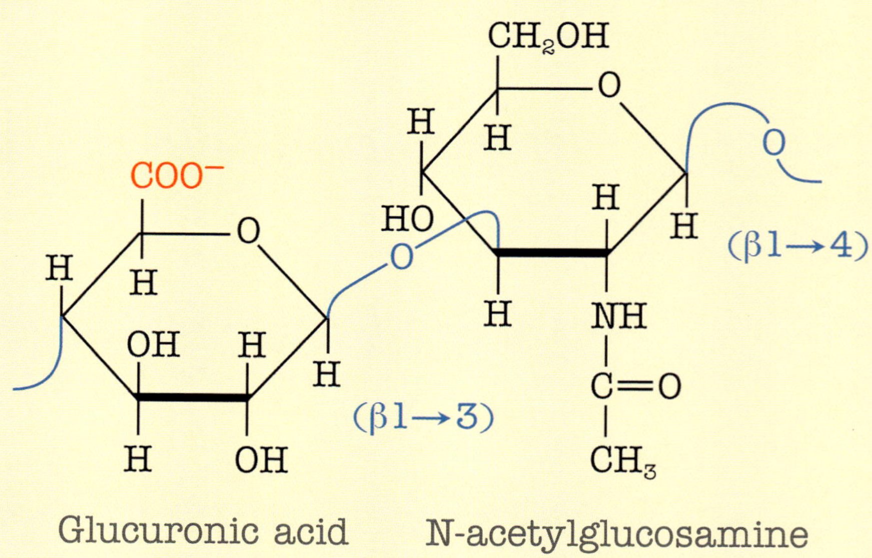

Thanks to its ability to absorb water molecules, hyaluronic acid maintains the hydration, the turgidity, the plasticity and the viscosity of the tissues. It acts as a binder and as a molecule that protects against impact preventing damage to the tissue cells from physical stress. In some specific cases, it acts as an efficient lubricant, for example in the synovial liquid.
The molecule of hyaluronic acid is extremely long: this characteristic allows it to create in the tissues large reticular structures that act as a matrix that is essential for maintaining the shape and the tone of the tissue; it can also act as a filter against the liberal diffusion into the tissues of specific substances or infecting agents.
Only substances with a molecular weight low enough to pass through the "links" in this reticular matrix will be able to spread freely in the tissue; all the substances with a greater molecular weight, such as bacteria or viruses, will be trapped in the net. It should be pointed out that many bacteria contain hyaluronidase, an enzyme that can split hyaluronic acid, which provides them with an entrance point.

Essential fatty acids

Saturated fatty acids are contained in milk-based products (cheese, butter, cream), in fatty meat, and in palm or coconut oil; they tend to raise the cholesterol level and consequently should not exceed 10% of the body's total caloric intake. Unsaturated fatty acids, on the other hand, reduce the blood cholesterol level. The monounsaturated fats are found in olive oil (oleic acid) and can account for up to 20% of the total calorie input in the diet.
Polyunsaturated fatty acids should account for approximately 7% of the total calories. They can be grouped into 2 families (omega-3 and omega-6) depending on the position of the double bond closest to the terminal methyl group of the fatty acid. The ratio of polyunsaturated acids in the diet should be omega-6:omega-3 = 5:1.
Some of them cannot be synthesized by animals and for this reason they are called "essential" or essential fatty acids (EFA); the only intake is in the diet *(Table 1.1)*. Linoleic acid is 18:2omega-6, and 18:3omega-3; it is used as a precursor for important polyunsaturated fatty acids, EPA, and DHA. These are produced in the liver[33]; in this organ, they are also incorporated in the lipoprotein LDL for transport in the circulatory cascade.
The presence of DHA in the body depends predominantly on the direct intake and to a lesser degree on the intake of its precursor.
In the eye, the essential fatty acids are involved in the transport of retinoids through the interphotoreceptor matrix[34] and are used to build cell membranes, increasing their fluidity. They contribute to the hemostatic and thromboembolic processes, and they are also behind the formation of the prostaglandins. They can be used intracellularly as a second messenger of the activation of the chinase protein kinase C.[35]

EPA and DHA are used in the construction of the cell membranes.

Table 1.1

Sources of essential fatty acids

	Omega-3	Omega-6
Salmon, mackerel, herring	✔✔	
Walnuts	✔	✔✔✔
Peanuts, pistachios, almonds		✔
Chick peas		✔
Sunflower seed oil		✔✔✔
Corn oil		✔✔✔
Wheatgerm oil	✔	✔✔✔
Linseed oil	✔✔✔	✔
Olive oil		✔

no check = no content; ✔ = low content; ✔✔ = medium conent; and ✔✔✔ = high content

DHA and EPA are found in considerable quantities in human breast milk.

The omega-3 are found in large quantities in fish (salmon, herring) and in some types of oil (linseed oil, for example). The omega-6 are found in large quantities in vegetable oils, such as sesame seed oil, borage or starflower oil, or primrose oil. The total requirements of essential fatty acids has not been precisely defined but must account for 1% to 2% of the daily caloric intake for adults and 3% for children. The use of skim milk will reduce the dietary intake and is associated with a growth deficiency in children. In the past, a deficit in essential fatty acids was observed in patients subjected to total drip feeding, which had a low fat content; this problem has been recognized and is now routinely corrected.

A lack of omega-3 fatty acids can cause sight damage.

A diet lacking omega-3 fatty acids in the animal model is associated with a visual deficiency, indicating that the polyunsaturated fatty acids contribute to the function of the photoreceptors.[36] In studies on humans, reductions in visual acuity and electroretinogram were observed.[37] A greater dietary intake increases the amount of polyunsaturated fatty acids in the cell membranes.

Carotenoids

Carotenoids are fat-soluble pigments found in plants for the most part. Their yellow, orange, and red colors are often masked by chlorophyll. They can be split into 2 groups: carotene and xanthophyll. Only some carotenes have been identified in human plasma: α-carotene, β-carotene, β-cryptoxanthin, and lycopene. Only the first 3 of these can be transformed into retinol (vitamin A). Xanthophylls are oxygenated derivatives of carotene. In human plasma, only luteine and zeaxanthin have been identified. These molecules cannot be transformed into vitamin A *(Table 1.2)*.

Luteine (L) and zeaxanthin (Z) are pigments contained in the cell body of the photoreceptors, and for this reason they are called "macular pigments" (MP). L and Z are 2 structural isomers, and L can be metabolized in Z. Other structure isomers of Z exist in the macula, RRZ, SSZ, and meso-Z; however, they cannot be measured in the plasma. It is assumed that meso-Z is a conversion product of L, which is found in the retina itself and is not of food origin. This hypothesis is also supported by the relative rarity of Z in food and its maximum concentration in the cones.[38] In plants, Z is produced in the presence of excess light and is eliminated following a return to the baseline conditions.

Luteine and zeaxanthin are the macular pigments.

The macular pigments have a dual function: protection of the oxidative photochemical damage and an improvement in the visual function as they absorb light in the blue-green frequency[39-41] before it reaches the substrates that can be oxidized in the photoreceptors and in the pigmented epithelium. Thanks to the presence of the hydroxyl radical at the end of the carotene chain, L

The macular pigments protect the eye from oxidative damage and improve visual function.

Table 1.2

Sources of carotenoids

Luteine and zeaxanthin	Egg yolk, pumpkin, zucchini, spinach, broccoli, Brussels sprouts, sweet peppers, saffron, goji berry, kiwi fruit, oranges, red apples, mango, peaches
Lycopene	Tomato, saffron, red apples, oranges, cucumber, apricot, pink grapefruit, grapes, papaya
Astaxanthin	Crustaceans, salmon
ß-carotene	Carrots, broccoli, sweet peppers, spinach, pumpkin, zucchini, mango, peach, apricot, oranges

L and Z neutralize the singlet oxygen and other possible radicals of oxygen with a mechanism called quenching.

and Z are positioned perpendicular to the cell membrane, which allows them to screen the light more efficiently.[42] The light that is more potentially damaging for the retina has a wavelength of 450 nm, which corresponds to the absorption peak of the macular pigments[43]; it has been calculated that the macular pigments reduce the incident light on the fovea by about 40%.[44]
Both L and Z are fairly resistant to destruction by oxidation. They neutralize the singlet oxygen[45] and other possible radicals of oxygen with a mechanism called quenching *(Figure 1.3)*. The excess energy in the singlet oxygen is transferred to the structure of the carotenoids, which is rich in electrons; this energy brings the carotenoid molecule into an unstable state called triplet (3Car). From the 3Car state, the molecule releases excess energy as heat and returns to the normal state as before (1Car). This is a physical mechanism, not chemical, and, consequently, the molecule's structure is not modified; the carotenoid remains intact and can be used repeatedly *(Table 1.3)*.

Figure 1.3

Quenching mechanism

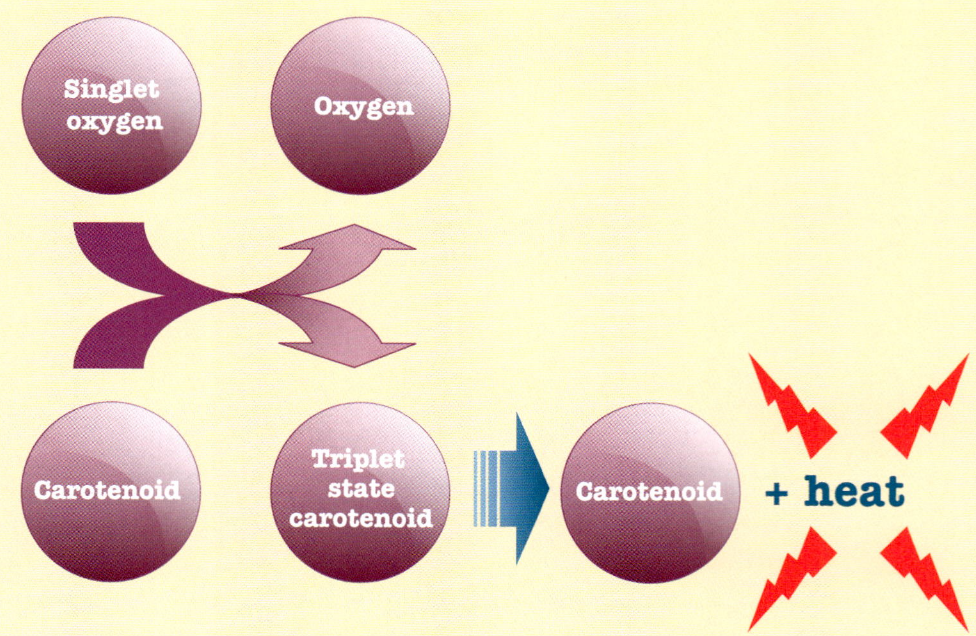

Table 1.3

Carotenoids listed according to their capacity for eliminating radicals (quenching)
Lycopene
Astaxanthin
ß-carotene
Zeaxanthin
Luteine

Moreover, the carotenoids can block the triplet state of oxygen. Thanks to their electron-rich structure, the carotenoids neutralize the free radicals by donating an electron or by forming covalent bonds with them.[46] However, this type of process involves the chemical structure of the molecule and leads ultimately to its destruction. The macular pigment molecules are extremely efficient in preventing the process of peroxidation of the membrane phospholipids.[47] Z is the most efficient in this function[48] because it has a greater number of double bonds than L. Even in solution, β-carotene, L, and Z have comparable antioxidant capacity; L is the most efficient in the cell systems for inhibiting the autooxidation of the cell lipids; Z is actually 50% more efficient in delaying the formation of hydroperoxides in the liposomes of phosphatidylcholine. Lycopene is the best at eliminating singlet oxygen.[49]

In vitro, Z incorporated in the phospholipid membrane modifies the structure and mechanically stabilizes it with a reduction of the water flow through it. Moreover, it reduces the products of the diffusion and the concentration of oxygen and can contribute to protecting the fatty acids from peroxidation. Many of the oxidation products of L and Z can be extracted from the retina, which suggests their role in protection against oxidative damage.[50] It has also been suggested that, in some way, the visual pigment may actually initiate the damage or activate a physiological cascade of events that may have damaging effects at a later stage.[51]

Carotenoids have been isolated from human breast milk,[52] and L and Z are found in large quantities in egg yolk and spinach but are absent from carrots. L is the carotenoid with the highest concentration in kiwi fruit, pumpkin, and spinach and is also found in saffron. Z is the rarest of the pigments and is found in green and orange peppers but not in the yellow and red varieties.[53] Gou qi zi (*Lycium barbarum*—goji berry) is a small red berry that originated in

China and contains the highest concentration of Z (more than 5 mg/100 g).[54] Animals are not able to synthesize carotenoids.

The quantity of macular pigment depends on the diet and is regulated genetically.

The quantity of macular pigment depends on the diet and is regulated genetically[55]; in fact, in the majority of people, but not all, the blood level of carotenoids rises following supplement intake.[56]

The concentration of lycopene is high in tomatoes and some tropical fruits such as papaya. Astaxanthin, a carotenoid with a powerful antioxidant effect, gives the red color to crustaceans and some fish such as salmon; these animals are unable to synthesize it. Their diet of zooplankton, which in turn are nourished by a diet of phytoplanktons, provides the necessary amounts.[57]

In plants, the carotenoids are conjugated with proteins to form carotenoproteins. Cooking food denatures them and releases the carotenoids, which can then be absorbed; at the same time, some are destroyed by the heat. The bioavailability of the carotenoids is correlated with the size of the food particles and their digestibility, with the introduction of fats, iron, oleic and linolenic acid, fiber, and total calories; fat absorbed with the diet improves the absorption. The bioavailability is limited by malabsorption syndromes and intestinal parassitosis, renal or hepatic disorders, alcohol consumption, or drugs that inhibit cytochrome P450.

Absorption of carotenoids.

In cultures of intestinal cells, carotenoids are absorbed with no receptor regulation; *in vivo*, the carotenoids are transported passively through the intestinal mucosa and incorporated in micelles consisting of lipids and biliary acids. In the liver, during the postprandial period, the carotenoids are incorporated in lipoproteins but not in a uniform manner: LDL preferentially carries β-carotene, while HDL carries L and Z. Compared to β-carotene, L and Z are found in lower concentrations in blood. Following supplement intake, the blood levels of carotenoids remain high.[58,59]

The concentration of macular pigment would appear to be higher in males than in females with equal blood concentrations of L and Z.[60]

The macular pigments are carried by a protein that binds to the xanthophylls and are accumulated through a bond with cytosolic tubulin.[61] There would appear to be a mechanism of active selective transport to the inside of the photoreceptors; in actuality, both pigments are found in all photoreceptors with a higher concentration of L in the rods and of Z in the cones. It would appear that there are also special concentration ratios between L and Z depending on the type of cone.[62]

In animal models, if the diet lacks carotenoids, a loss of the macular pigment is observed with a consequent defect in the cones due to a deterioration in the cell membranes and the accumulation of lipofuscine in the pigmented epithelium.

In humans,[63] the reduction in the macular pigment is associated with classical fluorangiographic alterations such as hyperfluorescence and the appearance of drusen.

With smokers there is a reduced carotenoid intake with the diet, and the blood concentration of carotenoids in smokers is low at any rate. It is thought that the oxidizing impact of smoke consumes the blood carotenoids, similar to the effect on vitamin C.

The retinal concentration of L and Z is reduced in smokers. It has been observed that eating egg yolks raises the total serum cholesterol levels but also increases the HDL level, not varying the risk index for ischemic heart disease. Eating eggs should therefore be a valid way of increasing L and Z intake. There are correlations, alhough extremely variable, between the dietary consumption of the various carotenoids, their blood concentrations, and the levels in the tissue. Through specific supplements, it is possible to modify the serum levels of the various carotenoids.[64] At the time of publication, there are no findings to support any toxic effect caused by L and Z intake.

Smokers have lower levels of carotenoids.

Retinol

Vitamin A was given this name because it was the first vitamin to be discovered. In nature, retinol is found only in animal tissue. However, plant tissue contains carotenoids that act as provitamins. There are 3 different forms of vitamin A: alcohol (retinol), aldehyde (retinaldehyde or retinal), and acid (retinoic acid). Retinol and retinal can be transformed into each other; retinol can be irreversibly transformed into retinoic acid.

Vitamin A has good heat resistance, and a percentage in excess of 70% remains intact after the food has been cooked. Prior to being absorbed, the esters of retinol must be hydrolyzed. The absorption of retinol occurs by means of a process of facilitated diffusion; however, in the event that the concentration of retinol is high, mechanisms of passive diffusion may also occur.

The absorption of retinol depends on the presence of lipids and bile acids. Carotenoids are absorbed in a quantity that varies between 5% and 50% through a mechanism of passive transport, which is also influenced by the presence of lipids.

Absorption of vitamin A.

The plasma levels of vitamin A are subjected to very precise homeostatic mechanisms and consequently its plasma concentration is kept between 40 and 80 µg/dl. If required, retinol will be released by the hepatocytes linked to alla retinol binding protein (RBP) and by the storage cells (adipocytes). In plasma, the retinol-RBP complex binds to transthyretin, which also carries the thyroid hormones, while retinol is conjugated with a number of plasma proteins. The carotenoids are transported by lipoproteins.

In plasma, there is a certain quantity of free retinol that would appear to be in equilibrium with the amount bonded to RBP. It is assumed that this can penetrate cells by means of a mechanism not mediated by receptors. Nevertheless, the EPR cells express a receptor for RBP that binds and carries the retinol with it. Once it enters the cell, retinol binds to cellular retinol binding protein (CRBP), a part of it becomes esterified, for storage or for conversion into the 2 active forms: retinoic acid and retinaldehyde. Inside EPR, CRPB is transported to the apex of the cell membrane on the side of the photoreceptors and retinol passes into the subretinal space where it binds to an interphotoreceptor protein that binds the retinol (IRBP) and where it becomes incorporated in the photoreceptors.

The recommended daily dose varies between 600 and 800 µg/dl. Retinol is found in a greater concentration in liver, eggs, and milk. Carotenoids are found in considerable quantities in vegetables with high pigment levels and in yellow/orange-colored fruits and vegetables.

Zinc deficiency reduces the synthesis of RBP, reduces the activity of the enzyme that releases retinol from its accumulated form, and decreases the conversion capacity of retinol in retinal.[65]

The levels of assumption of vitamin A are expressed in terms of retinol equivalent (RE) as follows: 1 RE =1 µg retinol = 6 µg β-carotene = 12 µg other carotenoids. At the time of publication, the daily recommended intake is 1000 RE for males and 800 RE for females; when breast-feeding, this should be increased by approximately 350 RE/day.

Vitamin A deficiency is a pathology observed frequently in developing countries and in places where access to a correct and well-balanced diet is difficult (famine, war fugitives, etc). Children are affected to a greater degree both during breast-feeding because the mothers are not eating sufficient nutrients and will be producing milk that lacks essential elements and in infancy because they are simply not getting enough food.

Deficiency and toxicity of vitamin A.

A reduced level of vitamin A in the eye will lead to lower efficiency of the goblet cells with initial symptoms of dry eye. A lack of vitamin A will then lead to night blindness, and in the more advanced stages in xerophthalmia, it will lead to the presence of a typical color of the conjunctiva (Bitot's spots) and finally with keratinization of the eye surface and keratomalacia. Integration is possible with retinyl-palmitate, retinyl-acetate, or β-carotene.

Cases of chronic toxicity associated with the continual use of nonexcessive doses of vitamin A are frequent; however, the doses are greater than the liver's accumulation capacity. β-carotene cannot cause an overdose of vitamin A because it cannot be converted into retinol at sufficient speed.

In smokers, consumption of high doses of β-carotene increases the risk of lung cancer.[66]

Intake of doses of vitamin A higher than 300 mg can lead to acute intoxication with nausea, vomiting, migraine, loss of coordination, and visual disturbances. Compared to acute toxicity, cases of chronic toxicity are more frequent as this condition can appear when daily doses are consumed in excess of the liver's capacity for storage or elimination; this occurs when people frequently consume food that is rich in vitamin A or excessively consume supplements. This will lead to the appearance of symptoms characterized by loss of appetite, muscle pain, anemia, hair loss, and a variety of neurological alterations. High doses of β-carotene supplements (>30 mg/day) will cause changes to the skin (carotenodermia) with the appearance of a yellow-orange pigmentation of the skin and mucosa, a phenomenon that will rapidly disappear once the dose of carotenoid has been reduced. For this reason, a maximum daily dose of 9 mg for males and 7.5 mg for women is recommended. Daily doses in excess of 30 mg/day would appear to have a teratogenic effect on the fetus. Consequently, vitamin A supplements should not be taken during pregnancy, with a recommendation of not exceeding a dose of vitamin A of 6 mg/day.

The biochemical cycle of visual function

Vitamin A is essential for the visual process and for cell differentiation; it is necessary for growth, reproduction, and the correct functioning of the immune system.
Retinaldehyde, which can also be formed from retinol by means of alcohol dehydrogenase, is part of the vision mechanism. Retinaldehyde (also known as retinal) in the 11-cis form is combined to a retinal protein, opsin, and forms rodopsin. Rodopsin is found in the membrane of the photoreceptor disks. When a photon interacts with 11-cis retinal, it acts as a catalyst for the conversion to all-trans-retinal, which determines a conformational change in opsin. The immediate consequence of this is a sort of steric block, with opsin losing its affinity for retinal. Rodopsin passes extremely rapidly through a series of highly unstable intermediates: pre-lumirodopsin (or bathorodopsin), lumirodopsin, metharodopsin I, and metharodopsin II, which is the active form of opsin *(Figure 1.4)*.
Rodopsin is a receptor that functions when coupled with a G-protein. When metharodopsin II is formed, the G-protein is activated.The G-protein of the visual cycle is called transducin. This activates a specific GTP phosphodiesterase that splits cGMP into GMP and causes a reduction in the concentration of cGMP. The rods contain numerous Na^+ channels, which are kept open, in conditions of darkness by high concentrations of cGMP. When the concentration of cGMP drops, the Na^+ channels along the cell membrane of the rods close, causing a variation in the membrane potential (hyperpolarization), and this generates an electric impulse. In the meantime, all-trans-retinal splits from opsin and is reduced by an NADPH-dependent dehydrogenase to all-trans-retinal, which is then recaptured by the pigmented epithelium and stored, following esterification. The all-trans-retinal is successively reconverted into 11-cis retinal through reactions of oxidation and isomerization *(Figure 1.5)*.

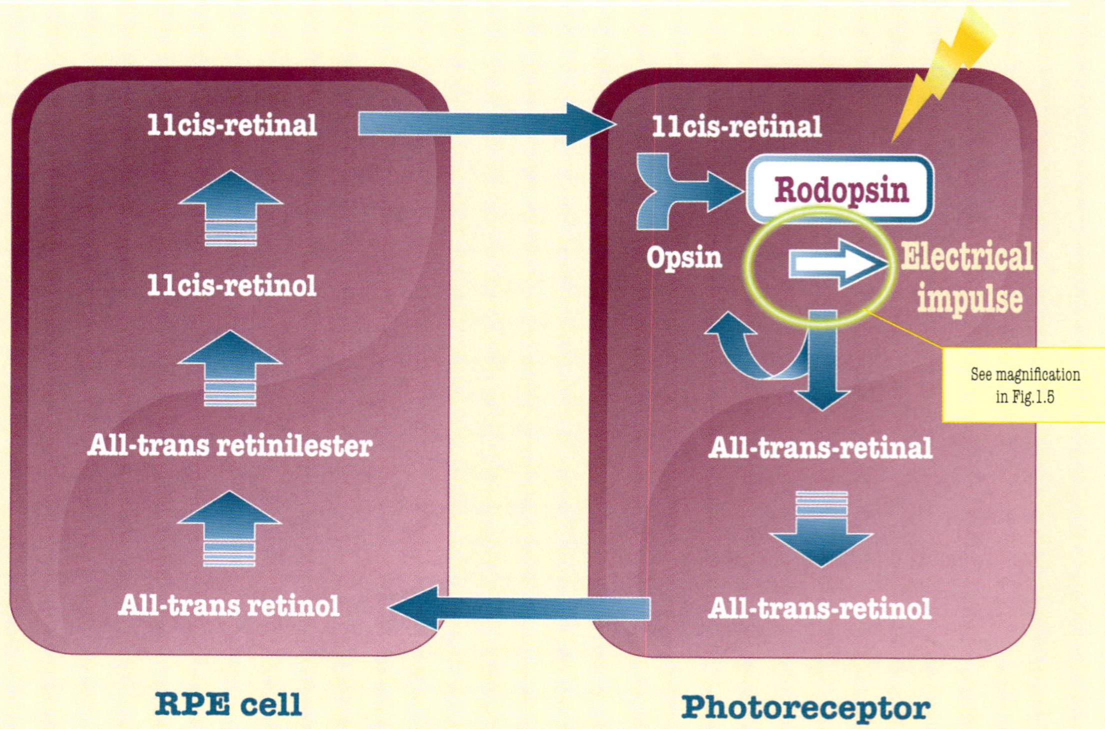

Figure 1.4

The biochemical cycle of the visual function

Figure 1.5

The biochemical cycle of the visual function (detail of Figure 1.4)

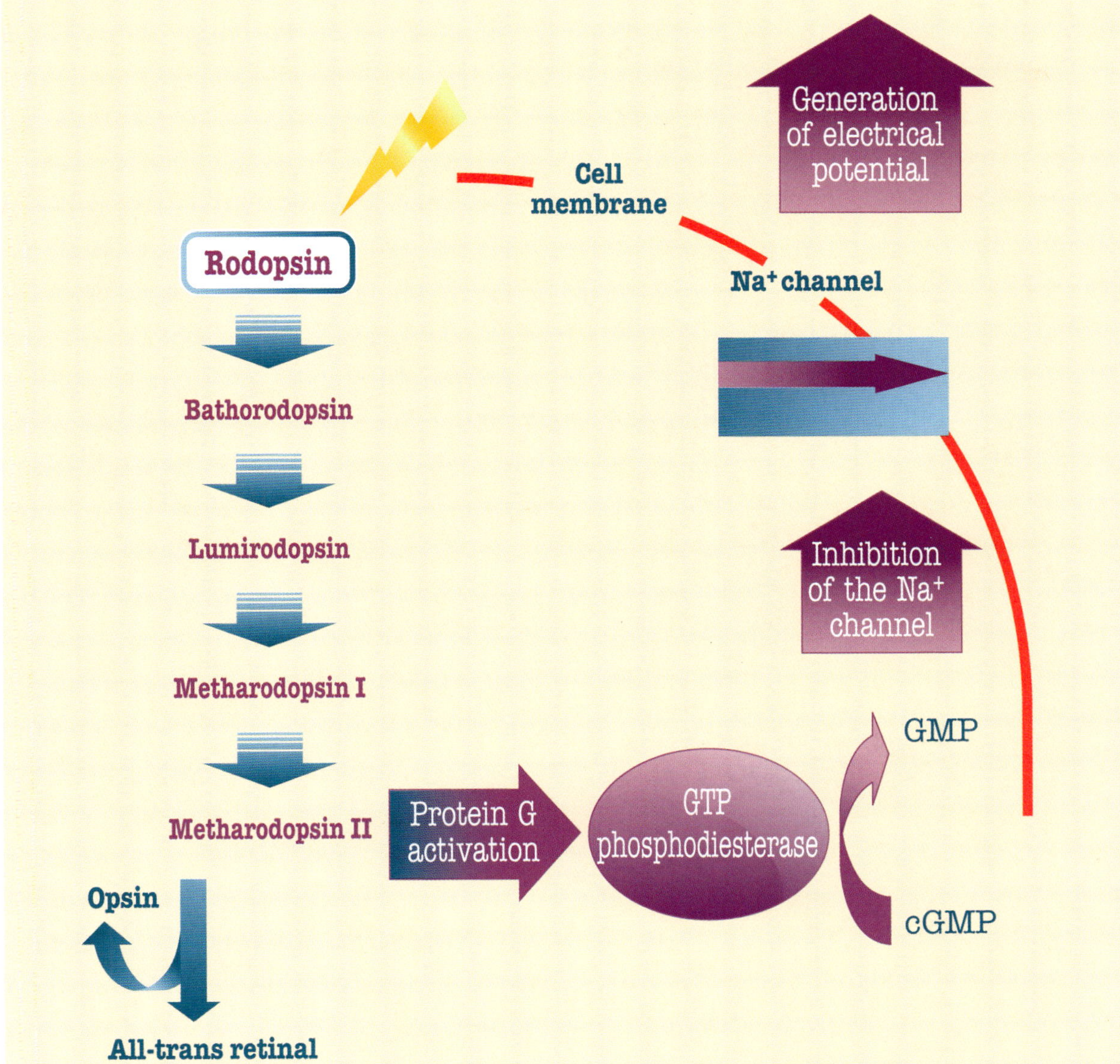

Oxidative stress and the **antioxidant systems**

Oxidative stress

In the eye, photochemical damage is the most common form of oxidative damage.

Free radicals can form even during normal metabolic processes.

The membrane lipids are structures sensitive to oxidation.

Exposure to the external atmosphere, to light, to toxic factors, and also to normal metabolic processes, including aging, activates a number of oxidative processes in the retina that lead to the formation of the so-called free radicals."[67]

Through the action of compounds such as these, oxidative damage can affect the cell structures, mainly the cell membranes (lipid peroxidation) and the enzyme systems. Light that reaches the macula can damage both the pigmented epithelium and the photoreceptors.[68]

An energy source and oxygen are needed for the formation of free radicals.

In the eye, the most common pathway of oxidative damage is photochemical oxidative damage. Light can activate molecular oxygen directly and form singlet oxygen. Light energy, particularly UV light, can be absorbed by sensitive molecules such as meta-hemoglobin and can contribute to the processes of peroxidation directly or through the release of iron.[69] Metal ions can interact with hydrogen peroxide (Fenton's reaction), producing the hydroxyl radical, which is an extremely reactive and dangerous type of oxygen *(Figure 2.1)*.

Oxidation-reduction reactions are ongoing inside every cell, as part of the normal metabolic events and also to control the damage from external stress factors. Oxygen is normally reduced to water without free radicals being produced; however, it can also accept an electron from a reducing agent, which will produce oxygen radicals, such as the superoxide anion, hydrogen peroxide, and hydroxyl radicals.

For example, the superoxide radical can be produced accidentally in the mitochondrial and microsomial respiratory chain because of the transfer of an electron directly to oxygen by the electron carriers.

In the RPE cells, many oxidative processes are linked to phagocytosis of the external segment of the photoreceptors. During phagocytosis, a superoxide anion is produced, and this can damage the cell directly or it can be converted into a hydroxyl radical.

The molecules in the retina that are most sensitive to oxidative damage are the polyunsaturated membrane lipids,[70] the cytochromes, the flavinic enzymes of the mitochondria, and free riboflavin to name but a few. Regarding the lipids, the higher the degree of unsaturation, the greater the sensitivity to oxidative damage. Lipid hydroperoxides are highly reactive, and they split rapidly into compounds that are toxic for the retina. High concentrations of omega-3 fatty acids do not alter the

Figure 2.1

Fenton's reaction

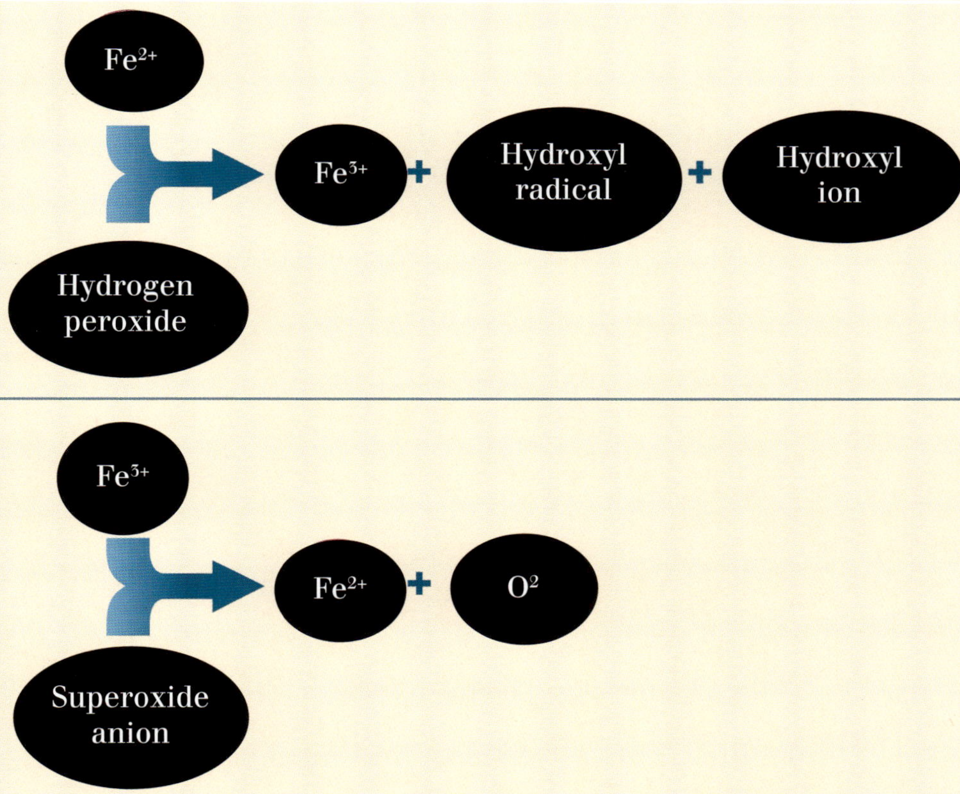

damage sensitivity of the external segment of the cones.[71] The macular region is sensitive to lipid peroxidation; the same does not appear to apply to the peripheral region, possibly due to its arrangement in fatty acids.[72] This sensitivity increases with age.

The antioxidant systems

Exposure to oxidative processes increases the concentration of antioxidant factors[73] as a protective measure *(Figure 2.2)*. The protection system against free radicals is guaranteed by the interaction

Figure 2.2

Defense against oxidative stress

Good	Bad
SOD & CAT	Singlet oxygen
GSH-Px & GSSG-Red	Hydrogen peroxide
Vit. C & Vit. E	
Luteine & zeaxanthine	
	Superoxide anion
	Hydroxyl radical
	Lipid peroxyl radical

between systems of endogenous origin (enzyme systems) and elements of exogenous origin introduced with the diet, with the role of enzyme cofactors, or a direct antioxidant action[74] (scavenging and quenching).

RPE is the most important tissue that protects the retina from oxidative damage; it contains an elevated number of antioxidant enzymes. These enzyme systems are found to a varying degree in all of our body tissues.

SOD, CAT, Glutathione.

In the extracellular ambience, in the cytoplasm, and in the mitochondria, the enzyme superoxide dismutase (SOD)[75] eliminates the superoxide anion and transforms it into hydrogen peroxide. This is then eliminated by catalase (CAT) contained in the peroxysomes *(Figure 2.3)*; alternately, it is eliminated by glutathione peroxydase (GSH-Px) with the elimination of glutathione, which is oxidized. Glutathione reductase (GSSG-Red) regenerates glutathione using *NADP*, an element in the normal - cell energetic processes *(Figure 2.4)*. This chain of enzymes is one of the metabolic defenses against oxidative damage of fundamental importance for the eye and defends the organ from the phototoxic effect.[76] It changes with age and under the effects of some pathologies.

Figure 2.3

Antioxidant enzymes

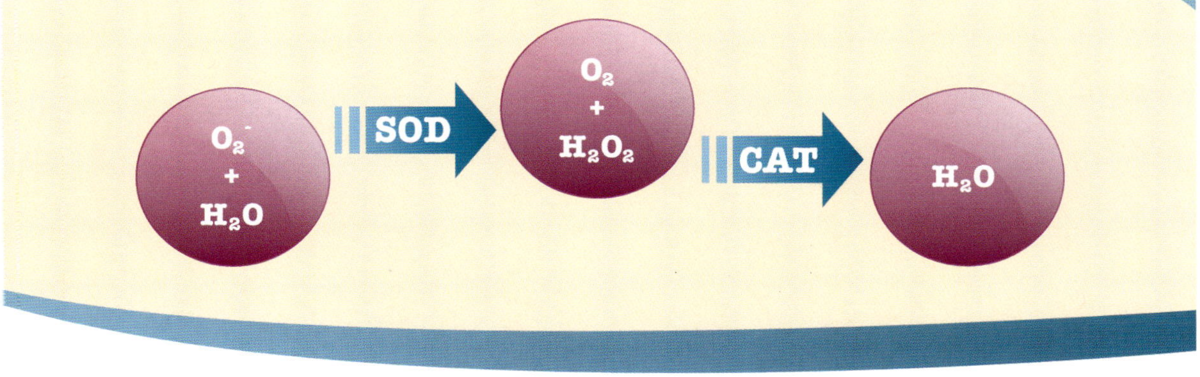

The corneal epithelium is permeable to oxygen and exposure to reactive oxygen intermediates (ROI). In addition to glycolysis and the Krebs Cycle, in this epithelium, glucose is used mainly in the hexose monofosfate pathway to produce NADPH[77] and keep the GSH-Px/GSSG-Red active. Even in the crystalline lens, redox is maintained mainly by glutathione.[78,79]

Vitamin E can neutralize the free radicals. This type of substance is called a scavenger. It takes an electron from the oxidized polyunsaturated fatty acids, passing from tocopherol to tocopheryl; it is later reactivated by vitamin C that passes from ascorbate to semidehydroascorbate. Exogenous dihydrolipoic acid (DHLA) improves the effect of ascorbate, regenerating it from dehydroascorbate[80] (*Figure 2.5*).

Vitamins C and E.

Even the macular pigments and, more generally, the carotenoids can act as scavengers. Scavenging is a chemical reaction; in addition to this function, they can perform the action called quenching, which neutralizes the ROI that provoke physical, not chemical, variations of the molecule. This is described in the specific chapter dedicated to the carotenoids.

For these systems to function, the availability of the component elements and their cofactors is crucial; all of these substances are introduced with the diet.

Figure 2.4

Antioxidant action of the enzymes that contain glutathione

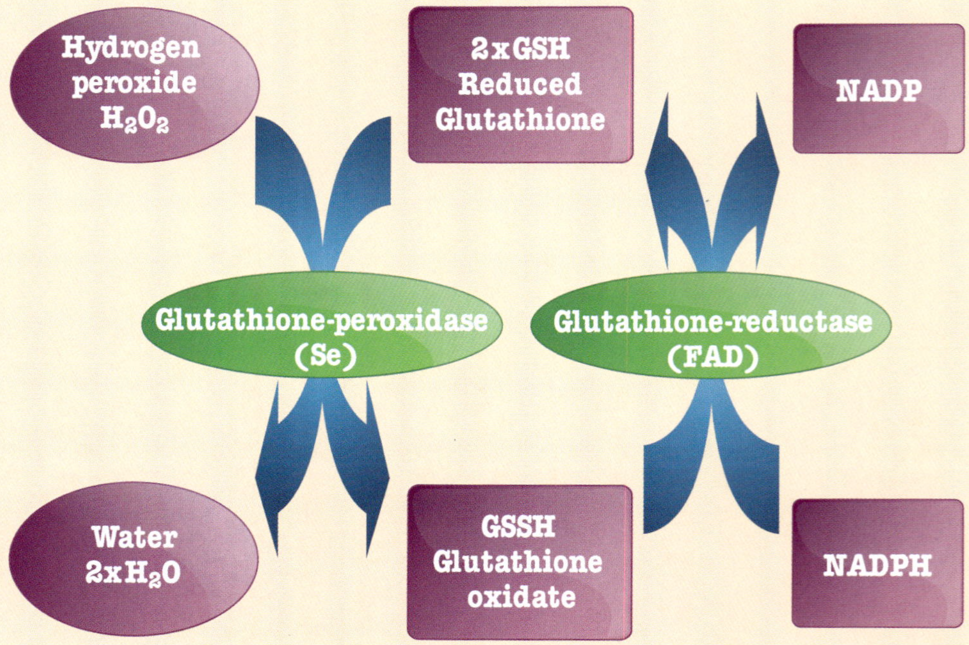

Se: Selenium, cofactor of the enzyme glutathione-peroxidase.

FAD: Flavina-adenin-dinucleotide, cofactor of the enzyme glutathione reductase.

Figure 2.5

Antioxidant action of the vitamins C and E

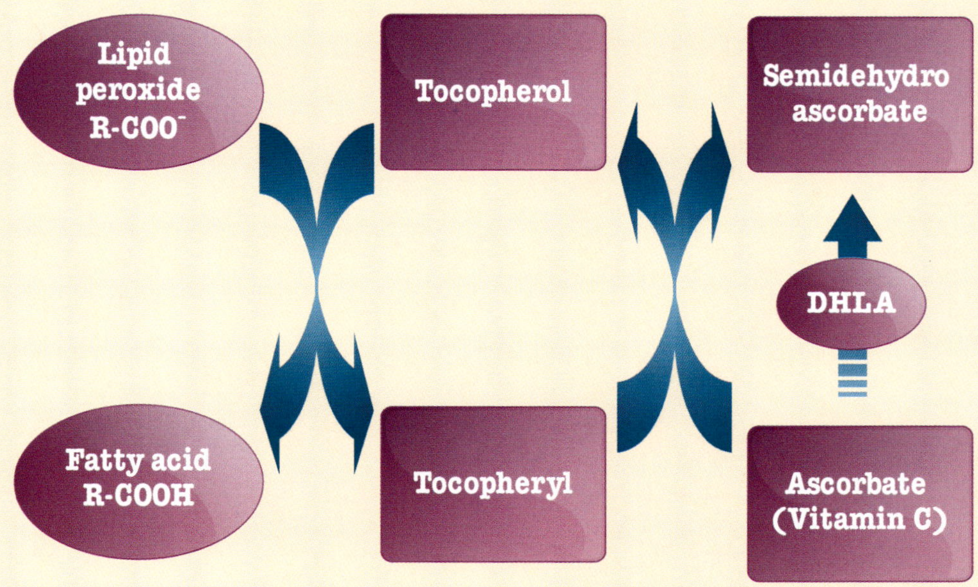

More detailed information

Vitamins

Vitamin C

Vitamin C is a water-soluble vitamin that is sensitive to heat and the effects of exposure to oxygen. It intervenes in the formation of collagen and protects the structure of tissues of mesenchymal origin.

Along with vitamin E, vitamin C protects against oxidative damage.

In the protection against oxidative damage, the role of vitamin C is linked to the role of vitamin E. It intervenes in the regeneration of vitamin E starting from the tocopheryl radical that is formed from the oxidation reaction of tocopherol following contact with lipoperoxides. Moreover, vitamin C can release electrons to the free radicals, stabilizing them. It also reduces the peroxidation of membrane DHA in the external segment of the photoreceptors. The RDA of vitamin C is 60 mg/day.

Large quantities of vitamin C are found in citrus fruits, apples, bananas, berries, tomatoes, potatoes, broccoli, sweet peppers, and other green and yellow vegetables. Vitamin C is water-soluble and will remain in the water used to cook food. It is rapidly absorbed by the intestine, and it increases the absorption of iron.

Considerable quantities of vitamin C are found in the eye and are actively transported by the plasma.

Chronic alcohol consumption will decrease the reserves of all the water-soluble vitamins, including vitamin C.

In animal models, a deficiency of vitamin C is responsible for damage to a retina subjected to intense light.

Ascorbate is oxidized when it is exposed to intense light; food supplements will protect against oxidative damage, will reduce the loss of photoreceptors following exposure to intense light, and will protect against DMLE.

Severe vitamin C deficiency causes scurvy.

A mild deficiency of vitamin C is associated with bleeding and gingivitis; more serious deficiency will cause scurvy, a condition associated with bleeding in the joints, asthenia, weight loss and irritability. Patients can actually die following convulsions or brain hemorrhage.

Conjunctival or eyelid hemorrhage and dry-eye syndrome can be observed in the eye. Long-term high-dose consumption of vitamin C is associated with the formation of kidney stones.

Vitamin E

Vitamin E is a mixture of the various tocopherols α, β, γ, and δ; α-tocopherol is considered to be the most active form.

Vitamin E is fat-soluble. It is an efficacious scavenger, an antioxidant that can neutralize the free radicals that form in the eye under phototoxic effect.[81] It, therefore, has a protective effect against damage to the retina caused by exposure to light. It also combats lipid peroxidation, particularly in the tissues rich in polyunsaturated fatty acids such as the retina.[82,83]

It is an efficacious scavenger.

The vitamin E requirement is greater if the diet contains a high quantity of unsaturated fatty acids. The RDA is 15 to 30 UI (8 to 10 mg).

Vitamin E is found in large quantities in whole wheat and whole cereals in general, soy, beans, nuts, broccoli, Brussels sprouts, broad green leaf vegetables, vegetable oils, and eggs.

Its absorption is similar to other fat-soluble vitamins. It reaches the circulation through the lymphatic system. Following intestinal absorption, it can be found in the kilomicrons and is then transported by the β-lipoproteins.

In the retina, the carotenoids and vitamin E have complementary distribution patterns correlated to the oxygen concentration: vitamin E is found in greater quantities in the external layers of the cones and the retina, where the concentration of oxygen is greater.

The levels of vitamin E are extremely high in the retina, higher in the RPE than the external segments of the photoreceptors.[84]

Vitamin E levels are very high in the retina.

There is an increase in the levels of vitamin E in the RPE of the macula in people who are 40 years or younger and decrease from age 60 or older. In the RPE of the outer retina, there is a slow but constant increase in the levels of vitamin E with age[85]; there is as much as 7 times more at 80 years of age than at 20.[86]

Vitamin E deficiency is a rare occurrence, although it may be observed in cases of severe malnutrition. In malabsorption syndromes, particularly in cases of steathorrea (celiac disease, cystic fibrosis), secondary deficiency may appear. Smoking reduces the level of vitamin E in the eye.[87]

Systemically, vitamin E deficiency leads to hemolysis, creatinuria, and deposits of ceroid substances in the muscle tissue, cerebellar ataxia, and peripheral neuropathy. A genetic deficiency of the protein that carries α-tocopherol also exists and this leads to progressive peripheral neuropathy, which results in ataxia (AVED syndrome). In the eye, this can lead to retinal degeneration in the macular area and is associated with the appearance of DMLE as a probable consequence of the accumulation of products of peroxidation.

A lack of vitamin E activates a degenerative process of the external segment of the photoreceptors, which will shorten. Subsequently, there is thinning of the external nuclear layer. Cones and rods are affected in the same way; a reduction in the cellular organelles is observed.

With a deficiency of vitamin E, the external segment of the photoreceptors degenerates.

When α-tocopherol is administered as a supplement, it is reduced to γ-tocopherol, which is more efficacious in eliminating nitrogen dioxide, one of the main oxidants in cigarette smoke that would appear to stimulate the production of VEGF in the pathogenesis of neovascularization.[88,89]

In vitro, α-tocopherol inhibits the proliferation of RPE cells with no cytotoxic effects.[90] The maximum effect is observed with the concentration of 100 μm, which is easily achieved with a standard oral administration. Vitamin E succinate, an ester, inhibits cell proliferation and migration without causing any cell toxicity.[91]

However, dietary supplements of vitamin E in smokers have led to an increased risk of brain hemorrhage, even though no increase in mortality has been observed.[92] Excessive doses of vitamin E lead to an alteration in cell-mediated immune responses.

Minerals

Zinc

Zinc plays a part in taste sensitivity, sensations of hunger and appetite, cell-mediated immunity, and wound healing. In children, a lack of zinc can lead to growth delay, loss of appetite, and alterations of taste sensitivity. In adults, the deficiency of this mineral leads to neurological alterations such as lethargy.

In metabolism, zinc improves the mobilization of retinol from the liver and is also used in the constitution of more than 100 enzymes, including carbonic anhydrase (accounting for 30% of the weight), alcohol dehydrogenase, CAT and SOD, and retinol dehydrogenase, an enzyme that is part of the regeneration cycle of the visual pigment.

Zinc is a cofactor of CAT.

In vitro, the activity of CAT is associated with the availability of zinc[93]: it appears to intervene in the regulation of transcription.[94] The presence of zinc improves the effect of the scavenger molecules for free radicals.[95] Zinc is a cofactor in the constitution of the extracellular matrix and is highly concentrated in the retina, the pigmented epithelium, and the choroid. It intervenes in the formation of the electric signal of the photoreceptors.[96]

An RDA of 7 to 10 mg/day of zinc is recommended. Zinc in food of animal origin has a greater bioavailability than zinc of plant origin; it can be found in wheat germ, brewers' yeast, pumpkin seeds, seafood (oysters), eggs, liver, beef, and lamb.

Chelated zinc is absorbed better than zinc sulfate. The absorption of zinc would appear to be under the homeostatic control and is correlated with the total calorie intake. In plasma, one-third of zinc is bonded weakly to albumin, and two-thirds is strongly bonded to globulin. Zinc is preferentially incorporated by the pigmented tissues in general. Recently, it was demonstrated that it is actively incorporated and retained by the RPE, the choroid, and other tissues of the retina.[97]

The risk of low blood zinc levels is higher in patients with cirrhosis or diabetes, in people affected by malabsorption syndromes, and in people taking diuretics. Zinc deficiency may be observed with diets that are rich in fiber or phytates in whole grain breads, in parasite infestations, with high levels of iron and calcium, with chronic consumption of alcohol, with malabsorption, with drip-feeding, during pregnancy, and during breast-feeding.

Zinc deficiency can lead to shunted development of the thymus gland and the lymphocytes.

A zinc deficiency can lead to stunted development of the thymus gland and the lymphocytes. A low serum zinc level is associated with the appearance of exudative DMLE.[98]

Zinc supplements.

Excessive supplements of zinc can lead to an increase in the concentration of metallothionine in the cells of the intestinal lumen. Metallothionine can bond strongly with copper, preventing its release into the circulatory cascade. Zinc should, therefore, be consumed with an appropriate quantity of copper.[99] Zinc serum levels increase following high supplement doses. Subjects with high levels of zinc frequently also have high triglyceride, total cholesterol and LDL cholesterol levels; no link with HDL cholesterol has been observed.[100] These findings underline how important it is to control the overall medical parameters when zinc supplements are being used. Ingestion of large doses of zinc can cause headache, nausea, stomach cramps, vomiting and diarrhea, and can lead to convulsions. High levels of zinc are toxic and can cause anemia.

Selenium

Selenium is a fundamental component of the enzyme glutathione peroxidase.

Selenium is a fundamental component of the enzyme glutathione peroxidase (GSH-Px), which belongs to the cells' antioxidant defense system. This enzyme catalyzes the degradation of the hydroperoxides, which form following oxidation of the polyunsaturated fatty acids in the cell membranes. It is also a component of the enzyme phospholipid hydroperoxide glutathione peroxidase (PHGSH-Px), which has an antioxidant action in the cell membrane.

Selenium facilitates the digestion and the absorption of lipids and improves the absorption of vitamin E. It also improves cellular antioxidant action and reduces the vitamin E requirement.

An RDA of 55 µg/day is recommended. The content of selenium in vegetables depends on the composition of the soil. In Italy, techniques have been used to integrate the soil content by fertilizing potato plants with organic selenium, resulting in products that have a selenium content that is 10 times greater at a very low cost.

Selenium is found in considerable quantities in wheat germ, durum wheat (rather than soft wheat), bran, broccoli, garlic, onions, and tomatoes. It is found in small quantities in fruits and vegetables. It is also found in fish (tuna, sardines, sole and cod) and seafood, red meat, liver, and eggs.

Selenium deficiency is observed in patients subjected to long-term drip treatments. An endemic deficiency can lead to a form of infantile cardiomyopathy. If ingested in large quantities, selenium can be toxic and lead to hair and nail loss. While this condition is extremely rare in the normal population, cases have been observed in people on mineral supplements who have ingested a dose of approximately 27 mg/day.

Copper

There is a large quantity of copper in the eye. It intervenes in the processes involved in the formation of the pigment, and its serum level increases in relation to the abnormalities of the RPE.

It is a component of SOD cytoplasmatic enzymes and some mitochondrial enzymes.

The RDA is 1.2 mg/day.

It is found in seafood and crustaceans, beans, nuts, chocolate, meat, whole grain wheat, and potatoes.

The dietary contribution of copper is conditioned by the presence of zinc and dietary fiber. It is absorbed by the proximal stretch of the small intestine, in proportion to the body's requirements. Ninety percent is bonded to ceruloplasmin in the blood, the remaining 10% to albumin and transcuprein.

Deficiency is rare and in general is associated with poor diet characterized by a low protein content.

Some age-related retinal alterations appear following a reduction in the activity of the copper-containing enzymes.[101]

Acute intoxication occurs following ingestion of more than 10 mg/day. The symptoms are nausea, vomiting, and diarrhea, and the most serious symptom is hemolytic anemia. In some cases, there may be neurological manifestations that may result in coma. Slow progressive accumulation can lead to the well-known Wilson's disease, which is normally a hereditary condition.

Manganese

Manganese is contained in the mitochondrial SOD enzyme and is essential for the constitution of bone tissue. The RDA is between 1.0 to 10.0 mg/day. Manganese is found in nuts, green broadleaf vegetables, fruit, beans (peas), beetroot, egg yolk, whole cereals, lyophilized coffee, tea, and cocoa powder.

Absorption of manganese is obstructed by calcium, phosphate, and soy proteins.

Symptoms of manganese deficiency have only been identified in volunteers subjected to purified diets.

Cases of toxicity are limited to subjects who have been mining metal. The symptoms are similar to Parkinsonism and Wilson's disease.

Other protective dietary elements

Bioflavonoids

Flavonoids or bioflavonoids are polyphenolic compounds contained largely in plants. They have a synergetic effect with vitamin C and are sometimes referred to as vitamin C2 or vitamin P. Several types of flavonoids can be found in the same plant. Their name is derived from the Latin word *flavus*, which means yellow. In angiosperm plants, they are found in the typical pigments of the flowers but are also found in the fruit and leaves. A specific group of flavonoids, the anthocyanines, are responsible for the red, blue, and purple colors of some plants and fruit. Other flavonoids, the flavons and flavonols, are not colored to the human eye but can be perceived by insects. Thanks to their color, these pigments can attract insects and animals and are essential mediators in pollination *(Table 2.1)*.

There are several classes of flavonoids. One of these includes the flavons, which are widespread throughout the plant world, generally speaking in herbs. Then, there are the isoflavons, which in contrast with the other flavonoids are colorless, have a fairly limited distribution, and are found exclusively in the bean and iris families. Special attention is paid to the isoflavons contained in soy, which would appear to have protective antitumor properties. In ophthalmology, genisteine, which acts an inhibitor of thyroxin kinase, is studied because of its properties in the treatment of neovascular DMLE. Flavonols, on the other hand, are commonly found in the plant kingdom,

Table 2.1

Sources of bioflavonoids

	GREEN TEA	DARK CHOCOLATE	RED WINE	FOREST FRUITS	CITRUS FRUITS	RED GRAPES	SOY	APPLES	ONIONS
Rutin			✔		✔	✔			
Esperidin					✔				
Quercetin			✔		✔	✔		✔	✔
Catechine	✔	✔	✔						
Polyphenols			✔						
Anthocyanosides				✔					
Isoflavons							✔		

generally in lignified angiosperm plants. The most well-known are quercetin and rutin. Unquestionably, the class containing anthocyan or anthocyanine are of greatest interest in ophthalmology.

Anthocyanines are present in varying quantities in all of the superior plants, particularly in fruit and blossoms but can also be found in leaves and roots, frequently in association with other pigments. Thanks to their antioxidant power, the anthocyanines protect plants from the damage caused by UV light. With exposure to large quantities of UV radiation, their production increases rapidly.

Flavonoids have the function of scavengers.

Flavonoids act as scavengers against superoxide anions, hydroxyl radicals, and singlet oxygen. They can interact with inflammatory processes where the key enzymes are cyclo-oxygenase and lipo-oxygenase, and they can inhibit the production, aggregation, and adhesiveness of the platelets.[102] They can also stabilize the membranes, reducing their fluidity.[103] In reference to the antioxidant mechanisms, there is mutual synergism between bioflavonoids and vitamins C and E. *In vivo*, the copresence of these substances is essential.[104]

They can act together with vitamin C.

Some flavonoids have demonstrated—*in vitro* and *in vivo*—their ability to slow or block neoplastic growth. It has been shown that the addition of vitamin C and vitamin E to an experimental animal's diet drastically reduces the probability it will develop forms of cancer when treated with carcinogenic agents. The same type of result was observed when the experimental animals were administered quercetin. A diet rich in fruits and vegetables—containing vitamins C and E, β-carotene, and bioflavonoids—reduces the probability of developing cancer. .

The specific flavonoids that are investigated to a greater degree are quercetin, rutin, diosmin, and esperidin. These compounds are also found in citrus fruits and are described as efficacious in reducing capillary permeability with antivaricose and antihemorrhoid activity. These are joined by the anthocyanosides found in blueberries, which are considered to be efficacious in the treatment of retinopathy and diabetic angiopathy and as a protector of the endothelium.

There are risks associated with the use of flavonoids during pregnancy.

In vitro experiments have shown that some flavonoids have the ability to provoke chromosome alterations of the MLL gene through the inhibitory action of topoisomerase II. This type of alteration is the same as that observed in a high percentage of acute infantile leukemias. It was probably this finding that suggested that bioflavonoids may play an important role in the incidence of this disease. Add to this the fact that the bioflavonoids can cross the placenta barrier, and this may expose the fetus to topoisomerase II activity in a delicate phase of the pregnancy. At the time of publication, there are no final conclusions, and it has been necessary to standardize the information leaflets attached to some medicinal specialties that contain flavonoids with the following warning: "*The safety of the drug during pregnancy has not been confirmed; consequently, the product should not be administered during pregnancy.*"[105]

Cooking will reduce and sometimes destroy flavonoids. These substances are absorbed by the intestinal tract, and any excess is eliminated with the urine or sweat. The symptoms of a

flavonoid deficiency are the same as those observed for the vitamin C deficiency (ie, fragile capillaries, hemorrhoids, and bleeding gums).
Given that the flavonoids can also be involved in the absorption of vitamin C, their deficiency can also lead to deficiency of vitamin C.

Ginkgo biloba

Ginkgo biloba is a plant of Chinese origin, often used as an ornamental plant or for the production of bonsai. The word *ginkgo* derives from the Chinese *Yin-Kwo* (silver fruit), the word *biloba* from the 2-lobed shape of the leaves.[106] The ginkgo plant was first mentioned in 2800 BC as a component of Chinese medicine. It was used in respiratory diseases, to improve cerebral function, and to prevent memory loss.
The fibrous internal part of the seeds is a delicacy in Asia and is part of the Chinese culinary tradition. It is traded under the name *"White Nuts."* In Japan, ginkgo seeds are added to many dishes (eg, chawanmushi) and used as a side dish. The doses of dry extract from ginkgo biloba used therapeutically oscillate between 112 and 200 mg/day.
Of the numerous substances contained in gingko biloba, the most important from a pharmacological point of view are the flavonoids and the triterpenic lactones (ginkgolitese and bilobalites),[107] ginketol, isigenketol, bilabetol, and ginkoloid, which have a vasodilating action with effects on the cerebrovascular functions and can act as a coadjuvant in Alzheimer's disease. Ginkgo is also used as a platelet anticlotting agent to improve circulation.

Ginko biloba assists in vasodilatation and anti-clotting action.

Its hemorheological properties are well known as are its action on the torsion capacity of the red corpuscles, which can be observed as an increase in the perfusion speed.

Hemo-rheological properties.

The therapeutic activity of the ginkgo biloba plant would appear to depend on its antioxidant activity and the antagonistic activity of the so-called platelet activating factor (PAF) of the active ingredients it contains.[108] In patients with diabetes mellitus, oral administration of this product improves the deformability of the erythrocytes and the blood viscosity, facilitating blood perfusion. Moreover, a clinically significant improvement is observed in the retinal flow of patients with Type II diabetes and retinopathy.[109]
EGb 761 (extract of ginkgo biloba 761) is the subject of numerous medical experiments. It contains a fraction of flavonoids (24% of the extract) and 6% terpenes (ginkgolites and bilobalites). It operates in many different organs and diverse conditions and exerts a protective effect against neurodegenerative and vascular disease.

EGb 761 would appear to regulate the metabolic functions.

In particular, it does not have a unidirectional effect, activating or inhibiting some of the mechanisms, but would appear to be a regulator that helps the organism adapt to the surrounding conditions or circumstances.[110]

It acts against the free radicals and protects against ischemic damage.

Gb 761 eliminates the free radicals of oxygen—primary (O_2^-, OH•) and secondary (ROO•). Oral administration of EGb 761 protects against lipoperoxidation and is also effective against conditions such as ischemia reperfusion following occlusion of the central retinal artery or ocular hypertony. Gb 761 protects the retina against ischemic damage, and zinc can integrate this effect, particularly when combined with other scavengers. EGb 761 has a dose-dependent protective effect against acute and chronic toxicity from chlorokine[111] and can be used to prevent the damage from chronic treatment.[112]

Ginkgo biloba has antioxidant, anti-apoptotic and cytoprotective effects.

Ginkgo biloba has antioxidant, antiapoptotic, and cytoprotective properties. For example, it protects against cataract,[113] and under experimental conditions, it protects the crystalline lens from damage induced by radiation.[114]

Ginkgo biloba would appear to be relatively safe to use with very few documented side effects (eg, moderate gastrointestinal disturbances and headache). Nevertheless, some recent cases of spontaneous hemorrhage were reported in subjects administered ginkgo biloba as a hypoemic agent[115] or intracranial hemorrhage[116] or subdural hemorrhage[117]; however, the doses were higher than those generally found in the products commercially available in Italy. The hemorrhage was blamed on the platelet anticlotting effect of ginkgo biloba[118] and the summation effect with other anticlotting agents such as aspirin. Therefore, it is not appropriate to prescribe ginkgo without examining the patient sufficiently.[119]

Until further information is available, caution should be used when ingesting ginkgo with some anticoagulant and anticlotting drugs.

Diet and **supplements**

A healthy lifestyle necessitates controlling the quality and quantity of food intake, regular physical activity, and no smoking. In Italy, in particular, it should be remembered that the *Mediterranean diet* is preferable over other dietary regimens because it can protect against many illnesses and diseases. Following this type of diet has enormous social-cultural importance, and apart from anything else, eating a healthy Mediterranean diet is actually a very pleasant experience. In normal healthy Italians, this type of diet can maintain low cholesterol and homocysteine levels, reducing the cardiovascular risk factors.[120] It is interesting that physical activity of benefit to the cardiovascular system is performed during leisure time and can sometimes be extremely tiring; however, a job or an occupation that involves heavy physical labor would appear to have no benefit at all.[121]

Unfortunately, the diet of Italians is not always very *Mediterranean*. There is a tendency to eat an excessive amount of protein and too much saturated fat compared to the amount of unsaturated fat; too much cholesterol is consumed and too little vitamin-rich food; and the amount of dietary fiber is very low. In other words, Italians eat too much meat and not enough fruit and vegetables.[122]

The Mediterranean diet is healthy but not adopted by the majority of people.

The *Guidelines for a Healthy Italian Diet* recommend weight control and physical activity; a greater quantity of cereals, legumes, fruits, and vegetables; restrictions on the quantity and quality of fats, a limited amount of carbohydrates; the right amount of water; a limit on the amount of salt; and well-controlled moderate alcohol consumption. Finally, it is recommended that the choice of food in the diet is varied.[123]

The *Guidelines for a Healthy Italian Diet* recommend that the choice of food in the diet is varied.

In other words, this simply means living a healthier lifestyle or something that is more conducive to man's needs. By choosing to tackle the problem in this way, it may prove to be useful to integrate the diet with vitamins, oligo-elements (trace elements), and with substances that have an antioxidant action and structural functions to increase the protective factors and reduce the risk factors.[124-126]

However, does an ideal model of a dietary supplement exist for the eye? It could prove useful for people who have a family history of dry eye, glaucoma, macular degeneration, etc; however, it could be a useful dietary addition in some precocious phases of disease. Vitamin A is essential for the production of rodopsin; however, β-carotene has been connected to an increased risk of lung cancer in smokers. Vitamins C and E form a powerful antioxidant system; lutein and zeaxanthin protect the ocular structures; selenium and zinc are components of powerful antioxidant enzymes; ginkgo biloba has vasodilatory and anticlotting properties: these latter molecules can rightly be included in a supplement treatment.[127]

Dietary deficiencies must always be integrated.

Can a pill replace a meal? Of course not. When the diet is insufficient, the food intake must be improved, and supplements are often essential for the treatment of serious forms of malnutrition. In developed countries, there should be no need for dietary supplements, at least where healthy people are concerned. Yet, the market for diet supplements is in continual expansion. Anyone who purchases supplements is usually looking for some form of protection from serious or debilitating diseases; some people are trying to improve their physical appearance but too many people listen to scientifically unfounded promises. Patients and doctors all have unrealistic expectations.

First of all, it is essential to move cautiously. Clearly, if there are deficiencies in the diet, these must be corrected; supplements cannot replace the variety of nutrients of a normal healthy diet. However, it should be said that if plants grow in soil lacking in nutrients, this will have a negative effect on the food chain and supplements may be essential. Moreover, if the patient is suffering from a disease caused by some deficiency, it must be treated with supplements.

Dietary supplements do not protect the body from the damage caused by stress, alcohol, and smoking. Natural does not mean harmless.

Evidence-based medicine states that doctors must base their decisions on fact. But what do the facts say?

If we take a look at our lifestyle, we should always be aware that dietary supplements do not protect against the negative effects of drinking alcohol and smoking; on the contrary, drinking alcohol and smoking may interfere with the normal absorption of nutrients. An increase in nutrients is not necessary to combat stress. As a result, supplements are not necessary, and stress should be treated with sleep and an increase in the hours dedicated to relaxation.

Another fact is that supplements are often derived from plants; however, this *natural* origin does not mean that they lack side effects. Moreover, while an *appropriate* vitamin intake is beneficial, a high-dose supplement can be dangerous. Once again, we should remember that the nutrients interact, and high doses can lead to the deficiency of another or camouflage the effects.

Oversupplementing can have side effects.

There are reliable studies that report the beneficial effect of dietary supplements in some patient categories affected by specific illnesses. In this chapter, these issues will be covered in detail. In many cases, it is not a question of supplements to overcome a deficiency, but overdosing with supplements.

How should we consider this problem? Unquestionably, we have to use common sense and pay close attention before acting, as should be the case for any scientific evaluation. If we come across an article on the subject, let us try to read something more than the title. We must try to understand whether the study design is adequate.

By reading the literature, we can check the validity of the studies.

We should remember that a single study is never enough; we must always try to find other studies on the same subject that will confirm or contradict the findings. We should not get excited about preliminary results but should accept them for what they are, until other studies validate them. Many studies are performed on animal models or even *in vitro,* and the results cannot always be applied to humans. It is essential to give the exact importance to the words and not jump to conclusions, but maintain a healthy form of skepticism.[128]

We should try to live a healthy lifestyle and add supplements only when necessary.
When we consider using a commercial supplement, we must control all aspects of its composition. First, we must consider the correspondence of the product's composition to the studies performed: the product might have a different concentration of the active ingredient, or there may be the conjugation with different molecules of the same ingredient or a similar, not the same, substance, or a different extract from the same plant. Always be aware of the phrase *"studies on this subject are still ongoing,"* which usually means that there are no studies to support the findings; the studies may actually exist but they have been conducted on patient groups that were too small or not representative of the population or the studies may not even have been published because they were conducted in an inappropriate manner. Finally, it should be remembered that dietary supplements will not give an immediate response to our health needs but will only provide results in the long-term.[129]

By examining the formulation of the supplements, we can control the correspondence with the formulation used in the studies.

Dry eye

Dry eye is defined as a disorder of the eye surface associated with a deficiency in the quantity or composition of the tears with or without excessive evaporation. It is characterized by hyperosmolarity of the tears and is accompanied by inflammation that can cause damage to the eye surface, visual symptoms, or discomfort. The pathologies of the eye surfaces can be dry eye syndromes (with a reduced quantity of water or increased evaporation) or other inflammatory diseases of the surface associated with the meibomian glands or the conjunctiva. The various types of dry eye can coexist in the same patient.[130]
Replacement therapy with artificial tears is the most widely used worldwide, but it is a palliative treatment and does not really treat the problem; it just relieves the symptoms. A number of therapeutic agents are currently being studied, and dietary treatment is among them.

Treatment with artificial tears is palliative.

A sufficient intake of protein, vitamin A, vitamin B6, vitamin C, potassium, and zinc might be essential for a normal lacrimal function. Excessive dietary fat, an incorrect amount of salt, high cholesterol, and the abuse of alcohol are associated with lacrimal dysfunction.
In the healthy, well-nourished population of our geographical area, there are no specific problems; nevertheless, people are advised to control the correct dietary intake of the macronutrients (protein, fats, and sugars); to increase the quantity of vitamin A (in vegetables), zinc, and folates (whole food and legumes); and ensure the appropriate intake of vitamin B6 (walnuts, bananas, beans) and vitamin C (citrus fruit). Alcohol and coffee should be eliminated while the consumption of salt should be reduced. It should be remembered that water is the predominant component of tears; as a result, the body should be hydrated appropriately with adequate fluid intake.[131]

For normal lacrimal function, it is important to introduce vitamins and liquids.

The administration of antioxidants improves the lacrimal function, improves the stability of the lacrimal film, and increases the number of the goblet cells. It has been suggested that this is due to

Omega-3 fatty acids contribute to inflammation control.

a reduction in oxidative stress; no one is certain whether the lacrimal film improves the conjunctiva or vice versa.[132] Vitamin A is essential for the good health of the mucosa; the goblet cells of the conjunctiva increase in numbers following the administration of vitamin A.[133] Vitamin C supplements lead to an increase in its concentration in the plasma and in tears; however, there would appear to be a limit on the concentration in tears; this would suggest that there is an active mechanism of control.[134] A combined therapy of vitamins A and B6 and primrose oil, which contains essential fatty acids, would appear to be useful.[135]

Control of inflammation associated with dry eye would appear to be crucial. PG-E1 is a prostaglandin with a powerful anti-inflammatory effect, necessary for its correct secretion by the salivary and lacrimal glands. The administration of its precursors, the essential fatty acids—linoleic acid (LA) and gamma-linoleic acid (GLA)—leads to an increase in the salivary and lacrimal concentration,[136,137] especially when associated with the simultaneous administration of vitamin C and vitamin B6.[138] Initially, a diet therapy was attempted in patients with Sjögren's syndrome. They were given supplements containing a high level of LA and GLA. An improvement in the plasma levels of PG-E1 was achieved, but no improvement in the objective ocular picture was observed.[139] Recently, the consumption of LA and GLA was evaluated in a randomized double-blind study in patients affected by rheumatoid arthritis, and this proved to be efficacious in the relief of the symptoms of dry eye, in addition to improving the indicators of inflammation present in the tears.[140]

One substance that is studied to a lesser degree is lactoferrin, a glycoprotein that is found in milk. It can supply a dietary support for the treatment of intestinal disorders associated with hyperpermeability, oxidative stress, and inflammation. Lactoferrin collects iron that is not bonded to proteins and prevents it from being chemically oxidized, thus reducing the damage from free radicals; it also prevents it from being used by bacteria.[141] When administered orally, it is absorbed by the superior gastrointestinal tract.[142] Lactoferrin is also found in tears; its concentration is lower in cases of dry eye and the concentration is directly correlated with the severity of the disease. The concentration is used as a diagnostic index.[143] These factors could form the basis for its use in the treatment of dry eye syndrome.

Vitreal degeneration

The vitreous is a gelatinous substance that modifies with age[144]; in myopic eyes, these modifications can be observed more precociously. There are 2 types of alteration: the collapse of the collagen fibers, a phenomenon called synchysis, and the creation of optically void cavities of vitreal fluidification, a phenomenon called syneresis. In these cavities, the collagen fibers form precipitates that are often described by the patients as floaters. The spaces of liquefaction are more extensive in older patients; the mechanism that causes them would appear to be associated with the fragmentation of the collagen molecules by an extracellular process.[145]

Recently, researchers have identified some enzymes in the vitreous, called the matrix metalloproteinase (MMP) which would appear to be involved in the degradation of vitreal collagen; their function is regulated by other enzymes called tissue inhibitor of metalloproteinases (TIMP).[146] Among the causes of vitreal hyaluronic acid degradation, the ROI play an important role.[147]

MMP and TIMP are involved in synchysis and vitreal sineresi.

The vitreous consists largely of water. Diuretic drugs taken to treat pathologies not necessarily associated with the eye will affect the aqueous component of the vitreous. The constant depletion of water and potassium tends to reduce the aqueous component of the vitreal mass, and, consequently, this alters the correct ratio between it and the fibrous component, in addition to encouraging the vitreo-retinal tractions. The straightforward rehydration of the vitreal gel encourages the re-expansion of the vitreal mass and reduces the movement of the broken fibrils inside the vitreal voids, permitting a considerable reduction in the perception of floaters, with an obvious improvement in the subjective phenomena.[148]

The collagen and the hyaluronic acid found in the vitreous are of endogenous origin and are not introduced with diet. The intake of their constituents (glucuronic acid, N-acetylglucosamine, glycine, proline, lysine) with the normal diet or with supplements should supply the necessary material for an adequate turnover of the constituents of the vitreous.

Consumption of precursors of collagen and hyaluronic acid can supply the material necessary for vitreal turnover.

Finally, in order to influence the evolution of the vitreal alterations, it is important to act on the control of MMP action and oxidative stress. Some substances such as ascorbate and leukocyanidine have a non-specific inhibitory action on MMP.[149]

The cataract

Age-related cataract is the most prevalent cause of blindness in the world. The development of a cataract is not only related to aging but also to lifestyle; smoking, for example, has a direct influence on its development.[150] Low income and a poor level of education are also important factors.[151] Around the world, cataract surgery is the most frequent operation in people over 65 years of age. This is an expensive procedure, even in the industrialized world[152] and is a critical factor in developing countries. It has been calculated that if the appearance of cataract was delayed by 10 years, it would translate into a 50% reduction in the need for surgery.[153]

Delaying the appearance of cataract reduces the need for surgery.

An important mechanism in the development of cataract is the oxidative damage produced by the particular metabolism of glucose in the crystalline lens on the sorbitol pathway[154]; damage to the epithelial cells and toxic factors also play important roles.

Therapies have been attempted in diabetic patients to block the aldose-reductase to reduce the accumulation of sorbitol. Other studies focused on the stimulation of the metabolism of glutathione and others used drugs in an attempt to protect the epithelial cells against H_2O_2. However, in all of these cases, the treatments were neither efficacious nor safe.[155] Aldose-redutase is strongly inhibited by quercetin (ie, a flavonoid). Given that the oxidative damage responsible for cataract is also due to

Quercetin influences the sorbitol pathway.

Oxidative damage is controlled by glutathione.

Lutein is the only carotenoid present in the crystalline.

insufficient levels of glutathione, the level and activity can be increased through the consumption of lipoic acid, vitamins C and E, and selenium; riboflavin is the precursor of flavina-adenin-dinucleotide (FAD), cofactor of glutathione-reductase. The relative deficiency of carotenoids can be supplemented.[156] For these reasons, numerous studies have focused on the dietary aspects.

Lutein is the only carotenoid found in the crystalline lens. An 8-year study followed and examined more than 36,000 professional American men between the ages of 45 and 75 years. All subjects were asked to complete a questionnaire regarding their diet. The subjects with a high dietary lutein intake had an 18% lower risk of developing a cataract.[157]

In a study conducted by the Beaver Dam group,[158] it was found that a high intake of lutein in middle age reduces the risk of cataract in old age by 60%; if consumed when young, the risk is reduced to 50%.

Regarding vitamin E, the consumption of high quantities with the diet is associated with a 42% reduction in the risk of cataract,[159] while high plasma levels of vitamin E would appear to have a direct relationship with a reduced risk; moreover, there would appear to be a dose-response ratio associated with vitamin E supplements.[160]

In a study conducted in Finland, the plasma levels of vitamin E were associated with precocious cortex opacity but not with nuclear opacity.[161]

Studies that focused specifically on vitamin supplements were also performed.

The Lens Opacities Case-Control study compared patients with cataract and controls; the study involved taking regular vitamin A supplements at least once a week for at least one year. In patients taking vitamin A supplements, a reduction of 55% of the cortex opacities and 40% of the mixed opacities was observed.[162] Consumption of multivitamin supplements also showed favorable correlation.

In another study[163] conducted by the Beaver Dam group, a modest intake of vitamin A was associated with a 40% reduction in the risk of a nuclear cataract; in smokers, multivitamin supplements resulted in a reduction in the risk by much as 50%.

The effects of supplementation with carotenoids has been studied.

In the Nurses' Health Study, a group of nurses was studied for 8 years. The consumption of total carotene was associated with a 27% reduction in the risk of cataract.[164]

The Physician's Health Study followed a group of doctors and studied the cardiovascular risk in relation to the consumption of aspirin and β-carotene. A substudy showed that the consumption of multivitamin supplements reduced the risk of cataract by 27% and that the risk decreased in direct proportion to the period of supplementation.[165]

Two studies of the Nutrition and Vision Project (NVP) highlighted the fact that supplementation with antioxidants protects the eye against cortex and nuclear opacities,[166] while vitamin E supplements and high doses of vitamins in the B group decreased the progression of cataract.[167] The Linxian study[168] was a randomized study on the use of vitamin supplements. The prevalence of nuclear cataract was 36% lower in subjects who consumed multivitamin supplements at doses equivalent to 3 times the RDA, containing riboflavin/niacin, but not other vitamins; however, there was an increased risk in the appearance of a posterior subcapsular cataract. The results of these studies would appear to point favorably to the idea of supplements with nutritional factors to produce a reduction in the risk of cataract. However, the Age-Related Eye Disease Study (AREDS), which involved high-dose supplements of vitamin C, vitamin E, and β-carotene with or without zinc and copper, following a 7-year follow-up period did not demonstrate any apparent effect of the supplements on the risk of cataract development.[169]

Even though there are sufficient epidemiological indications regarding a reduction in the risk of cataract in subjects who assume antioxidants, supplements should not be recommended until there is clear proof regarding the efficacy of this type of therapy.[170]

The AREDS trial has not shown any advantage in its supplementation model for cataract.

Glaucoma

A reduction in the intraocular pressure (IOP) in the treatment of glaucoma can contribute to preventing nerve damage in patients with suspected glaucoma and prevent or delay the progression of the damage in patients diagnosed with glaucoma; the reduction in IOP will not protect all patients.

The first aspect to be considered is the control of IOP. The synthesis of abnormal GAG of the trabeculate has been associated with an altered deflux of the aqueous humor in glaucoma and therefore an increase in IOP. Vitamin C and glucosamine sulfate can influence the GAG synthesis process.

Forskolin (extracted from ***Coleus forskohlii***) was used topically in the past to reduce IOP. Intramuscular injections of ***Salvia miltiorrhiza*** were administered, and these improved the visual acuity and the peripheral vision of glaucoma patients. Other potential nutrients are lipoic acid, vitamin B12, and melatonin.[171] High doses of vitamin C administered locally or systemically can reduce the IOP, even though the effect is clinically irrelevant.[172]

Used topically, vitamin C and forskolin reduce the IOP.

One second important aspect is vascular. In many patients with glaucoma, an altered regulation of the blood flow to the optic nerve may be extremely damaging, even when the IOP does not increase. The vascular control can be implemented with the administration of systemic magnesium and improved with the consumption of dark chocolate and omega-3 fatty acids.[173]

Ginkgo biloba is a possible drug for use in the treatment of glaucoma. It improves central and peripheral blood flow, reduces the vasospasm, reduces the blood viscosity, has antioxidant activity, inhibits the platelet-activating factor (PAF), and apoptosis.[174] It improves the diastolic flow speed in the ophthalmic artery[175] and would appear to improve the values of the visual field.[176] It has also demonstrated a protective capacity against nerve death induced by glutamate.[177] The pre-treatment and the precocious treatment with EGb 761 have demonstrated a neuroprotector effect in animal models with chronic glaucoma.[178]

Ginkgo biloba is a powerful drug for the treatment of glaucoma.

The most recent aspect of glaucoma therapy is neuroprotection. This can be defined as the use of therapeutic agents that prevent, delay, or annul the death of the neurons following a primary insult and independent of the insult itself.

Glaucoma is a chronic disease that normally has a slow progression; the initial damage usually occurs in the axon of the nerve as opposed to the cell bodies. As a result, it may lend itself to neuroprotection similar to the types that have proved efficacious in the treatment of amyotrophic lateral sclerosis and Alzheimer's or Parkinson's disease.[179]

Epigallocatechin gallate is a promising neuro-protector.

A powerful flavonoid extract from green tea has been used to treat the cognitive deficits associated with these pathologies: epigallocatechin gallate.[180] For many years, extracts of ginkgo biloba have been used. Generally speaking, the same substance can be used to attenuate the damage from oxidative stress in age-related macular degeneration (AMD) and in glaucoma.[181]

Forskolin, in synergy with neurotrophins, improves the survival of the retinal ganglions.

The paper by Meyer and Franke, published in the journal *Neuron*, highlighted forskolin's ability to improve the survival of the retinal ganglion cells in synergy with the neurotrophins.

Choline has a neuroprotective effect and improves the visual function.

Phosphatidylcholine (or lecithin) is a complex phospholipid present in the cell membranes and in the myelin-coated nerve structures. It is a substance found in soy and used in the food industry as a thickening agent. Its main constituent, choline, was studied specifically for use in glaucoma.[182] It is administered orally or by injection in the form of cyticholine; the oral formulation provides an excellent bioavailability. Following absorption, it is split into its components cytidine and choline, which are distributed throughout the body and pass through the blood-brain barrier to reach the central nervous system. Here it stimulates the synthesis of phosphatidylcholine and stimulates the action of some neurotransmitters such as dopamine.[183] In this way, it exerts a neuroprotective effect under conditions of hypoxide cerebral ischemia and even in glaucoma where an improvement in visual function was observed.[184-186]

Age-related macular degeneration

The prevalence of lesions as predisposing factors to AMD increase with age and the prevalence of full-blown AMD is lower than the predisposing lesions and increases with age.

In industrialized countries, AMD is the most common cause of legal blindness in patients over 55 years of age.[187-189] The prevalence of the disease is destined to increase, if only for the increase in the average age of the population.[190]

AMD is defined as a degenerative disorder that affects people who are older than 50. In the early stages, it is characterized in the macular zone of soft drusen and hypo- or hyperpigmentation, and in the later stages, it is characterized by geographical atrophy (dry maculopathy), chorioretinal neovascularization with or without the detachment of the RPE, and finally, scarring in the area of the macula (wet maculopathy).[191]

Numerous epidemiological studies have been performed in an attempt to identify the risk factors, the most famous being Framingham, Beaver Dam,[151,158,239] Rotterdam,[204] and Blue Mountain.[207] Despite the fact that these were studies performed on populations that differed in terms of genetics, lifestyles, and living environments, some general conclusions can be drawn: the prevalence of lesions that may lead to AMD increases with age and the prevalence of full-blown AMD is lower than the number of patients with predisposing factors and increases with age.

Some risk factors are evident: age (ie, the aging process that affects the body) creates the substrate for the subsequent damage caused by AMD. In some studies, it appears that women would appear to be more susceptible.[192] AMD is observed more frequently in women who have had at least one child; exogenous estrogen supplements in the postmenopause period would appear to play a protective role. The use of oral estrogens would appear to alter the relationship between the plasma lipids with an increase in total cholesterol and also HDL with an improvement in the distribution of the macular pigments and vitamin E throughout the organism.[193] There are genetic factors associated with race. The disease is less common in the Black and Asian populations than in the white populations. There would appear to be a genetic predisposition[194,195] to AMD with autosomic dominant transmission. Lately, some chromosome loci have been discovered that are associated with the atrophic form of the disease.[196] Studies of families[197] and identical (monozygotic) twins[198-200] confirmed a greater incidence of AMD in an affected person's relatives, which would suggest a hereditary factor. The high intake of saturated fats and cholesterol is associated with a high risk of AMD, for the mechanisms linked to the circulation, and for the fat deposited along Bruch's membrane. Moderate consumption of red wine (which has a high phenol content) would appear to provide moderate protection.[201]

Smoking is an important risk factor.

Cigarette smoke is not strictly a dietary factor; it is more a behavioral event. Nevertheless, it is a fairly certain risk factor that can be eliminated. Smoking exposes the eye to a greater level of oxidation, provokes hypoxia, and reduces the choroidal blood flow. In smokers, high concentrations of the lipid peroxidation products are found in the blood and the exhaled air. The activity of the enzymes that protect the erythrocytes is reduced, and it seems that smoke reduces the density of the macular pigment.[202] The risk of developing neovascular AMD[203] and possibly the atrophic form[204] is very high in people who smoke more than 20 to 25 cigarettes each day, particularly when they are women. There is an increased risk even when fewer than 20 cigarettes are smoked each day. Exsmokers have a slightly increased risk, which will remain higher even 15 to 20 years after they have stopped. Passive smoking is also associated with an increased risk, although the risk is not statistically significant.[205-207]

There is no correlation between smoking and the early appearance of symptoms of AMD.[208]

No clear correlation has been observed between the presence of cataract and AMD; however, an increase in the progression of AMD has been observed following cataract surgery.[209] The connection between being overweight and AMD is interesting. People who are obese have an altered in-

AMD can be triggered by oxidative stress, altered choroidal circulation and the degeneration of Bruch's membrane.

take of macular pigment and it should be remembered that the adipose tissue is the main storage tissue of these pigments. An increase in BMI (ie, the proportion of fat) will influence the quantity of macular pigment available for the retina. Obese subjects have a lower concentration of serum carotenoids[210] and a relative deficiency of retinal macular pigments that may be a risk for the progression of AMD.[211]

There are several suggestions regarding the pathogenesis of AMD that do not mutually exclude each other but more probably they are integrated. Oxidative stress, altered choroidal circulation, and degeneration of Bruch's membrane are all possible causes.

Aging is associated with oxidative damage and is probably also a consequence. The retina is exposed to high levels of radiation, and it contains numerous photosensitive molecules such as lipofuscin. Phagocytosis of the external segments of the photoreceptors by the RPE produces H_2O_2. Through the chorîdal circulation, the retina receives a large quantity of oxygen and there is high consumption with the risk of free radicals being produced. The cell membranes of the photoreceptors are extremely rich in polyunsaturated fatty acids, which are the ideal substrate for oxidative damage.[212] Lipid peroxidation occurs through the formation of radicals of oxygen (ROI) following metabolic reactions or photo-oxidation. The increase in the oxidative stress and/or the reduction in the possibility of defense caused by a lack of dietary antioxidants contribute to the onset of AMD.

AMD may be a vascular disease caused by mechanisms associated with atherosclerosis. The choroid shows a diet- and age-related increased resistance to flow. If the resistance of the cerebral circulation is less than the resistance of the choroid, hypofusion may occur that could cause the atrophic form of the disease.[213] Many of the risk factors for cardiovascular disease are common to AMD. Among the most recent discoveries is hyperhomocysteinemia, which is a clinical condition associated with vascular alterations, loss of the endothelium's antithrombotic function, and induction of an environment that favors coagulation. It was recently associated with the neovascular but not with the atrophic form of AMD.[214]

With age, Bruch's membrane loses its ability to transport nutrients because of the increased amount of lipid deposits inside.[215] Moreover, the function of RPE becomes less efficient, provoking the formation of drusen.[216] In response to metabolic stress or a reduced oxygen intake, RPE may release vascular growth factors and stimulate neovascular formations. Calcification and fragmentation of the Bruch's membrane would appear to facilitate the growth of neovascular membranes with the subsequent development of exudative AMD.[217] RPE can modulate the neoformation of choroidal capillaries.[218]

Antioxidants would appear to have a protective role.

There is no doubt that the pathogenesis of AMD is multifactorial. This is all that can be confirmed. At the time of publication, however, we are aware of many mechanisms that are the basis of this disease, with oxidative damage leading the way.

Numerous epidemiological studies based on questionnaires[219,220] and clinical findings have highlighted the protective role against the damage caused by some of these antioxidants, vitamins,

oligoelementi, and macular pigments. Any dietary treatment of AMD must include components that are involved in the protection mechanisms: substances that have an antioxidant action or that are part of enzyme systems as main-players or cofactors.
Supplementing with vitamin E alone has been analyzed in a number of different studies but no benefit on the progression or the prevalence of AMD was demonstrated.[221,222] Supplementing with vitamin C proved to be efficacious in the reduction of damage from radiation[223]; however, its action in AMD was studied alongside other antioxidants. Vitamin C acts with vitamin E, reactivating it following the elimination of the free radicals.
People who have high blood levels of antioxidants, carotenoids in particular, run a lower risk of developing AMD.[224] A correlation was found between high serum levels of vitamin C, L and Z, and a high dietary intake of fish with a reduction in the level of homocysteine.[225]
Supplementation with carotenoids, particularly the macular pigments, through diet reduces the quantity of light that reaches the photoreceptors[226] and is associated with a reduced risk of AMD.[227]
The research on new molecules with antioxidant activity led to other carotenoids being studied. It was discovered that the activity of astaxanthin is 4 times greater than lutein.
Experimental studies have shown that the molecule can cross the blood-retinal barrier and will concentrate in the retina. It has antioxidant activity in the lipid membrane.[228]
It is one of the main carotenoids in the macula of Japanese quail.[229] Its protective effects in lipoperoxidation were observed in a group of healthy humans following oral administration.[230]
The main source of lycopene is tomato, and it is one of the few substances that can be measured in normal human serum. It has a protective antioxidant effect on RPE cell cultures[231] even though it is less effective as a filter of blue light.[232] It inhibits the accumulation of lipofuscin in RPE cells.[233] Different types of carotenoids consumed as part of the diet do not interfere with each other's activity in the determination of the serum concentration.[234]
There is no clear evidence demonstrating the risks provoked by the oral administration of high doses of L and lycopene; long-term findings are not available.[235] Moreover, regarding the risk of lung cancer associated with the consumption of β-carotene, it is recommended to not exceed a dose in excess of 6 mg/day of L and Z; dietary carotenoids are considered to be much safer than supplements.[236,237]
Zinc supplements alone are associated with a lower incidence of predisposing factors to AMD but not to full-blown AMD.[238,239] Following zinc supplements, no short-term protective effect to AMD was observed in the second eye of a patient affected by exudative AMD[240]; however, in patients who were treated with zinc, there was a lower average sight loss when affected by AMD.
With the appropriate diet, it is possible to reduce a certain number of risk factors.[241]
At the time of publication, AREDS is the most important and comprehensive study performed on nutritional factors and the evolution of age-related ocular diseases. Twenty-two reports have been published and many of them refer to AMD.

The majority of studies examine the antioxidant properties of the carotenoids: a high blood level has been shown to protect against AMD.

The AREDS study.

The first reports define the study[242] and describe the risk factors associated with cataract[243] and AMD.[244]

In report o. 8,[245] the effects of high levels of zinc and antioxidants were studied in 3640 patients. The patients were administered 500 mg of vitamin C, 400 UI vitamin E, and 15 mg β-carotene associated with 80 mg of zinc and 2 mg of copper. The subjects with large soft drusen or advanced DLME in one eye (those are most at risk) had lower progression of the disease.

These findings pointed toward the benefits of antioxidant supplements in subjects who are at risk.

According to report No. 11,[246] through the projection of the population, it is possible to forecast that over a 5-year period, approximately 8 million people in the United States will be at risk and approximately 1.3 million will develop neovascular AMD if not given dietary supplements.

The AREDS study emphasized the importance of supplements in the prevention of AMD; however, when this study began, no studies had been performed on antioxidants such as lutein. Reports No. 20[247] and No. 22[248] indicated that there is a direct relationship between the consumption of an elevated quantity of L and Z and omega-3 fatty acids and a reduced risk of developing neovascular AMD; L and Z are also associated with a reduced risk of geographical atrophy and drusen. The study AREDS-2 is examining the effects of combined supplements of L and Z with EPA+DHA.

The mechanism of angiogenesis involved in exudative AMD is one interesting aspect of diet therapy.

The mechanism of angiogenesis involved in exudative AMD is one interesting aspect of diet therapy.

Angiogenesis is a process that is strictly regulated in time and space, controlled by multiple growth factors and proangiogenic cytokines, and modulated by a group of inhibitors of neovascularization that have the opposite effect.[249,250]

Recent studies identified vascular endothelial growth factor (VEGF) as the most important mediator of ocular angiogenesis, physiological or otherwise.[251-255] VEGF plays a role in both diabetic retinopathy and in AMD,[256-258] although it does not appear to be the only mediator involved.

VEGF necessary for ocular angiogenesis is produced at a local level[259,260]; in the case of exudative AMD, it would appear that VEGF is produced by damaged RPE cells.[261,262]

VEGF binds to the high affinity receptors[263] that have tyrosine-kinase function[264,265] mainly located in the endothelial cells.[266,267] Genisteine, a flavonoid, is a powerful inhibitor of tyrosine-kinase and *in vitro* has been able to block VEGF.[268,269]

The antioxidant vitamins A, C, and E have a protective action in age-related macular damage. Zinc and selenium have important roles in the antioxidant cell metabolism and mechanisms; however, researchers are not as familiar with the behavior of copper. The carotenoids are protective for the macular area, and the omega-3 fatty acids are essential for the structural functions.[270] Numerous studies have been completed to investigate the protection offered by these molecules. Generally speaking, patients with low serum levels of these nutrients are at a greater risk of developing AMD. A high serum level of a group of antioxidants would appear to have greater efficacy than the individual substances.[271,272]

Therapy based on these substances must have a specific rationale[273,274]; high serum levels of some of these minerals are toxic and we only know some of the side effects of some vitamins.[275] For example, in a recent study, the consumption of β-carotene appears to be correlated with a deterioration of AMD.[276]

Retinitis pigmentosa

Retinitis pigmentosa (RP) is the most common cause of blindness among children and young people, with a prevalence of 1:4000.

RP indicates a group of pathologies characterized by night blindness in children and young people; there is a progressive loss of the visual field in the early years, only central vision remains in later years, and the problem progresses as far as blindness.

The electroretinogram will be altered, and the performance of the receptors decreases long before the appearance of the symptoms. It can involve the eye alone, or it can be part of a more complex systemic syndrome. More than 45 genes connected to the disease have been identified. At the time of publication, there is no treatment for RP; however, researchers are studying dietary methods involving the prescription of vitamin A and fatty acids to slow down the progression of the disease.[277]

Supplementing with vitamin A, lutein, and DHA has been studied.

The effects of lutein supplements have been studied in a series of randomized studies. In one study, lutein administered for 48 weeks had a positive effect on the central visual field and slowed-down the natural loss of the expected visual functions.[278] However, in another study, no changes were observed.[279]

Vitamin A proved to be efficacious at high doses (15,000 UI/dl), but in the same study, high doses of vitamin E had adverse effects.[280] It could be that vitamin E inhibits the absorption or the transport of vitamin A. The safety of prolonged administration of vitamin A in patients with RP has been tested; a dose below 25,000 UI/dl can be considered to be safe in patients between the ages of 18 and 54 years. Monitoring the liver function and controlling serum vitamin A are recommended.[281]

In an animal model of RP, high doses of antioxidants reduce the oxidative damage to the cones, increase their density, and preserve the function.[282]

In some forms of RP with dominant transmission, a low level of DHA was detected in the membranes of the erythrocytes. This was associated with an alteration of the lipid metabolism, which could damage the retina.[283] The level of erythrocyte DHA is directly correlated with the loss of the visual field. DHA and high-dose vitamin A supplements did not change the natural progression of the disease; however, a greater dietary intake of omega-3 slowed down the damage to the visual field in the first 2 years.[284,285]

Prematurity and infancy

Oxidative stress plays an important role in the development of retinopathy in prematurity (ROP).

Early supplementing with long-chain fatty acids (LCPUFA) improves the cognitive development of premature babies, but also reduces pathological retinal angiogenesis, which would suggest a role in ROP control.

Between 5% to 7% of babies are born prematurely (ie, prior to the 37th week of pregnancy). Prematurity is the major cause of newborn death, morbidity, and long-term disability.[286] The percentage survival for preterm births has improved considerably thanks to developments in perinatal assistance and the efforts made to reduce the newborn's respiratory distress. The majority of deaths are due to lung immaturity, respiratory distress, and its complications and outcomes.[287] In order to deal with the respiratory problems, premature babies are exposed to potentially damaging concentrations of oxygen and intense light (by newborn standards) in the neonatal intensive care unit.

Premature babies are at an extremely high risk of strabismus and refractive defects[288]; however, the problem that causes most concern for the ophthalmologist is retinopathy of prematurity (ROP). The protocols include periodic controls every 1 to 2 weeks for low-weight premature babies starting from the 31st week from conception to the 4th week after birth.[289]

Oxidative stress plays an important role in the development of ROP but is also a factor in other major problems of prematurity, such as bronchopulmonary dysplasia or hypoxic/ischemic encephalopathy. Unfortunately, premature babies are not frequently exposed to pathologies caused by oxidative stress but they also have an extremely immature immune system.[290] Oxygen affects the onset of oxidative stress: newborn babies with a low Apgar score and who are artificially ventilated with oxygen show a much greater and persistent index of oxidative stress (the reduced/oxidized glutathione ratio) compared to babies who are breathing room air.[291] Limited use of oxygen, steroid therapy, changes to the blood transfusion protocols, reduced exposure to light, and the administration of dietary factors are possible strategies of preventive intervention[292]; essential fatty acids and the carotenoids have a structural and protective function.

The long-chain polyunsaturated fatty acids (LCPUFA)—a group that includes the omega-3s—are structural components of the cell membranes (there is a considerable quantity in the brain and the retina) and they are precursors in the synthesis of eicosanoids (prostaglandins, prostacyclines, thromboxans and leukotrienes) and useful in the control of cell and tissue function.[293,294] Human milk contains this type of fatty acid; until recently, formula milk did not contain LCPUFA supplements but now the formulas are supplemented with amino-aids and LCPUFA for full- and premature babies[295] with concentrations that differ depending on the baby's age, as the requirements for these substances change.[296]

These supplements contribute to improving the visual, mental, immune, and psychomotory functions.[297] Early addition of LCPUFA supplements will improve the cognitive development of premature babies[298] and will also reduce pathological retinal angiogenesis, suggesting a role in the control of ROP.[299]

Carotenoids are found in the colostrum of human milk; mothers who have breastfed in the past will have a higher concentration with subsequent children.[300] The concentration of lutein is 2 to 3 times greater than β-carotene. Specific active transport mechanisms would appear to be involved.[301] The concentration patterns of the various carotenoids contained in milk varies from country to country and is associated with the diet and the mother's state of nourishment[302]; the pattern of each individual mother changes during the breastfeeding period.[303] Lutein has a trophic effect on the retina and a protective action against the damaging effects of blue light; the most important source of lutein for babies is mother's milk. Premature babies will require a greater amount of nutrients as they will not benefit from the period of maximum transfer across the placenta of energy and nutrients that occurs during the final weeks of pregnancy.[304]

Lutein has a trophic function on the retina and a protective action against damage from blue light.

Lutein can protect lipids from peroxidation[305] and this led to the idea of associating the integration of omega-3 with lutein. Supplements of lutein and omega-3 are administered to the preterm baby and in the formula-fed full-term baby to supply important structural elements, increase the antioxidant capacity, and generally implement the defense mechanisms to improve growth and resistance to any damage from the environment.

The association of omega-3 and lutein supplements in the premature baby and the formula-fed full-term baby increases the antioxidant capacity.

Recommendations to the chef

The researchers who have examined and investigated the eyes and nutrition have asked numerous questions. Do the eye and its structures need specific nutrients in order to function correctly? Can a deficiency or supplements affect the natural progression of diseases? Last, do any nutritional elements have a protective or even curative effect? The studies that we read would all seem to confirm that the answer to these questions is very definitely, "yes." Unfortunately, they have not clarified the effects and the limits of the substances studied, but they indicate the substances that we should take into consideration.

Our normal diet should contain a sufficient quantity of fruit and vegetables, more than one portion every day. When choosing vegetables, we should opt for those that are rich in carotenoids because of the structural function and the antioxidant ability. The first choice is lutein, which is found in the retina and in the crystalline lens. This substance is found in cauliflower, broccoli, spinach, sweet peppers, and, generally speaking, in all the dark green broad-leafed vegetables. It should be pointed out that cooking the vegetables will release the carotenoids for absorption but it will also destroy some of them; as a result, both raw and cooked vegetables should be eaten. Moreover, dietary fat improves the absorption, so adding oil to the vegetables, particularly if rich in unsaturated fatty acids, is highly recommended.

Include a sufficient quantity of fruit and vegetables with antioxidant properties.

If we prefer something fresh and somewhat exotic, lutein can be found in mango, papaya, and kiwi as well as in our home-grown peaches or saffron. The best source of lycopene is the tomato. Astaxanthine is found in crustaceans and salmon, animals that accumulate large quantities of this substance from their diet.

Fish and nuts contain omega-3 fatty acids.

Large quantities of vitamin C are found in citrus fruit.

Selenium's content in vegetables depends on the composition of the soil.

In foods of animal origin, fish—especially salmon, mackerel, and herring—contain high quantities of polyunsaturated omega-3 fatty acids; if nothing better is available, tinned tuna fish is an acceptable alternative. The omega-3 and the omega-6 fatty acids are found in hazelnuts, walnuts, and in some oils. The oils that contain the greatest quantities of omega-3 are flax or linseed oils, while corn and sunflower seed oils contain high quantities of omega-6; the omega-6 are also found in olive oil, which also contains large quantities of oleic acid, which is a monounsaturated fat. Vitamin E is also found in vegetable oils; this vitamin is generally found in large quantities in whole grain cereals, beans, hazelnuts, broccoli, Brussels sprouts, green broad-leaf vegetables, and eggs.

Vitamin A is found in liver, eggs, and milk; its precursor, β-carotene, is found in pumpkin, zucchini, carrots, highly-colored vegetables, and fruits and vegetables that are yellow-orange in color.

Large quantities of vitamin C are found in citrus fruits; tomatoes; potatoes; broccoli; sweet peppers; green and yellow vegetables; and fruits such as apples, bananas, and berries. Vitamin C is hydrosoluble and is found in the water used to cook the food. Citrus fruit and berries, strawberries, and blueberries in particular, also contain large quantities of bioflavonoids. These foods should normally be eaten raw because cooking will reduce or completely destroy the quantity of flavonoids. Despite this, green tea and dark (not milk) chocolate are excellent sources of gallates. Red wine in moderation is a good source of phenols, even though it also contains alcohol which may sometimes have undesirable effects.

Phosphatidicholine (or lecithin) is found in large quantities in soy and is used in the food industry as a thickening agent; it is used in the production of ice cream, chocolate, margarine, and mayonnaise and is also found in beer yeast, egg yolks, liver, and wheat germ.

Zinc contained in food of animal origin has a greater bioavailability with respect to zinc present in vegetables. It is found in seafood (oysters in particular), eggs, liver, beef, and lamb. For vegetarian diets, it is present in wheat germ, beer yeast, and pumpkin seeds.

Selenium deserves a special mention. It is found in fish (tuna, sardines, sole, cod) and seafood, red meat, liver, and eggs. In Italy, the most important source of selenium is wheat and its derivatives, particularly durum wheat; pasta contains a greater quantity than bread. Its content in vegetables depends on the composition of the land. For this reason, products cultivated in enriched soil are now commercially available.

Recently, market demand has driven the food industry toward research for specific product qualities. A number of staple food products are being studied to integrate them with additional functional characteristics (ie, supplement them with specific ingredients that can have a positive effect on health). They are called functional foods and have been enriched with vitamins and minerals during the production phases and during the successive industrial processing. Potatoes enriched with selenium is one example; another is vitamin-enriched corn flakes. These foods are considered to be healthy, but they are consumed with no medical supervision. In the future, we will find an increasing number of these products in the supermarkets.

Another aspect of the food industry's research is the attention paid to the antioxidant properties of the vegetables' total antioxidant capacity (TAC). This does not depend only on the type and species of the fruit but also on the intraspecific genetic differences. The objective is to select from successive generations (through genetic manipulation with grafts or other means) a quality of fruit with excellent properties that can be part of a healthy diet.

Notes on the supplements

What is a supplement?

At the time of publication, there is much confusion regarding the definition of this type of product, even in terms of the governing legislation.
The European Health Product Manufacturers (EHPM) defines a supplement as a preparation consisting of or containing nutrients and/or other edible substances that can be used to supplement the normal diet. These are products that will supply substances not found in sufficient quantity with the normal diet. There are 2 ways of administering these substances: the first involves a dose that is sufficient to prevent deficiency-linked diseases, and the second, in a broad sense, involves a dose that will prevent the onset of the visible symptoms but will also contribute to the body's good health and resistance to disease. One typical example of the latter is the antioxidant supplement administered in doses greater than the RDA for the population.

Can a supplement be classed as a medicinal drug?

Can a supplement be classified as a medicinal drug?

We need to distinguish between drug and food. The presentation of the product (ie, the label) must contain the information for a specific drug, indicating which illnesses it treats or prevents; this type of information is forbidden for food. The information on a drug must also indicate the side effects; again, this does not apply to dietary supplements.
Dietary products are similar to the supplements.
As defined in the *Italian Official Gazzette*, the dietary foods for special medical purposes (DFSMP) should be administered in the diet (the entire diet or just part of it) for clinical reasons to a patient who shows signs of alterations, disturbances, or disorders in the ability to consume, digest, absorb, metabolize, or excrete the common food or specific nutrients. In these patients, a well-balanced food intake cannot be achieved simply by modifying the normal dietary regimen, by replacing with other foods, or with a combination of both.
The DFSMP may be incomplete in nutritional terms supplied with a standard formulation or be a supplied formula that has been adapted for a specific illness, disturbance, or pathological state and cannot be used as a sole source of nutrition.
The formulation of the DFSMP must be based on reliable medical and food science principles. They must have a manufacturer's guarantee and be safe for human consumption, and they must be healthy and respond efficaciously to specific nutritional needs of the individual group of patients, on the basis of well-recognized scientific data.

The main difference between these and food supplements is that they must carry the information *"Indicated for the dietary requirements of patients affected by..."* specifying the name of the illness, the disturbance, or the pathological state the product is being used to treat.
Once again, while the dietary products by law must have a certain nutritional objective and the relative information must be carried on the label, the food supplements do not carry any diet-oriented indication. Food supplements and enriched products must not be considered to be "dietetic" as they were not conceived to satisfy nutritional requirements or specific physiological conditions.
The food supplement, therefore, is not a medicinal drug nor a dietary food preparation but a food product that can be administered as a tablet, capsule, powder or liquid; it consists largely of nutri-

Table 3.1

The table shows the presence of some components of dietary supplements available on the Italian market and produced by pharmaceutical companies dedicated to ophthalmology.

Brand name	Manufacturer	Carotenoids				Vitamins			EFA	
		L	Z	A	β	B	C	E	Ω3	Ω6
Kronek	SOOFT					+				
Lutein ofta	SOOFT	+								
Lutein omega3	SOOFT	+					+	+	+	
Macular active	SOOFT	+					+	+		
Myoops	SOOFT	+			+			+		
Maxiven	BIOOS						+		+	
Tioretin fast/slow	BIOOS					+	+	+		
Vitreoxigen	BIOOS						+	+		
Medilar	BAUSCH&LOMB					+	+	+	+	+
Ocuvite preservision	BAUSCH&LOMB				+		+	+		
Preservision 3	BAUSCH&LOMB	+	+				+	+	+	
Trofinerv	BAUSCH&LOMB					+		+	+	
Trofinerv antiox	BAUSCH&LOMB				+	+	+	+	+	+
Vasopt	BAUSCH&LOMB							+		
Azyr	SIFI	+	+	+			+	+		
Epinerve	SIFI									
Vitreoclar	SIFI							+		
Chiton	ALFA INTES					+			+	+
Pre astig	ALFA INTES				+		+	+		
Retinovit forte	ALFA INTES				+			+		
Meralut	THEA	+	+		+					

Key to Table 3.1

L: **lutein**
Z: **zeaxanthin**
A: **astaxanthin**
β: **β-carotene or vitamin A**
Ru: **rutin**
Pm: **maritime pine extract**
An: **anthocyanoside**
Ge: **genisteine**
Fo: **forskolin**
Eg: **epigallocatechin gallate**
al: **other bioflavonoids**
Col: **choline**
Ac lip: **lipoic acid**
AA: **amino acids**
NAG: **N-acetyl glucosamine**

ents, micronutrients and other edible substances that are taken in unitary doses. Their objective is to supplement the normal diet (with no medical objectives or specific dietetic ends). Their use aims to optimize the quantity of the specific substance in the diet, supplying substances that are of dietary interest with a protective or trophic effect and improve the body's metabolism and the physiological activities. *Table 3.1* lists some of the main food supplements produced by companies operating in the field of ophthalmology in Italy. The components but not the doses are specified. Obviously, according to the definition of food supplement, we have not specified the pathologies for which these food supplements were developed to treat.

	Oligominerals			Bioflavonoids							Ginkgo Biloba	CoQ_{10}	Col	Lipoic Acid	AA	NAG
	Zn	Cu	Se	Ru	Pm	An	Ge	Fo	Eg	al.						
				+				+								
	+	+														
	+	+									+					
						+										
				+	+						+					
							+							+		
				+		+				+	+				+	
	+															
	+	+														
	+	+														
	+	+	+													
	+	+									+					
	+	+														
									+							
										+					+	
	+	+														+
	+	+	+													
										+						
						+										

References

1. Cahkravarti S. The cornea through the eyes of knock-out mice. *Exp Eye Res.* 1965;4:349.
2. Meek KM, Fullwood NJ. Corneal and scleral collagens—a microscopist prospective. *Micron.* 2001;32:261-274.
3. Farrel RA, McCalley RL. Corneal transparency. In: Albert DN, Jacobiek FA, eds. *Principles and practice of ophthalmology*. Philadelphia, PA: WB Saunders; 2000:629-644.
4. Freeman IL. Collagen polymorphism in mature rabbit cornea. *Invest Ophthalmol Vis Sci.* 1978;17:171-177.
5. Scott JE. Proteoglycan: collagen interactions and corneal ultrastructure. *Biochem Soc Trans.* 1991;19:877-881.
6. Fatt I. Hydraulic flow conductivity of the vitreous gel. *Invest Ophthalomol Vis Sci.* 1977;16:565-568.
7. Scott JE. The chemical morphology of the vitreous. *Eye.* 1992;6:553-555.
8. Nishikawa S, Tamai M. Ultrastructure of hyaluronic acid and collagen in the human vitreous. *Curr Eye Res.* 1996;15(1):37-43.
9. Bishop PN, McLeod D, Reardon A. The role of glycosaminoglycans in the structural organization of mammalian eyes. *Invest Ophthalmol Vis Sci.* 1999;40:2173-2178.
10. Bishop PN. Structural macromolecules and supramolecular organisation of the vitreous gel. *Prog Retin Eye Res.* 2000;19(3):323-344.
11. Theccharis AD, Papageorgakopoulou N, Feretis E, Theocharis DA. Occurrence and structural characterization of versican-like proteoglycan in human vitreous. *Biochimie.* 2002;84(12):1237-1243.
12. Duncan G, Wormstone IM, Davies PD. The aging human lens: structure, growth, and physiological behaviour. *Br J Ophthalmol.* 1997;81(10):818-823.
13. Kuriyama H, Sasaki K, Fukuda M. Studies on diabetic cataract in rats induced by streptozotocin. II. Biochemical examinations of rat lenses in relation to cataract stages. *Ophthalmic Res.* 1983;15(4):191-197.
14. Abraham AG, Condon NG, West Gower E. The new epidemiology of cataract. *Ophthalmol Clin North Am.* 2006;19(4):415-425.
15. Ottonello S, Foroni C, Carta A, et al. Oxidative stress and age related cataract. *Ophthalmologica.* 2000;214:78-85.
16. Spector A. Oxidation and cataract. *Ciba Found Symp.* 1984;106:48-64.
17. Rennie MJ. Teasing out the truth about collagen. *J Physiol.* 1999;15(521 Pt 1):1.
18. Sommer F, Kobuch K, Brandl F, et al. Ascorbic acid modulates proliferation and extracellular matrix accumulation of hyalocytes. *Tissue Eng.* 2007;13(6):1281-1289.
19. Smith K, Rennie MJ. New approaches and recent results concerning human-tissue collagen synthesis. *Curr Opin Clin Nutr Metab Care.* 2007;10(5):582-590.
20. Becquet F, Goureau O, Soubrane G, Coscas G, Courtois Y, Hicks D. Superoxide inhibits proliferation and phagocytic internalization of photoreceptor outer segments by bovine retinal pigment epithelium in vitro. *Exp Cell Res.* 1994;212(2):374-382.
21. Masters C. Omega-3 fatty acids and the peroxisome. *Mol Cell Biochem.* 1996;165(2):83-93.
22. Reinboth JJ, Gautschi K, Munz K, Eldred GE, Remé CE. Lipofuscin in the retina: quantitative assay for an unprecedented autofluorescent compound (pyridinium bis-retinoid, A2-E) of ocular age pigment. *Exp Eye Res.* 1997;65(5):639-643.
23. Wihlmark U, Wrigstad A, Roberg K, Nilsson SE, Brunk UT. Lipofuscin accumulation in cultured retinal pigment epithelial cells causes enhanced sensitivity to blue light irradiation. *Free Radic Biol Med.* 1997;22(7):1229-1234.
24. Brunk UT, Wihlmark U, Wrigstad A, Roberg K, Nilsson SE. Accumulation of lipofuscin within retinal pigment epithelial cells results in enhanced sensitivity to photo-oxidation. *Gerontology.* 1995;41(Suppl 2):201-212.
25. Holz FG, Sheraidah G, Pauleikhoff D, Bird AC. Analysis of lipid deposits extracted from human macular and peripheral Bruch's membrane. *Arch Ophthalmol.* 1994;112(3):402-406.
26. Capaccioli S, Nucci C, Quattrone A, Carella E. Apoptosi in oftalmologia: monografie della Società Oftalmologica Italiana, Ed. INC, 1998.
27. Del Priore LV, Kaplan HJ, Hornbeck R, Jones Z, Swinn M. Retinal pigment epithelial debridement as a model for the pathogenesis and treatment of macular degeneration. *Am J Ophthalmol.* 1996;122(5):629-643.
28. Daemen F. Vertebrate rod outer segment membranes. *Biochim Biophis Acta.* 1973;300:255-288.
29. Van Nieuwenhoven FA, Van der Vusse GJ, Glatz JF. Membrane-associated and cytoplasmic fatty acid-binding proteins. *Lipids.* 1996;31 Suppl:S223-227.
30. Glatz JF, van Nieuwenhoven FA, Luiken JJ, Schaap FG, van der Vusse GJ. Role of membrane-associated and cytoplasmic fatty acid-binding proteins in cellular fatty acid metabolism. *Prostaglandins Leukot Essent Fatty Acids.* 1997;57(4-5):373-378.
31. Chen H, Anderson RE. Comparison of uptake and incorporation of docosahexaenoic and arachidonic acids by frog retinas. *Curr Eye Res.* 1993;12(9):851-860.
32. Bazan NG, Rodriguez De Turco EB, Gordon WB. Supply, uptake and retention of docosahexanoic acid by the developing and mature retina and brain. Paper presented at: Lipids, learning and the brain: fats in infant formulas; 103rd Ross conference on pediatric research; Adelaide, South Australia; 1993.
33. Scott BL, Bazan NG. Membrane docosahexaenoate is supplied to developping brain and retina. *Proc Natl Acad Sci USA.* 1989;86:2903-2907.
34. Chen Y, Houghton LA, Brenna JT, Noy N. Docosahexaenoic acid modulates the interactions of the interphotoreceptor retinoid-binding protein with 11-cis-retinal. *J Biol Chem.* 1996;271(34):20507-20515.
35. Grammatikos SI, Subbaiah PV, Victor TA, Miller WM. Diverse effects of essential (n-6 and n-3) fatty acids on cultured cells. *Cytotechnology.* 1994;15(1-3):31-50.
36. Keys SA, Boley E, Zimmerman WF. A model membrane system to investigate antioxidants in bovine rod outer segments. *Exp Eye Res.* 1997;64(3):313-321.
37. Bjerve KS. Omega 3 fatty acid deficiency in man: implications for the requirement of alpha-linolenic acid and long-chain omega 3 fatty acids. *World Rev Nutr Diet.* 1991;66:133-142.
38. Bone RA, Landrum JT, Hime GW, Cains A, Zamor J. Stereochemistry of the human macular carotenoids. *Invest Ophthalmol Vis Sci.* 1993;34(6):2033-2040.
39. Handelman GJ, Dratz EA, Reay CC, van Kuijk JG. Carotenoids in the human macula and whole retina. *Invest Ophthalmol Vis Sci.* 1988;29(6):850-855.
40. Davies NP, Morland AB. Macular pigments: their characteristics and putative role. *Prog Retin Eye Res.* 2004;23(5):533-559.
41. Schalch W. Carotenoids in the retina—a review of their possible role in preventing or limiting damage caused by light and oxygen. *EXS.* 1992;62:280-298.
42. Snodderly DM, Handelman GJ, Adler AJ. Distribution of individual macular pigment carotenoids in central retina of macaque and squirrel monkeys. *Invest Ophthalmol Vis Sci.* 1991;32(2):268-729.
43. Hammond BR, Wooten BR, Snodderly DM. Protection of the retina by macular pigment. *Invest Ophthalmol Vis Sci* 1996;37:3062.
44. Snodderly DM, Auran JD, Delori FC. The macular pigment II. Spatial distribution in primate retinas. *Invest Ophthalmol Vis Sci.* 1984;25:674-685.
45. Di Mascio P, Devasagayam TP, Kaiser S, Sies H. Carotenoids, tocopherols and thiols as biological singlet molecular oxygen quenchers. *Biochem Soc Trans.* 1990;18(6):1054-1056.
46. Nolan J, Neelam K. Carotenoids. In: Eperjesi F, Beatty S, eds. *Nutrition and the eye.* New York, NY: Elsevier; 2006:91-99.
47. Krinsky NI, Deneke SM. Interaction of oxygen and oxy-radicals with carotenoids. *J Natl Cancer Inst.* 1982; 69(1):205-210.
48. Handelman GJ, Snodderly DM, Krinsky NI, Russett MD, Adler AJ. Biological control of primate macular pigment. Biochemical and densitometric studies. *Invest Ophthalmol Vis Sci.* 1991;32(2):257-267.
49. Young AJ, Lowe GM. Lycopene as the most effective biological carotenoid singlet oxygen quencher. *Arch Biochem Biophis.* 1989;274:532-538.
50. Khachik F, Bernstein PS, Garland DL. Identification of lutein and zeaxanthin oxidation products in human and monkey retinas. *Invest Ophthalmol Vis Sci.* 1997;38(9):1802-1811.
51. Crabtree DV, Adler AJ. Is beta-carotene an antioxidant? *Med Hypotheses.* 1997;48(2):183-187.

52. Khachik F, Spangler CJ, Smith JC Jr, Canfield LM, Steck A, Pfander H. Identification, quantification, and relative concentrations of carotenoids and their metabolites in human milk and serum. *Anal Chem.* 1997;69(10): 1873-1881.
53. Sommerburg O, Keunen JE, Bird AC, van Kuijk FJ. Fruits and vegetables that are s for lutein and zeaxanthin: the macular pigment in human eyes. *Br J Ophthalmol.* 1998;82(8):907-910.
54. Lei Z, Leung I, Tso MOM, Lam KW. The identification of diapalmityl zeaxanthin as the major carotenoid in gou qi zi high pressure liquid chromatography and mass spectrometry. *J Ocul Pharm Ther*. 1999;15:557-560.
55. Hammond BR Jr, Fuld K, Curran-Celentano J. Macular pigment density in monozygotic twins. *Invest Ophthalmol Vis Sci.* 1995;36(12):2531-2541.
56. Hammond BR Jr, Johnson EJ, Russell RM, et al. Dietary modification of human macular pigment density. *Invest Ophthalmol Vis Sci.* 1997;38(9):1795-1801.
57. Pece A, Marabottini N. Terapia medica e antiossidanti. In: Pece A, Lanzetta P, ed. *La terapia della degenerazione maculare legata all'età*. Savona, Italia: Dogma; 2003.
58. Parker RS. Absorption, metabolism, and transport of carotenoids. *FASEB J.* 1996;10(5):542-551.
59. Ribaya-Mercado JD, Ordovas JM, Russell RM. Effect of beta-carotene supplementation on the concentrations and distribution of carotenoids, vitamin E, vitamin A, and cholesterol in plasma lipoprotein and non-lipoprotein fractions in healthy older women. *J Am Coll Nutr.* 1995; 14(6):614-620.
60. Hammond BR Jr, Curran-Celentano J, Judd S, et al. Sex differences in macular pigment optical density: relation to plasma carotenoid concentrations and dietary patterns. *Vision Res.* 1996;36(13):2001-2012.
61. Bernstein PS, Balashov NA, Tsong ED, Rando RR. Retinal tubulin binds macular carotenoids. *Invest Ophthalmol Vis Sci.* 1997;38:167-175.
62. Bone RA, Landrum JT, Fernandez L, Tarsis SL. Analysis of the macular pigment by HPLC: retinal distribution and age study. *Invest Ophthalmol Vis Sci.* 1988;29(6): 843-849.
63. VandenLangenberg GM, Brady WE, Nebeling LC, et al. Influence of using different s of carotenoid data in epidemiologic studies. *J Am Diet Assoc.* 1996;96(12):1271-1275.
64. Snodderly DM, Shen B, Land RI, Krinsky NI. Dietary manipulation of plasma carotenoid concentrations of squirrel monkeys (Saimiri sciureus). *J Nutr.* 1997;127(1):122-129.
65. Underwood BA, Arthur P. The contribution of vitamin A to public health. *FASEB J.* 1996;10:1040-1048.
66. Omenn GS. Chemoprevention of lung cancers: lessons from CARET, the beta-carotene and retinol efficacy trial, and prospects for the future. *Eur J Cancer Prev.* 2007;16(3):184-191.
67. Florence TM. The role of free radicals in disease. *Aust N Z J Ophthalmol.* 1995;23(1):3-7.
68. Snodderly DM. Evidence for protection against age-related macular degeneration by carotenoids and antioxidant vitamins. *Am J Clin Nutr.* 1995;62(6 Suppl):1448S-1461S.
69. Ito T, Nakano M, Yamamoto Y, Hiramitsu T, Mizuno Y. Hemoglobin-induced lipid peroxidation in the retina: a possible mechanism for macular degeneration. *Arch Biochem Biophys.* 1995;316(2):864-872.
70. Comporti M. Lipid peroxidation: biopathological significance. *Mol Aspects Med.* 1993;14(3):199-207.
71. Remé CE, Malnoë A, Jung HH, Wei Q, Munz K. Effect of dietary fish oil on acute light-induced photoreceptor damage in the rat retina. *Invest Ophthalmol Vis Sci.* 1994;35(1):78-90.
72. van Kuijk FJ, Buck P. Fatty acid composition of the human macula and peripheral retina. *Invest Ophthalmol Vis Sci.* 1992;33(13):3493-3496.
73. Tate DJ Jr, Miceli MV, Newsome DA. Phagocytosis and H_2O_2 induce catalase and metallothionein gene expression in human retinal pigment epithelial cells. *Invest Ophthalmol Vis Sci.* 1995;36(7):1271-1279.
74. Savouré N. Free radicals. *Allerg Immunol (Paris).* 1993;25(10):404-407.
75. Behndig A, Svensson B, Marklund SL, Karlsson K. Superoxide dismutase isoenzymes in the human eye. *Invest Ophthalmol Vis Sci.* 1998;39(3):471-475.
76. Ogawa T, Ohira A, Amemiya T. Manganese and copper-zinc superoxide dismutases in the developing rat retina. *Acta Histochem* 1997 Mar;99(1):1-12.
77. Geroski DH, Edelhouser H, O Brien WJ. Hexose-monophosphate shunt response to diamide in the component layers of the cornea. *Exp Eye Res.* 1978;26:611-619.
78. Ottonello S, Foroni A, Carta A, et al. Oxidative stress and age related cataract. *Ophthalmologica.* 2000;214:78-85.
79. Harding JJ, Crabbe MJC. The lens: development, proteins, metabolism an cataract. In: Davson H, ed. *The eye.* Vol II. New York, NY: New York Academic Press; 1984:207-492.
80. Stoyanovsky DA, Goldman R, Darrow RM, Organisciak DT, Kagan VE. Endogenous ascorbate regenerates vitamin E in the retina directly and in combination with exogenous dihydrolipoic acid. *Curr Eye Res.* 1995;14(3):181-189.
81. Aonuma H, Koide K, Masuda K, Watanabe I. Retinal light damage: protective effect of alpha-tocopherol. *Jpn J Ophthalmol.* 1997;41(3):160-167.
82. el-Hifnawi el-S, Lincoln DT, Dashti H. Nutritionally induced retinal degeneration in rats. *Nutrition.* 1995;11(5 Suppl):705-707.
83. el-Hifnawi el-S, Lincoln DT, Dashti H. Effects of vitamin E on the retina and retinal pigment epithelium of IRCS rats. *Nutrition.* 1995;11(5 Suppl):576-581.
84. Stephens RJ, et el. Vitamin E distribution in ocular tissues following long term dietary depletion and supplementation as determined by microdissection and gas chromatography-mass spectrometry. *Exp Eye Res.* 1988;47:237-245.
85. Friedrichson T, Kalbach HL, Buck P, van Kuijk FJ. Vitamin E in macular and peripheral tissues of the human eye. *Curr Eye Res.* 1995;14(8):693-701.
86. Organisciak DT, Berman ER, Wang HM, Feeney-Burns L. Vitamin E in human neural retina and retinal pigment epithelium: effect of age. *Curr Eye Res.* 1987;6(8):1051-1055.
87. Handelman GJ, Packer L, Cross CE. Destruction of tocopherols, carotenoids, and retinol in human plasma by cigarette smoke. *Am J Clin Nutr.* 1996;63(4):559-565.
88. Tuder RM, Flook BE, Voelkel NF. Increased gene expression for VEGF and the VEGF receptors KDR/Flk and Flt in lungs exposed to acute or to chronic hypoxia: modulation of gene expression by nitric oxide. *J Clin Invest.*1995;95(4):1798-1807.
89. Teikari JM, Laatikainen L, Rapola JM, et al. Retinal vascular changes following supplementation with alpha-tocopherol or beta-carotene. *Acta Ophthalmol Scand.* 1998;76(1):68-73.
90. Mojon D, Boscoboinik D, Haas A, Bohnke M, Azzi A. Vitamin E inhibits retinal pigment epithelium cell proliferation in vitro. *Ophthalmic Res.* 1994;26(5):304-309.
91. Sakamoto T, Hinton DR, Kimura H, Spee C, Gopalakrishna R, Ryan SJ. Vitamin E succinate inhibits proliferation and migration of retinal pigment epithelial cells in vitro: therapeutic implication for proliferative vitreoretinopathy. *Graefes Arch Clin Exp Ophthalmol.* 1996;234(3):186-192.
92. The Alpha-Tocopherol, Beta Carotene Cancer Prevention Study Group. The effect of vitamin E and beta carotene on the incidence of lung cancer and other cancers in male smokers. *N Engl J Med.* 1994;330(15): 1029-1035.
93. Tate DJ, Miceli MV, Newsome DA, Alcock NW, Oliver PD. Influence of zinc on selected cellular functions of cultured human retinal pigment epithelium. *Curr Eye Res.* 1995;14(10):897-903.
94. Tate DJ Jr, Miceli MV, Newsome DA. Zinc induces catalase expression in cultured fetal human retinal pigment epithelial cells. *Curr Eye Res.* 1997;16(10):1017-1023.
95. Kim SY, Kwak JS, Shin JP, Lee SH. The protection of the retina from ischemic injury by the free radical scavenger EGb 761 and zinc in the cat retina. *Ophthalmologica.* 1998;212(4):268-274.
96. Wu SM, Qiao X, Noebels JL, Yang XL. Localization and modulatory actions of zinc in vertebrate retina. *Vision Res.* 1993;33(18):2611-2616.
97. Newsome DA, Oliver PD, Deupree DM, Miceli MV, Diamond JG. Zinc uptake by primate retinal pigment epithelium and choroid. *Curr Eye Res.* 1992;11(3):213-217.
98. Ishihara N, Yuzawa M, Tamakoshi A. Antioxidants and angiogenetic factor associated with age-related macular degeneration (exudative type). *Nippon Ganka Gakkai Zasshi.* 1997;101(3):248-251.
99. Cousins RJ. Metallothionein—aspects related to copper and zinc metabolism. *J Inherit Metab Dis.* 1983;6(Suppl 1):15-21.
100. Hiller R, Seigel D, Sperduto RD, et al. Serum zinc and serum lipid profiles in 778 adults. *Ann Epidemiol.* 1995;5(6):490-496.

101. Olin KL, Morse LS, Murphy C, et al. Trace element status and free radical defense in elderly rhesus macaques (Macaca mulatta) with macular drusen. *Proc Soc Exp Biol Med.* 1995;208(4):370-377.
102. Harborne JB, Williams CA. Advances in flavonoid research since 1992. *Phytochemistry.* 2000;55:481-504.
103. Arora A, Byram TM, Nair MG, Strasburg GM. Modulation of liposomal membrane fluidity by flavonoids and isoflavonoids. *Arch Biochem Biophis.* 2000;373:102-109.
104. Liao KL, Yin MC. Individual and combined antioxidant effect of seven phenolic agents in human eritrocite membrane ghosts and phosphatidilcoline membrane system: importance of the partition coefficient. *J Agric Food Chem.* 2000;48:2266-2270.
105. Ministero della Salute. Bioflavonoidi: tanto rumore per nulla. Bollettino d'informazione sui farmaci, anno IX numero 5, sett-ott 2002:37-39.
106. Van Beek TA, Bombardelli E, Morazzoni P, Peterlongo F. Gingko biloba. *Fitoterapia.* 1998;69:195-244.
107. Curtis-Prior P, Vere D, Fray P. Therapeutic value of Ginkgo biloba in reducing symptoms of decline in mental function. *J Pharm Pharmacol.* 1999;51:535-541.
108. Miller LG. Herbal medicinals. Selected considerations focusing on known or potential drug-herb interactions. *Arch Intern Med.* 1998;158:2200-2211.
109. Huang SY, Jeng C, Kao SC, Yu JJ, Liu DZ. Improved haemorrheological properties by Ginkgo biloba extract (Egb 761) in type 2 diabetes mellitus complicated with retinopathy. *Clin Nutr.* 2004;23(4):615-621.
110. Christen Y, Maixent JM. What is Ginkgo biloba extract EGb 761? An overview-from molecular biology to clinical medicine. *Cell Mol Biol (Noisy-le-grand).* 2002;48(6):601-611.
111. Kim SY, Kwak JS, Shin JP, Lee SH. The protection of the retina from ischemic injury by the free radical scavenger EGb 761 and zinc in the cat retina. *Ophthalmologica.* 1998;212(4):268-274.
112. Droy-Lefaix MT, Vennat JC, Besse G, Doly M. Effect of Gingko biloba extract (EGb 761) on chloroquine induced retinal alterations. *Lens Eye Toxic Res.* 1992;9(3-4):521-528.
113. Thiagarajan G, Chandani S, Harinarayana Rao S, Samuni AM, Chandrasekaran K, Balasubramanian D. Molecular and cellular assessment of ginkgo biloba extract as a possible ophthalmic drug. *Exp Eye Res.* 2002;75(4):421-430.
114. Ertekin MV, Koçer I, Karslioglu I, et al. Effects of oral Ginkgo biloba supplementation on cataract formation and oxidative stress occurring in lenses of rats exposed to total cranium radiotherapy. *Jpn J Ophthalmol.* 2004;48(5):499-502.
115. Rosenblatt M, Mindel J. Spontaneous hyphema associated with ingestion of Ginkgo biloba extract (Letter). *N Engl J Med.* 1997;336:1108.
116. Cupp MJ. Herbal remedies: adverse effects and drug interactions. *Am Fam Physician.* 1999:59:1239-1245.
117. Rowin J, Lewis SL. Spontaneous bilateral subdural hematoma associated with chronic ginkgo biloba ingestion. *Neurology.* 1996;46:1775-1776.
118. Gilbert GJ. Ginkgo biloba (Letter). *Neurology.* 1997;48:1137.
119. Miller LG, Freeman B. Possible subdural hematoma associated with ginkgo biloba. *J Herb Pharmacother.* 2002;2(2):57-63.
120. Sofi F, Vecchio S, Giuliani G, et al. Dietary habits, lifestyle and cardiovascular risk factors in a clinically healthy Italian population: the "Florence" diet is not Mediterranean. *Eur J Clin Nutr.* 2005;59(4):584-591.
121. Sofi F, Capalbo A, Marcucci R, et al. Leisure time but not occupational physical activity significantly affects cardiovascular risk factors in an adult population. *Eur J Clin Invest.* 2007; 37(12):947-953.
122. Sofi F, Innocenti G, Dini C, et al. Low adherence of a clinically healthy Italian population to nutritional recommendations for primary prevention of chronic diseases. *Nutr Metab Cardiovasc Dis.* 2006;16(6):436-444. Epub 2006 Jan 18.
123. Istituto Nazionale di Ricerca per gli Alimenti e la Nutrizione. Linee guida per una sana alimentazione italiana. Revisione 2003.
124. Brown NA, Bron AJ, Harding JJ, Dewar HM. Nutrition supplements and the eye. *Eye.* 1998;12(Pt 1):127-133.
125. van der Hagen AM, Yolton DP, Kaminski MS, Yolton RL. Free radicals and antioxidant supplementation: a review of their roles in age-related macular degeneration. *J Am Optom Assoc.* 1993;64(12):871-878.
126. Kaminski MS, Yolton DP, Jordan WT, Yolton RL. Evaluation of dietary antioxidant levels and supplementation with ICAPS-Plus and Ocuvite. *J Am Optom Assoc.* 1993;64(12):862-870.
127. Bartlett H, Eperjesi F. An ideal ocular nutritional supplement? *Ophthalmic Physiol Opt.* 2004;24(4):339-349.
128. Duyff RL. Resources: more about healtful eating. In: *American Dietetic Association Complete Food and Nutrition Guide. 3rd ed.* Hoboken, NJ: Wiley & Sons; 2006:617-635.
129. Supplements: use and abuse. In: Duyff RL, ed. American Dietetic Association. 3rd ed. Hoboken, NJ: Wiley & Sons; 2006:590-614.
130. Bron AJ. Classification and diagnosis of dry eye syndromes. Atti congresso: FERMO... l'occhio secco, settembre 2006.
131. Caffery BE. Influence of diet on tear function. *Optom Vis Sci.* 1991;68(1):58-72.
132. Blades KJ, Patel S, Aidoo KE. Oral antioxidant therapy for marginal dry eye. *Eur J Clin Nutr.* 2001;55(7):589-597.
133. Sommer R, Green WR. Goblet cell response to vitamine A treatment for corneal xerophthalmia. *Am J Ophthalmol.* 1982;100:399-403.
134. Choy C, Benzie I, Cho P. Antioxidants in tears and plasma: Inter-relationships and effect of vitamin C supplementation. *Curr Eye Res.* 2003;27(1):55-60.
135. Shreeve CM. Treating the dry eye. *Ophthalm Opt.* 1982;25:650-651.
136. Horrobin DF, Campbell A. Sjogren's syndrome and the sicca syndrome: the role of prostaglandin E1 deficiency. Treatment with essential fatty acids and vitamin C. *Med Hypotheses.* 1980;6(3):225-232.
137. Aragona P, Giuffrida S, Bucolo C, et al. Tear PGE1 levels in dry eye patients after treatment with essential fatty acids. *Invest Ophthalmol Vis Sci.* 2001;42(suppl):259.
138. Horrobin DF, Campbell A, McEwen CG. Treatment of the Sicca syndrome and Sjögren's syndrome with E.F.A., pyridoxine and vitamin C. *Prog Lipid Res.* 1981;20:253-254.
139. Oxholm P, Manthorpe R, Prause JU, Horrobin D. Patients with primary Sjögren's syndrome treated for two months with evening primrose oil. *Scand J Rheumatol.* 1986;15(2):103-108.
140. Barabino S, Rolando M, Camicione P, et al. Systemic linoleic and gamma-linolenic acid therapy in dry eye syndrome with an inflammatory component. *Cornea.* 2003;22(2):97-101.
141. Weinberg ED. The therapeutic potential of lactoferrin. *Expert Opin Investig Drugs.* 2003;12(5):841-851.
142. Troost FJ, Saris WH, Brummer RJ. Orally ingested human lactoferrin is digested and secreted in the upper gastrointestinal tract in vivo in women with ileostomies. *J Nutr.* 2002;132(9):2597-2600.
143. Ohashi Y, Ishida R, Kojima T, et al. Abnormal protein profiles in tears with dry eye syndrome. *Am J Ophthalmol.* 2003;136(2):291-299.
144. Sebag J. Age-related changes in human vitreous structure. *Graefes Arch Clin Exp Ophthalmol.* 1987;225(2):89-93.
145. Los LI, van der Worp RJ, van Luyn MJ, Hooymans JM. Age-related liquefaction of the human vitreous body: LM and TEM evaluation of the role of proteoglycans and collagen. *Invest Ophthalmol Vis Sci.* 2003;44(7):2828-2833.
146. Plantner JM, et al. Matrix metalloproteinases and metalloproteinase inhibitors in human interphotoreceptor matrix and vitreous. *Curr Eye Res.* 1998;17:132-140.
147. Takahashi K, Arai K, Hayashi S, Tanaka Y. Degree of degraded proteoglycan in human vitreous and the influence of peroxidation. *Nippon Ganka Gakkai Zasshi.* 2006;110(3):171-179.
148. Filippello M, Picardo V, Stagni E. Fisiopatologia del corpo vitreo. *Reading in Oftalmologia*, anno XIII n° 3/2003.
149. Plantner J. Membrane type-1 matrix metalloproteinase in human ocular tissues. *Curr Eye Res.* 1997;16:925-929.
150. Age-Related Eye Disease Study Research Group. Risk factors associated with age-related nuclear and cortical cataract: a case-control study in the Age-Related Eye Disease Study, AREDS Report No. 5. *Ophthalmology.* 2001;108(8):1400-1408.

151. Klein R, Klein BE, Jensen SC, Moss SE, Cruickshanks KJ. The relation of socioeconomic factors to age-related cataract, maculopathy, and impaired vision: the Beaver Dam Eye Study. *Ophthalmology.* 1994;101(12):1969-1979.
152. Steinberg EP, Javitt JC, Sharkey PD, et al. The content and cost of cataract surgery. *Arch Ophthalmol.* 1993;111(8):1041-1049.
153. Taylor A. Association between nutrition and cataract. *Nutr Rev.* 1989;107:670-676.
154. Kuriyama H, Sasaki K, Fukuda M. Studies on diabetic cataract in rats induced by streptozotocin. II. Biochemical examinations of rat lenses in relation to cataract stages. *Ophthalmic Res.* 1983;15(4):191-197.
155. Carsten HM, Walter S. Nutritional supplement to prevent cataract formation. In: Augustine A, ed. Nutrition and the eye. Dev Ophthalmol. Basel, Karger, 2005;38:103-119.
156. Head KA. Natural therapies for ocular disorders, part two: cataracts and glaucoma. *Altern Med Rev.* 2001;6(2):141-166.
157. Brown L, Hankinson SE, Seddon JM, et al. A prospective study of carotenoid intake and cataracts among U.S. Men. (Abstract Number 213) Presented at the Annual Meeting of the Society for Epidemiologic Research; Chicago, IL; 1998.
158. Lyle BJ, Mares-Perlman JA, Klein BEK, et al. Antioxidant intake and risk of incident age-related nuclear cataracts in the Beaver Dam Eye Study. *Am J Epidemiol.* 1999;149:801-809.
159. Leske MC, Chylack LT Jr, Wu S. The lens opacities case-control study: risk factors for cataract. *Arch Ophthalmol.* 1991;109: 244-251.
160. Leske MC, Chylack LT, He Q, et al. Antioxidant vitamins and nuclear opacites. *Ophthalmology.* 1998;105: 831-836.
161. Rouhiainen P, Rouhiainen H, Salonen JT. Association between low plasma vitamin E concentration and progression of early cortical lens opacities. *Am J Epidemiol.* 1996;144:496-500.
162. Leske MC, Chylack LT Jr, Wu S. The lens opacities case-control study:risk factors for cataract. *Arch Ophthalmol.* 1991;109:244-251.
163. Mares-Perleman JA, Klein BEK, et al. Relationship between lens opacities and vitamin and mineral supplement use. *Ophthalmology.* 1994;101:315-325.
164. Hankinson SE, Stampfer MJ, Seddon JM, et al. Nutrient intake and cataract extraction in women: a prospective study. *BMJ.* 1992;305(6849):335-339.
165. Seddon JM, Christen WG, Manson JE, et al. The use of vitamin supplements and the risk of cataract among U.S. male physicians. *Am J Public Health.* 1994;84:788-792.
166. Jacques PF, et al. Long-term nutrient intake and early age-related nuclear lens opacities. *Arch Ophthalmol.* 2001;119:1009-1019.
167. Jacques PF, et al. Long-term nutrient intake and 5-year change in nuclear lens opacities. *Arch Ophthalmol.* 2005;123:517-526.
168. Sperduto RD, Hu TS, Milton RC, et al. The Linxian cataract studies: two nutrition intervention trials. *Arch Ophthalmol.* 1993;111(9):1246-1253.
169. Age-Related Eye Disease Study Research Group. A randomized, placebo-controlled, clinical trial of high-dose supplementation with vitamins C and E and beta carotene for age-related cataract and vision loss: AREDS report no. 9. *Arch Ophthalmol.* 2001;119(10):1439-1452.
170. Kottler UB, Dick HB, Augustin AJ. Is a cataract avoidable? Current status with special emphasis on the pathophysiology of oxidative lens damage, nutritional factors, and the ARED study. *Ophthalmologe.* 2003; 100(3):190-196.
171. Head KA. Natural therapies for ocular disorders, part two: cataracts and glaucoma. *Altern Med Rev.* 2001;6(2):141-166.
172. Linner E. The pressure lowering effect of ascorbic acid in ocular hypertension. *Acta Ophthalmologica.* 1969;47:685-689.
173. Mozaffarieh M, Flammer J. A novel perspective on natural therapeutic approaches in glaucoma therapy. *Expert Opin Emerg Drugs.* 2007;12(2):195-198.
174. Ritch R. Potential role for ginkgo biloba extract in the treatment of glaucoma. *Med Hypotheses.* 2000;54(2): 221-235.
175. Chung HS, Harris A, Kristinsson JK, et al. Ginkgo biloba estract increases ocular blood flow velocity. *J Ocul Pharmacol Ther.* 1999;15:233-240.
176. Levene RZ. Low tension glaucoma: a critical review and new material. *Surv Ophthalmol.* 1980;24:621-664.
177. Dubey AK, Shankar PR, Upadhyaya D, Deshpande VY. Ginkgo biloba—an appraisal. *Kathmandu Univ Med J (KUMJ).* 2004;2(3):225-229.
178. Hirooka K, Tokuda M, Miyamoto O, et al. The Ginkgo biloba extract (EGb 761) provides a neuroprotective effect on retinal ganglion cells in a rat model of chronic glaucoma. *Curr Eye Res.* 2004;28(3):153-157.
179. Goldberg I. Is this neuroprotective drug good for my glaucoma patients? Some key factors in clinical decision-making. *Can J Ophthalmol.* 2007;42(3):418-420.
180. Weinreb O, Mandel S, Amit T, Youdim MB. Neurological mechanisms of green tea polyphenols in Alzheimer's and Parkinson's diseases. *J Nutr Biochem.* 2004;15(9):506-516.
181. Zhang B, Osborne NN. Oxidative-induced retinal degeneration is attenuated by epigallocatechin gallate. *Brain Res.* 2006;1124(1):176-187.
182. Grieb P, Rejdak R. Pharmacodynamics of citicoline relevant to the treatment of glaucoma. *J Neurosci Res.* 2002;67(2):143-148.
183. Secades JJ, Lorenzo JL. Citicoline: pharmacological and clinical review, 2006 update. Methods. *Find Exp Clin Pharmacol.* 2006;28(Suppl B):1-56.
184. Virno M, Pecori-Giraldi J, Liguori A, De Gregorio F. The protective effect of citicoline on the progression of the perimetric defects in glaucomatous patients (perimetric study with a 10-year follow-up). *Acta Ophthalmol Scand Suppl.* 2000;(232):56-57.
185. Pecori Giraldi J, Virno M, Covelli G, Grechi G, De Gregorio F. Therapeutic value of citicoline in the treatment of glaucoma (computerized andautomated perimetric investigation). *Int Ophthalmol.* 1989;13(1-2):109-112.
186. Rejdak R, Toczołowski J, Kurkowski J, et al. Oral citicoline treatment improves visual pathway function in glaucoma. *Med Sci Monit.* 2003;9(3): PI24-PI28.
187. O'Shea JG. Age-related macular degeneration: a leading cause of blindness. *Med J Aust.* 1996; 165(10):561-564.
188. Rosenberg T, Klie F. The incidence of registered blindness caused by age-related macular degeneration. *Acta Ophthalmol Scand.* 1996;74(4):399-402.
189. Balatsoukas DD, Sioulis C, Parisi A, Millar GT. Visual handicap in south-east Scotland. *J R Coll Surg Edinb.* 1995;40(1):49-51.
190. Evans J, Wormald R. Is the incidence of registrable age-related macular degeneration increasing? *Br J Ophthalmol.* 1996;80(1):9-14.
191. Bird AC, Bressler NM, Bressler SB, et al. An international classification and grading system for age-related maculopathy and age-related macular degeneration. The International ARM Epidemiological Study Group. *Surv Ophthalmol.* 1995;39 (5):367-374.
192. O'Shea JG. Age-related macular degeneration. *Postgrad Med J.* 1998;74(870):203-207.
193. The Eye Disease Case-Control Study Group. Risk factors for neovascular age-related macular degeneration. *Arch Ophthalmol.* 1992;110(12):1701-1708.
194. Silvestri G, Johnston PB, Hughes AE. Is genetic predisposition an important risk factor in age-related macular degeneration? *Eye.* 1994;8(Pt 5):564-568.
195. Silvestri G. Age-related macular degeneration: genetics and implications for detection and treatment. *Mol Med Today.* 1997;3(2):84-91.
196. Klein ML, Schultz DW, Edwards A, et al. Age-related macular degenerationL clinical features in a large family and linkage to chromosome 1q. *Arch Ophthalmol.* 1998;116(8):1082-1088.
197. Seddon JM, Ajani UA, Mitchell BD. Familial aggregation of age-related maculopathy. *Am J Ophthalmol.* 1997;123(2):199-206.
198. Klein ML, Mauldin WM, Stoumbos VD. Heredity and age-related macular degeneration: observations in monozygotic twins. *Arch Ophthalmol.* 1994;112(7):932-937.
199. Meyers SM, Greene T, Gutman FA. A twin study of age-related macular degeneration. *Am J Ophthalmol.* 1995;120(6):757-766.
200. Meyers SM. A twin study on age-related macular degeneration. (2). *Trans Am Ophthalmol Soc.* 1994;92:775-843.

201. Obisesan TO, Hirsch R, Kosoko O, Carlson L, Parrott M. Moderate wine consumption is associated with decreased odds of developing age related macular degeneration in NHANES1. *J Am Ger Soc.* 1998;46:1-7.
202. Hammond BR Jr, Wooten BR, Snodderly DM. Cigarette smoking and retinal carotenoids: implications for age-related macular degeneration. *Vision Res.* 1996; 36(18):3003-3009.
203. Tamakoshi A, Yuzawa M, Matsui M, Uyama M, Fujiwara NK, Ohno Y. Smoking and neovascular form of age related macular degeneration in late middle aged males: findings from a case-control study in Japan. Research Committee on Chorioretinal Degenerations. *Br J Ophthalmol.* 1997;81(10):901-904.
204. Vingerling JR, Hofman A, Grobbee DE, de Jong PT. Age-related macular degeneration and smoking. The Rotterdam Study. *Arch Ophthalmol.* 1996;114(10):1193-1196.
205. Christen WG, Glynn RJ, Manson JE, Ajani UA, Buring JE. A prospective study of cigarette smoking and risk of age-related macular degeneration in men. *JAMA.* 1996;276(14):1147-1151.
206. Seddon JM, Willett WC, Speizer FE, Hankinson SE. A prospective study of cigarette smoking and age-related macular degeneration in women. *JAMA.* 1996; 276(14):1141-1146.
207. Smith W, Mitchell P, Leeder SR. Smoking and age-related maculopathy. The Blue Mountains Eye Study. *Arch Ophthalmol.* 1996;114(12):1518-1523.
208. Delcourt C, Diaz JL, Ponton-Sanchez A, Papoz L. Smoking and age-related macular degeneration. The POLA Study. Pathologies Oculaires Liées à l'Age. *Arch Ophthalmol.* 1998;116(8):1031-1035.
209. Gibson JM, Shaw DE, Rosenthal AR. Senile cataract and senile macular degeneration: an investigation into possible risk factors. *Trans Ophthalmol Soc UK.* 1986; 105(Pt 4):463-468.
210. Hammond BR Jr, Ciulla TA, Snodderly DM. Macular pigment density is reduced in obese subjects. *Invest Ophthalmol Vis Sci.* 2002;43(1):47-50.
211. Nolan J, O'Donovan O, Kavanagh H, et al. Macular pigment and percentage of body fat. *Invest Ophthalmol Vis Sci.* 2004;45(11):3940-3950.
212. Al Taje R, Nolan J, Neelam K. Age related macular degeneration. In: Eperjesi F, Beatty S, eds. Nutrition and the eye. New York, NY: Elsevier; 2006:187-201.
213. Friedman E. A hemodynamic model of the pathogenesis of age-related macular degeneration. *Am J Ophthalmol.* 1997;124(5):677-682.
214. Axer-Siegel R, Bourla D, Ehrlich R, et al. Association of neovascular age-related macular degeneration and hyperhomocysteinemia. *Am J Ophthalmol.* 2004;137(1): 84-89.
215. Huang JD, Presley JB, Chimento MF, Curcio CA, Johnson M. Age-related changes in human macular Bruch's membrane as seen by quick-freeze/deep-etch. *Exp Eye Res.* 2007;85(2): 202-218.
216. Ishibashi T, et al. Formation of drusen in the human eye. *Am J Ophthalmol.* 1986;102:342-353.
217. Spraul CW, Lang GE, Grossniklaus HE, Lang GK. Characteristics of drusen and changes in Bruch's membrane in eyes with age-related macular degeneration: histological study. *Ophthalmologe.* 1998;95(2):73-79.
218. Sakamoto T, Sakamoto H, Murphy TL, et al. Vessel formation by choroidal endothelial cells in vitro is modulated by retinal pigment epithelial cells. *Arch Ophthalmol.* 1995;113(4):512-520.
219. Ajani UA, Willett WC, Seddon JM. Reproducibility of a food frequency questionnaire for use in ocular research. Eye Disease Case-Control Study Group. *Invest Ophthalmol Vis Sci.* 1994;35(6):2725-2733.
220. Smith W, Mitchell P, Reay EM, Webb K, Harvey PW. Validity and reproducibility of a self-administered food frequency questionnaire in older people. *Aust N Z J Public Health.* 1998;22(4):456-463.
221. Chew EY, Clemons T. Vitamin E and the age-related eye disease study supplementation for age-related macular degeneration. *Arch Ophthalmol.* 2005;123(3):395-396.
222. Taylor HR, Tikellis G, Robman LD, McCarty CA, McNeil JJ. Vitamin E supplementation and macular degeneration: randomised controlled trial. *BMJ.* 2002;325 (7354):1-2.
223. Organisciak DT, Jiang YL, Wang HM, Bicknell I. The protective effect of ascorbic acid in retinal light damage of rats exposed to intermittent light. *Invest Ophthalmol Vis Sci.* 1990;31(7):1195-1202.
224. Eye Disease Case-Control Study Group. Antioxidant status and neovascular age-related macular degeneration. *Arch Ophthalmol.* 1993;111(1):104-109.
225. Seddon JM, Gensler G, Klein ML, Milton RC. C-reactive protein and homocysteine are associated with dietary and behavioural risk factors for age-related macular degeneration. *Nutrition.* 2006;22(4):441-443.
226. Landrum JT, Bone RA, Joa H, Kilburn MD, Moore LL, Sprague KE. A one year study of the macular pigment: the effect of 140 days of a lutein supplement. *Exp Eye Res.* 1997;65(1):57-62.
227. Eye Disease Case-Control Study Group. Seddon JM, Ajani UA, Sperduto RD, et al. Dietary carotenoids, vitamins A, C, and E, and advanced age-related macular degeneration. *JAMA.* 1994;272(18):1413-1420.
228. Shibata A, Kiba Y, Akati N, Fukuzawa K, Terada H. Molecular characteristics of astaxanthin and beta-carotene in the phospholipids monolayer and their distributions in the phospholipid bilayer. *Chem Phys Lipids.* 2001;113(1-2):11-22.
229. Toomey MB, McGraw KJ. Modified saponification and HPLC methods for analyzing carotenoids from the retina of quail: implications for its use as a nonprimate model species. *Invest Ophthalmol Vis Sci.* 2007;48(9): 3976-3982.
230. Karppi J, Rissanen TH, Nyyssönen K, et al. Effects of astaxanthin supplementation on lipid peroxidation. *Int J Vitam Nutr Res.* 2007;77(1):3-11.
231. Chichili GR, Nohr D, Frank J, et al. Protective effects of tomato extract with elevated beta-carotene levels on oxidative stress in ARPE-19 cells. *Br J Nutr.* 2006;96(4):643-649.
232. Junghans A, Sies H, Stahl W. Macular pigments lutein and zeaxanthin as blue light filters studied in liposomes. *Arch Biochem Biophys.* 2001;391(2):160-164.
233. Sundelin SP, Nilsson SE. Lipofuscin-formation in retinal pigment epithelial cells is reduced by antioxidants. *Free Radic Biol Med.* 2001;31(2):217-225.
234. Tyssandier V, Cardinault N, Caris-Veyrat C, et al. Vegetable-borne lutein, lycopene, and beta-carotene compete for incorporation into chylomicrons, with no adverse effect on the medium-term (3-wk) plasma status of carotenoids in humans. *Am J Clin Nutr.* 2002;75(3):526-534.
235. Shao A, Hathcock JN. Risk assessment for the carotenoids lutein and lycopene. *Regul Toxicol Pharmacol.* 2006;45(3):289-298.
236. Krinsky NI, Johnson EJ. Carotenoid actions and their relation to health and disease. *Mol Aspects Med.* 2005;26(6):459-516.
237. Johnson EJ. The role of carotenoids in human health. *Nutr Clin Care.* 2002;5(2):56-65.
238. Mares-Perlman JA, Klein R, Klein BE, et al. Association of zinc and antioxidant nutrients with age-related maculopathy. *Arch Ophthalmol.* 1996;114(8):991-997.
239. Vanden Langenberg GM, Mares-Perlman JA, Klein R, Klein BE, Brady WE, Palta M. Associations between antioxidant and zinc intake and the 5-year incidence of early age-related maculopathy in the Beaver Dam Eye Study. *Am J Epidemiol.* 1998;148(2):204-214.
240. Stur M, Tittl M, Reitner A, Meisinger V. Oral zinc and the second eye in age-related macular degeneration. *Invest Ophthalmol Vis Sci.* 1996;37(7):1225-1235.
241. Richer SP. Is there a prevention and treatment strategy for macular degeneration? *J Am Optom Assoc.* 1993;64(12):838-850.
242. Age-Related Eye Disease Study Research Group. The Age-Related Eye Disease Study (AREDS): design implications. AREDS report no. 1. *Control Clin Trials.* 1999;20(6):573-600.
243. Age-Related Eye Disease Study Research Group. Risk factors associated with age-related nuclear and cortical cataract: a case-control study in the Age-Related Eye Disease Study, AREDS Report No. 5. *Ophthalmology.* 2001;108(8):1400-1408.
244. Age-Related Eye Disease Study Research Group. Risk factors associated with age-related macular degeneration. A case-control study in the age-related eye disease study: Age-Related Eye Disease Study Report Number 3. *Ophthalmology.* 2000;107(12):2224-2232.
245. Age-Related Eye Disease Study Research Group. A randomized, placebo-controlled, clinical trial of high-dose supplementation with vitamins C and E, beta carotene, and zinc for age-related macular degeneration and vision loss: AREDS report no. 8. *Arch Ophthalmol.* 2001;119(10):1417-1436.

246. Bressler NM, Bressler SB, Congdon NG, et al, Age-Related Eye Disease Study Research Group. Potential public health impact of Age-Related Eye Disease Study results: AREDS report no. 11. *Arch Ophthalmol.* 2003;121(11):1621-1624.
247. SanGiovanni JP, Chew EY, Clemons TE, et al. The relationship of dietary lipid intake and age-related macular degeneration in a case-control study: AREDS Report No. 20. *Arch Ophthalmol*. 2007;125(5):671-679.
248. Age-Related Eye Disease Study Research Group, SanGiovanni JP, Chew EY, Clemons TE, et al. The relationship of dietary carotenoid and vitamin A, E, and C intake with age-related macular degeneration in a case-control study: AREDS Report No. 22. *Arch Ophthalmol.* 2007;125(9):1225-1232.
249. Polverini PJ. The pathophysiology of angiogenesis. *Crit Rev Oral Biol Med.* 1995;6(3):230-247.
250. Casey R, Li WW. Factors controlling ocular angiogenesis. *Am J Ophthalmol.* 1997;124(4):521-529.
251. Pe'er J, Folberg R, Itin A, Gnessin H, Hemo I, Keshet E. Vascular endothelial growth factor upregulation in human central retinal vein occlusion. *Ophthalmology.* 1998;105(3):412-416.
252. Mathews MK, Merges C, McLeod DS, Lutty GA. Vascular endothelial growth factor and vascular permeability changes in human diabetic retinopathy. *Invest Ophthalmol Vis Sci.* 1997;38(13):2729-2741.
253. Aiello LP, Avery RL, Arrigg PG, et al. Vascular endothelial growth factor in ocular fluid of patients with diabetic retinopathy and other retinal disorders. *N Engl J Med.* 1994;331(22):1480-1487.
254. Tolentino MJ, Miller JW, Gragoudas ES, et al. Vascular endothelial growth factor is sufficient to produce iris neovascularization and neovascular glaucoma in a nonhuman primate. *Arch Ophthalmol*. 1996;114(8):964-970.
255. Frank RN. Growth factors in age-related macular degeneration: pathogenic and therapeutic implications. *Ophthalmic Res.* 1997;29(5):341-353.
256. Tolentino MJ, Miller JW, Gragoudas ES, et al. Intravitreous injections of vascular endothelial growth factor produce retinal ischemia and microangiopathy in an adult primate. *Ophthalmology.* 1996;103(11):1820-1828.
257. Ozaki H, Hayashi H, Vinores SA, Moromizato Y, Campochiaro PA, Oshima K. Intravitreal sustained release of VEGF causes retinal neovascularization in rabbits and breakdown of the blood-retinal barrier in rabbits and primates. *Exp Eye Res.* 1997;64(4):505-517.
258. Pe'er J, Folberg R, Itin A, Gnessin H, Hemo I, Keshet E. Upregulated expression of vascular endothelial growth factor in proliferative diabetic retinopathy. *Br J Ophthalmol.* 1996;80(3):241-245.
259. Webb NJ, Bottomley MJ, Watson CJ, Brenchley PE. Vascular endothelial growth factor (VEGF) is released from platelets during blood clotting: implications for measurement of circulating VEGF levels in clinical disease. *Clin Sci (Colch).* 1998;94(4):395-404.
260. Burgos R, Simó R, Audí L, et al. Vitreous levels of vascular endothelial growth factor are not influenced by its serum concentrations in diabetic retinopathy. *Diabetologia.* 1997;40(9):1107-1109.
261. Kliffen M, Sharma HS, Mooy CM, Kerkvliet S, de Jong PT. Increased expression of angiogenic growth factors in age-related maculopathy. *Br J Ophthalmol.* 1997;81(2):154-162.
262. Amin R, Puklin JE, Frank RN. Growth factor localization in choroidal neovascular membranes of age-related macular degeneration. *Invest Ophthalmol Vis Sci.* 1994;35(8):3178-3188.
263. Fournier E, Birnbaum D, Borg JP. Receptors for factors of the VEGF (Vascular Endothelial Growth Family). *Bull Cancer.* 1997;84(4):397-405.
264. Galland F, Karamysheva A, Pebusque MJ, et al. The FLT4 gene encodes a transmembrane tyrosine kinase related to the vascular endothelial growth factor receptor. *Oncogene.* 1993;8(5):1233-1240.
265. Borg JP, deLapeyrière O, Noguchi T, Rottapel R, Dubreuil P, Birnbaum D. Biochemical characterization of two isoforms of FLT4, a VEGF receptor-related tyrosine kinase. *Oncogene.* 1995;10(5):973-984.
266. Ferrara N. The role of vascular endothelial growth factor in pathological angiogenesis. *Breast Cancer Res Treat.* 1995;36(2):127-137.
267. Takagi H, King GL, Aiello LP. Identification and characterization of vascular endothelial growth factor receptor (Flt) in bovine retinal pericytes. *Diabetes.* 1996;45(8):1016-1023.
268. Lutty G, Grunwald J, Majji AB, Uyama M, Yoneya S. Changes in choriocapillaris and retinal pigment epithelium in age-related macular degeneration. *Mol Vis.* 1999;5:35.
269. Ablonczy Z, Crosson CE. VEGF modulation of retinal pigment epithelium resistance. *Exp Eye Res.* 2007; 85(6):762-771.
270. Brown NA, Bron AJ, Harding JJ, Dewar HM. Nutrition supplements and the eye. *Eye.* 1998;12(Pt 1):127-133.
271. Eye Disease Case-Control Study Group. Antioxidant status and neovascular age-related macular degeneration. *Arch Ophthalmol*. 1993;111(1):104-109.
272. West S, Vitale S, Hallfrisch J, et al. Are antioxidants or supplements protective for age-related macular degeneration? *Arch Ophthalmol.* 1994;112(2): 222-227.
273. Eichenbaum JW. Vitamins for cataracts and macular degeneration. *J Ophthalmic Nurs Technol.* 1996;15(2):65-67.
274. Jacob RA, Burri BJ. Oxidative damage and defense. *Am J Clin Nutr.* 1996;63(6):985S-990S.
275. Mayne ST. Beta-carotene, carotenoids, and disease prevention in humans. *FASEB J.* 1996;10(7):690-701.
276. Parisi V, Tedeschi M, Gallinaro G, et al. Carotenoids and antioxidants in age-related maculopathy italian study: multifocal electroretinogram modifications after 1 year. *Ophthalmology*. 2008;115(2):324-333.
277. Hartong DT, Berson EL, Dryja TP. Retinitis pigmentosa. *Lancet.* 2006;368(9549):1795-1809.
278. Bahrami H, Melia M, Dagnelie G. Lutein supplementation in retinitis pigmentosa: PC-based vision assessment in a randomized double-masked placebo-controlled clinical trial. *BMC Ophthalmology.* 2006;6:23.
279. Aleman TS, Duncan JL, Bieber ML, et al. Macular pigment and lutein supplementation in retinitis pigmentosa and Usher syndrome. *Invest Ophthalmol Vis Sci.* 2001;42: 1873-1881.
280. Berson EL, et al. A randomized trial of vitamin A and vitamin E supplementation for retinitis pigmentosa. *Arch Ophthalmol.* 1993;111:761-772.
281. Sibulesky L, et al. Safety of <7500 RE (<25,000 IU) vitamin A daily in adults with retinitis pigmentosa. *Am J Clin Nutr.* 1999;69:656-663.
282. Komeima K, et al. Antioxidants reduce cone cell death in a model of retinitis pigmentosa. *PNAS.* 2006;103: 1130-1135.
283. Simonelli F, Manna C, Romano N, Nunziata G, Voto O, Rinaldi E. Evaluation of fatty acids in membrane phospholipids of erythrocytes in retinitis pigmentosa patients. *Ophthalmic Res.* 1996;28(2):93-98.
284. Berson EL, Rosner B, Sandberg MA, et al. Clinical trial of docosahexaenoic acid in patients with retinitis Pigmentosa receiving vitamin A treatment. *Arch Ophthalmol.* 2004;122(9):1297-305.
285. Berson EL, Rosner B, Sandberg MA, et al. Further evaluation of docosahexaenoic acid in patients with retinitis pigmentosa receiving vitamin A treatment: subgroup analyses. *Arch Ophthalmol.* 2004;122(9):1306-1314.
286. Bonn D. Keeping the stork at bay until the time is right. *Lancet.* 1998;351:576.
287. Cartlidge PHT, Jones HP, Stewart JH, et al. Confidential enquiry into deaths due to prematurity. *Acta Paediatrica.* 1999;88:220-223.
288. Gorman WA, Fallon M, Kelly M, et al. The Dublin outcome for low birth-weight infants. *Irish Medical Journal.* 1996;89:186-187.
289. Reynolds JD, Dobson V, Quinn GE, et al. Evidente based screening criteria for retinopathy of prematurity: natural history data from the CRYO ROP and LIGHT ROP studies. *Arch Ophthalmol.* 2002;120(11):1470-1476.
290. Dani C, Cecchi A, Bertini G. Role of oxidative stress as physiopathologic factor in the preterm infant. *Minerva Pediatr.* 2004;56(4):381-394.
291. Vento M, Asensi M, Sastre J, García-Sala F, Pallardó FV, Viña J. Resuscitation with room air instead of 100% oxygen prevents oxidative stress in moderately asphyxiated term neonates. *Pediatrics.* 2001;107(4):642-647.
292. Di Biasie A. Evidence-based review of retinopathy of prematurity prevention in VLBW and ELBW infants. *Neonatal Netw.* 2006;25(6):393-403.
293. Neuringer M, Connor WE. n-3 Fatty acids in the brain and retina: evidence for their essentiality. *Nutr Rev.* 1986;44:285-294.
294. Weber PC, Fischer S, von Schacky C, Lorenz R, Strasser T. Dietary omega-3 polyunsaturated fatty acids and eicosanoid formation in man. In: Simopoulos AP, Kifer RR, Martin RE, eds. *Health effects of polyunsaturated fatty acids in seafoods*. Orlando, FL: Academic Press; 1986:49-60.

295. Uauy R, Hoffman DR. Essential fat requirements of preterm infants. *Am J Clin Nutr.* 2000;71(1 Suppl): 245S-50S.
296. Hay WW. Early postnatal nutritional requirements of the very preterm infant based on a presentation at the NICHD-AAP workshop on research in neonatology. *J Perinatol.* 2006;26(Suppl 2):S13-S18.
297. Fleith M, Clandinin MT. Dietary PUFA for preterm and term infants: review of clinical studies. *Crit Rev Food Sci Nutr.* 2005;45(3):205-229.
298. Henriksen C, Haugholt K, Lindgren M, et al. Improved cognitive development among preterm infants attributable to early supplementation of human milk with docosahexaenoic acid and arachidonic acid. *Pediatrics.* 2008;121(6):1137-1145.
299. Connor KM, SanGiovanni JP, Lofqvist C, et al. Increased dietary intake of omega-3-polyunsaturated fatty acids reduces pathological retinal angiogenesis. *Nat Med.* 2007;13(7):868-873.
300. Patton S, Canfield LM, Huston GE, Ferris AM, Jensen RG. Carotenoids of human colostrums. *Lipids.* 1990;25(3):159-165.
301. Gossage CP, Deyhim M, Yamini S, Douglass LW, Moser-Veillon PB. Carotenoid composition of human milk during the first month postpartum and the response to beta-carotene supplementation. *Am J Clin Nutr.* 2002;76(1):193-197.
302. Canfield LM, Clandinin MT, Davies DP, et al. Multinational study of major breast milk carotenoids of healthy mothers. *Eur J Nutr.* 2003;42(3):133-41.
303. Schweigert FJ, Bathe K, Chen F, Büscher U, Dudenhausen JW. Effect of the stage of lactation in humans on carotenoid levels in milk, blood plasma and plasma lipoprotein fractions. *Eur J Nutr.* 2004;43(1):39-44.
304. Jewell VC, Northrop-Clewes CA, Tubman R, Thurnham DI. Nutritional factors and visual function in premature infants. *Proceedings of the Nutrition Society.* 2001;60:171-178.
305. Sujak A, Gabrielska J, Grudzinski W, Borc R, Mazurek P, Gruszecki WI. Lutein and zeaxanthin as protectors of lipid membranes against oxidative damage: the structural aspects. *Arch Biochem Biophys.* 1999;371(2):301-307.

Acronyms

1Car	Carotenoid to the normal state
3Car	Carotenoid to the triplet state

A

AMD	Age-related macular degeneration
AREDS	Age-related eye disease study
ARMD	Age-related macular degeneration
AVED syndrome	Ataxia with vitamin E deficiency

B

BMI	Body mass index

C

CAT	Catalase
cGMP	Cyclic guanosine monophosphate
CRBP	Cellular retinol-binding protein
Cu	Copper

D

DFSMP	Dietary foods for special medical purposes
DHA	Docosahexaenoic acid
DHLA	Dihydrolipoic acid

E

EFA	Essential fatty acids
EGb 761	Extract of ginkgo biloba 761
EPA	Eicosapentaenoic acid
ERG	Electroretinogram

F

FABP	Fat acid binding protein
FAD	Flavin adenine dinucleotide

G

GAG	Glycosaminoglycan
GLA	Gamma-linolenic acid
GMP	Guanosine monophosphate
GSH-Px	Glutathione-peroxidase
GSH-Red	Glutathione-reductase
GSSG-Red	Glutathione-reductase
GTP phosphohydrolase	Guanosine triphosphate phosphohydrolase

I

IOP	Intraocular pressure
IRBP	Interphotoreceptor retinoid-binding protein

L

L	Luteine
LA	Linoleic acid
LDL	Low-density lipoprotein

M

meso-Z	meso zeaxanthin
MLL	Myeloid/lymphoid leukemia
MMP	Matrix metalloproteinase
MP	Macular pigment

N

NADH	Nicotinamide-adenine-dinucleotide
NADP	Nicotinamide-adenine-dinucleotide phosphate
NADPH	Hydrogenated nicotinamide-adenine-dinucleotide phosphate
Na-K pump	Sodium-potassium pump

O

O_2^{-}	Superoxide anion radical
OH•	Hydroxyl radical

P

PAF	Platelet-activating factor
PG-E1	Prostaglandin E1

R

RBP	Retinol binding protein
RE	Retinol equivalent
RNA	Ribonucleic acid
ROI	Reactive oxygen intermediates
ROO•	Peroxyl radical
RP	Retinitis pigmentosa
RPE	Retinal pigment epithelium

S

Se	Selenium
SOD	Superoxide dismutase

T

TIMP	Tissue inhibitor of metalloproteinases

U

UV	Ultraviolet

V

VEGF	Vascular endothelial growth factor

Z

Z	Zeaxanthin
Zn	Zinc

Part III

Mauro Febbrari Defendente

Good Cheer at the Table

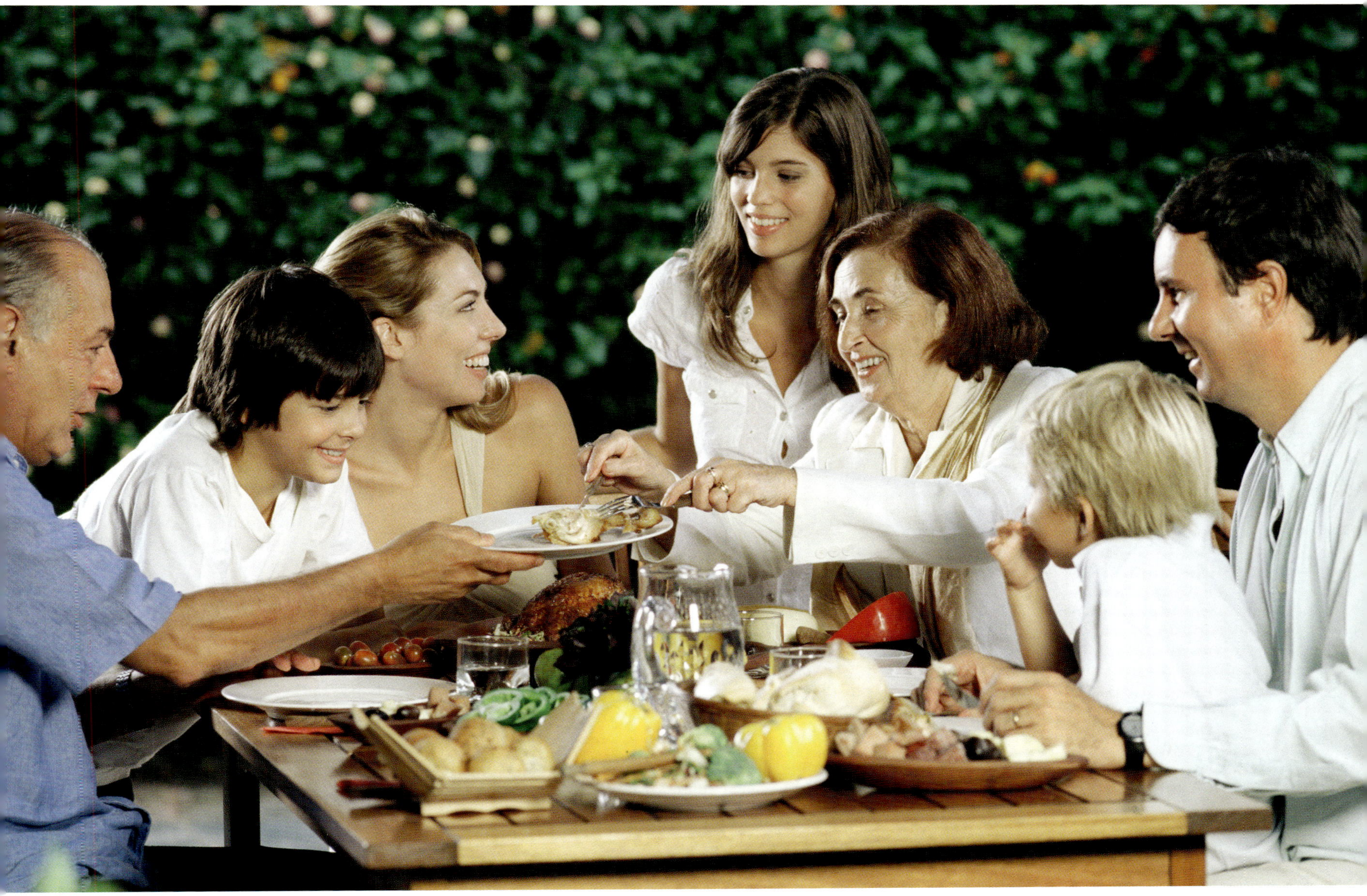

Good cheer at the table

The very latest research studies confirm that food is involved in the regulation of mechanisms that control mood, attention, memory, aggression, and the transmission of nervous impulses.

Consumption of food is influenced by numerous exogenous and endogenous factors that often interact; primarily, we should remember that the quantity and the quality of food—and here we must include the organoleptic characteristics of food—have an enormous influence on appetite.

The endogenous factors are split into hormonal, metabolic, and nervous impulses and are associated with complex neuronal systems that process and integrate the peripheral central afferent nerves.

The fundamental physiologic moments of eating are hunger and fullness. The former condition, hunger, not to be confused with appetite, is the perception of a true necessity of the body with regard to a quantitative and/or qualitative lack of nutrients; fullness is the sensation of satisfaction for the food demand and supply. The consumption of food and the hunger/fullness modulations are controlled principally by the hypothalamus, although extrahypothalmic structures are also involved in this complex system, in particular nuclei at the base and in some areas of the gray matter of the encephalic trunk.

The regulatory systems include actions of numerous mediators (neurotransmitters and neuropeptides) belonging to the catecholaminergic and serotoninergic pathways and the peptidergic systems with a stimulating or inhibiting effect on appetite.

In this way, by biologically orchestrating the neuronal connections, the neurotransmitters determine our mood and our emotions. These are the main protagonists of our feelings of happiness and our good mood; our mood is influenced by how we mentally interpret an event, by our physical condition, but above all by food.

Food is involved in the regulation of the mechanisms that control mood, attention, memory, aggression, and the transmission of nervous impulses.

Wurtman, a well-known neuroendocrinologist from the Massachussetts Institute of Technology, was certainly one of the first to attribute importance of the neurotransmitters in mood control, hunger, and food compulsions.

These molecules are "manufactured" by the nerve cells starting from the substances introduced to the body through the consumption of food. It is therefore clear that the first modification of this complex chain originates with the bioavailability of supplied food. Emotions and moods are created at the dining table, it is no secret that we eat to fuel our bodies with the essential ingredients for physical wellness and good humor as well as satisfying our senses of taste, smell, and sight, and augmenting the pleasure associated with conviviality.

At the dining table, emotions and moods are created.

Almost all senses (mainly taste, smell, sight, and touch) are involved in the definition of the degree of pleasure associated with food and, therefore, they are directly involved in the phases of hunger and fullness.

The control systems of nutritional behavior are closely connected to the central taste pathways; almost all of our senses are involved (namely taste, smell, sight, and touch) in the definition of the degree of pleasure associated with the food and, therefore, they have a direct influence in the phases of hunger and fullness. This is why we eat when the food served to us is appetizing and also why we stop when it no longer is.
The cerebral "observations" have shown that each nerve cell can have thousands of connections with other neurons; and all the cerebral activities, such as thought, memory, and consciousness, are possible thanks to the connections between the various brain cells.
The neurotransmitters consist principally of amino acids and vitamins and are the protagonists of these processes They exalt the existence of a direct connection between our diet and the production of neurotransmitters, and their presence, of suitable or unsuitable quality and quantity, has a direct influence on our emotional state.
The neurotransmitters allow us to perceive pleasure when we do the things we enjoy most during the day.
Because there are several of these activities, what follows is an analysis of the principles with a description of the effects on mood and stress management.

Serotonin regulates mood, aggression, sexual behavior, pain sensitivity, and the circadian sleep-wake cycle; it enhances a feeling of wellness by inducing relaxation.

Serotonin: This is a neurotransmitter with a wide range of functions as it acts on the central nervous, cardiovascular, respiratory, and gastrointestinal systems.
It regulates mood, aggression, sexual behavior, pain sensitivity, and the circadian sleep-wake cycle; it encourages wellness by inducing relaxation.
It is one of the main agents responsible for the pleasure sensations that accompany the consumption of food such as pasta, bread, pizza, and chocolate, sensations that can be so pleasurable that they actually create addictions. One typical example is the premenstrual period in women where the consumption of these foods, rich in tryptophan, a precursor of serotonin, leads to cravings caused by the accumulation of the neurotransmitter reduced under hormonal influence.

Dopamine controls pleasure, gratification, euphoria, and motivation.

Dopamine: This is the main neurotransmitter for the "emotional brain" as it plays an essential role in our ability to perceive pleasure and gratification, acting on the system that has the biological function of providing us with positive reinforcement, the gratification for an experience that allows us to perceive pleasure. It controls pleasure, gratification, euphoria, and motivation.

The endorphins can inhibit the perception of pain and are also responsible for sensations of pleasure.

Endorphins: These are also known as endogenous opioids and can inhibit the perception of pain. They create a feeling that can be likened to omnipotence. These are also the substances responsible for the feelings of pleasure associated with physical exercise; the sensations can sometimes be so strong that people can develop an addiction to a sporting activity. The endorphins and dopamine are also the agents responsible for the sensations of pleasure during sex. Even the taumaturgical power of laughing and good humor derive largely from the consequent production of endorphins.

Gamma-aminobutyrric acid: Gamma-aminobutyrric acid (GABA) induces peace and tranquility, and its inhibitory action is extremely important in the development of anxiety because it makes the neurons refractory to excessive excitation stimuli. In subjects affected by anxiety and/or panic attacks, there is a large reduction in the levels of GABA also because many anxiolytic drugs act on its receptors.

GABA induces peace and tranquility.

Acetylcholine: This modulates memory and learning, influences the circadian cycle, and regulates the transmission of nerve impulses.

These are just some of the agents involved, and there are many others: the stimulatory transmitters galanine, norepinephrine, and NPY, and the inhibitors leptin, insulin, bombesin, and somatostatin. We are aware how extremely important their role is for our psychophysical well-being and how their reduced performance is also associated with high stress levels.
It goes without saying that a large number of substances contribute to maintaining the delicate biochemical balance in our bodies, including vitamins, mineral salts, antioxidants, and lipids, substances that can be easily assimilated through the correct diet of fruits, vegetables, cereals, extra virgin olive oil, oily fish, beans, egg yolks, honey, almonds and walnuts, aromatic herbs, and good quality wine (preferably red).
In humans, evolution has selected the foods that are the most suitable and rich in nutritional ingredients that he requires to live better, locally sourced from the surrounding habitat.
Man does not need to travel far. Just observe how the mind positions pleasure from food and health into 2 separate categories that lie poles apart: hedonism on the one hand and denial on the other. Nothing could be further from the truth because eating well is therapeutic; however, it means abiding by the rules, knowledge, coherence, and continuity, a sort of "gastrosophy" where we take a "behavioral cultural pyramid" into account. If this system is respected, it does not lead to denials or demonizations, but only to dietary rules.

Eating well is extremely therapeutic, where "well'" means respecting the rules, knowledge, coherence, and continuity.

Gastrosophy and its rules

Gastrosophy, the collection of behavioral attitudes to food, is one of the main aspects for transforming a boring and useless diet consisting of denial, weighing, calorie counting, and transitional results (with rapid inversion of the outcome) into some sort of group of rules and regulations to be applied to one's lifestyle and everyday routine. The plan should be to pay attention to certain criteria, areas that are sometimes taken for granted and usually ignored. Knowledge, coherence, and continuity mean not eliminating food to regain our figures and our health but eliminating the alibis and the excuses that we "feed" ourselves with everyday.

Gastrophy is one of the fundamental aspects for transforming a boring and useless diet into simple and not-so-simple rules to be included in one's lifestyle, in the everyday routine.

Gastrosophy provides the option of initiating a project that respects digestive chemistry, which will lead to a reduction in the causes of aging (such as peroxidation) or illness, the results of the inefficient use of the immunity system.

We can get a glimpse of a group of rules where denials and demonizations are excluded with "living badly to die well" being replaced with "forbidden to forbid."

On a daily basis, we are responsible for the answers that we can give to counter the external and sometimes highly provocative stimuli from food, from the overwhelming social pace, on vacation, in Italy and abroad.

Nothing is more important than the hormonal activity and its circadian cycle in terms of metabolic chemistry. This explains why some foods are recommended at specific times of the day and not simply when we want to eat them.

Skipping breakfast is a big mistake.

For the insulin curve, a test performed in the morning when the insulin levels are high, anything we eat is permitted at this time of the day (this is why we should never skip breakfast). However, dieticians and nutritionists will recommend simple and/or complex carbohydrates at lunchtime and not in the evening. Vice versa, parathormone (PTH), which controls the introduction of calcium into the bones, is higher from the afternoon onward; as a result, meals with a high calcium content are recommended in the evening.

It should be mentioned that octopus, squid, oysters, anchovies, mackerel, salmon, herrings, frogs and mussels contain from a high to a discrete concentration of calcium and are the ideal replacement for cheese, an "arrogant" and less healthy store of calcium.

Chew slowly to avoid unnecessary distension of the stomach.

CHEW SLOWLY, as this allows for the minimum time necessary for digestion to be relayed to the brain (20 minutes). It also avoids distending the stomach unnecessarily (mechanical hunger), and it positions us as the protagonists taking part in an important gesture, namely bringing food to the mouth and creating memories that reiterate the emotions associated to a particular food, even in different forms.

Fullness is guaranteed. The slow pace of the gestures and the procedures allow sight and smell to play a satisfying sensory role prior to mastication, the final act of this conclusive pleasure. We can safely state, "Food is eaten by the eyes."

Monothematic actions reduce the abdominal bloating and the digestion times.

MONOTHEMACITY is another topic of fundamental importance for wellness; it reduces abdominal distention and the digestion time with obvious organoleptic improvements.

Some examples? Try eating just fish or just meat throughout a meal, from the hors d'oeuvres to the starter to the main course.

Cheese should be served at a separate meal. It is wrong to serve it at the end of a meal containing other forms of protein.

Vegetables should not be mixed. In a meal, they should all be cooked or all be raw. So following vegetable soup or minestrone, only cooked vegetables should be served.

Vegetables: all cooked or all raw.

Fruit should always be seasonal and should not be mixed. Fruit salad should be all berries, citrus (oranges, mandarins, etc), tropical-summer, apples (there are 42 types of apple), or a "minestrone" of melons.

We should avoid eating fruit with protein due to the fact that their relationship causes indigestion (for example, ham and melon, milk and fruit, or fruit after a protein-filled dinner); ham and melon take a long time to digest and the melon has a tendency to cause indigestion.

Avoid fruit with proteins.

Other bad associations? The most common are those that refer to carbohydrates: bread and pasta to mop-up sauce (a spoon is much more elegant), breadsticks nibbled while we wait for our pizza to be ready, or typical of North Italy (Veneto and Lombardy regions), polenta and bread or a side dish of potatoes.

One last piece of advice: we should eat 5 portions of fruits and vegetables every day. Fruit should be eaten on its own or a short time before any other food. As a result, all the preparations based on milk/fruit should be controlled/restricted.

Part IV

Lucio Buratto and Natalya Ushakova

With the collaboration of

Riccardo De Prà

Good Food Recipes

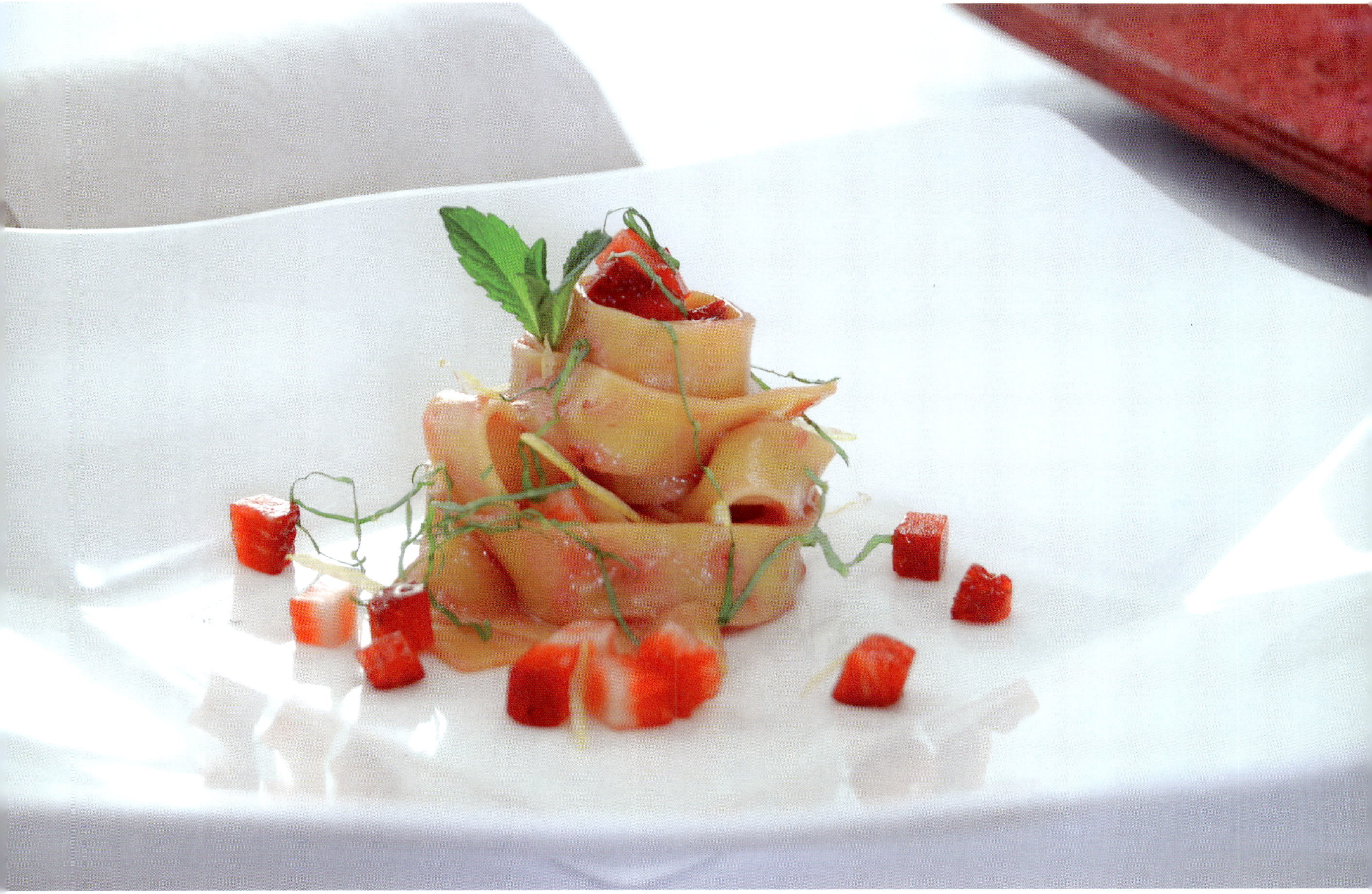

Quality and safety when eating

A healthy nutritious diet involves the use of good quality food. What do we mean by this? We should be eating good quality ingredients that are produced properly, preserved correctly, and prepared with attention. For example, fruits and vegetables should be eaten fresh; if they are stored in the fridge or in a basket in the kitchen for a long period of time, they can lose some or a large part of their nutritional value.

They should be eaten when fresh. They must be of guaranteed origin. The ideal scenario would be to pick them straight from the plant or the vegetable patch or purchase them from someone who has just picked them. However, this is the period of mass consumption, and this will become increasingly difficult. Organic products are also preferable.

The large supermarkets (and many of the smaller ones) offer fruit and vegetables with a highly inviting appearance; unfortunately, it should be pointed out that this produce is frequently picked when still unripe and not mature. It is then stored and allowed to mature just before it is displayed on the sales counter. Unfortunately, it is not "ripe" and does not possess all the nutritional characteristics that it should have in theory. Moreover, if a piece of fruit looks "beautiful and perfect," this will mean that during the production it will have been subjected to several anti-parasite treatments. In nature, an apple is never smooth and perfect. It should at least be washed carefully.

The origin of the meat should be checked. The products must be fresh and properly preserved before consumption.

Fish requires even closer inspection: it is better to eat deep frozen fish of certain origin as opposed to fresh fish where the "freshness" can be extremely dubious. As there is no such thing as a fish of certain origin, I would recommend "poor" fish (sardines, anchovies, mackerel, gray mullet) fished locally rather than a sea-bass farmed in Denmark.

Regarding food that has been canned, bottled, or stored in other ways, always check the expiration date and always try to purchase the products in stores that have a rapid turnover. It is more likely that these products will be fresh. However, it is worthwhile to remember that canned products are preserved thanks to the acidity of natural substances such as vinegar or to a heat-sterilization process. In both of these cases, the vitamins will be denatured so these products should be used as little as possible.

Other simple but important norms include not leaving cooked foods to cool outside of the fridge for more than 1 to 2 hours (just 1 in summertime) and without being covered. It is extremely important to try to cool cooked food that will not be eaten immediately as quickly as possible. By cooling, we mean a temperature of around 37.4°F, considerably lower than what we normally consider cold, which is a temperature lower than our body temperature —the perfect medium for bacterial proliferation!

Before eating food that has already been cooked, it must be reheated thoroughly.

When food is stored in the refrigerator, contact between different foods should be avoided; cooked food should be stored in closed containers; eggs should be stored in the original carton.

Do not defrost foods of animal origin at room temperature; they should be defrosted in the refrigerator or in the microwave, or they should be cooked while frozen.
Homemade preserves should be prepared with maximum care and attention paid to hygiene in order to avoid the proliferation of microorganisms that are extremely dangerous for health, particularly if they contain raw materials of animal origin. If you are not familiar with preparation and preservation techniques, it would be best not to bother trying.

Culinary preparations are infinite because each recipe can change the quantity and the quality of the contents.
In this part of the book, we decided to include recipes that have nutritional value for the eye and for sight, and we have ranked them indicatively with a star rating: a three-star recipe has an excellent value for the eye; one star indicates a low value.

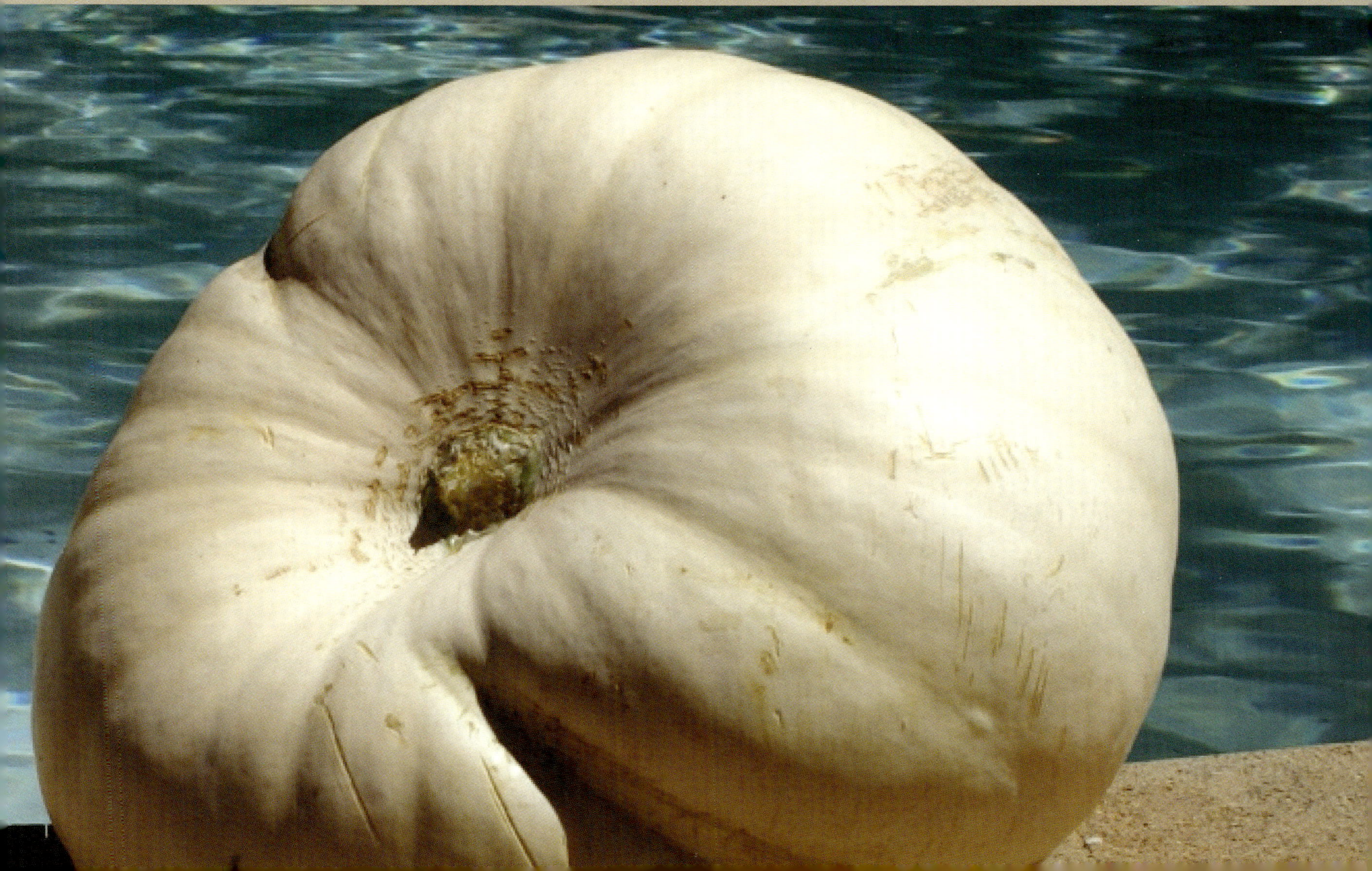

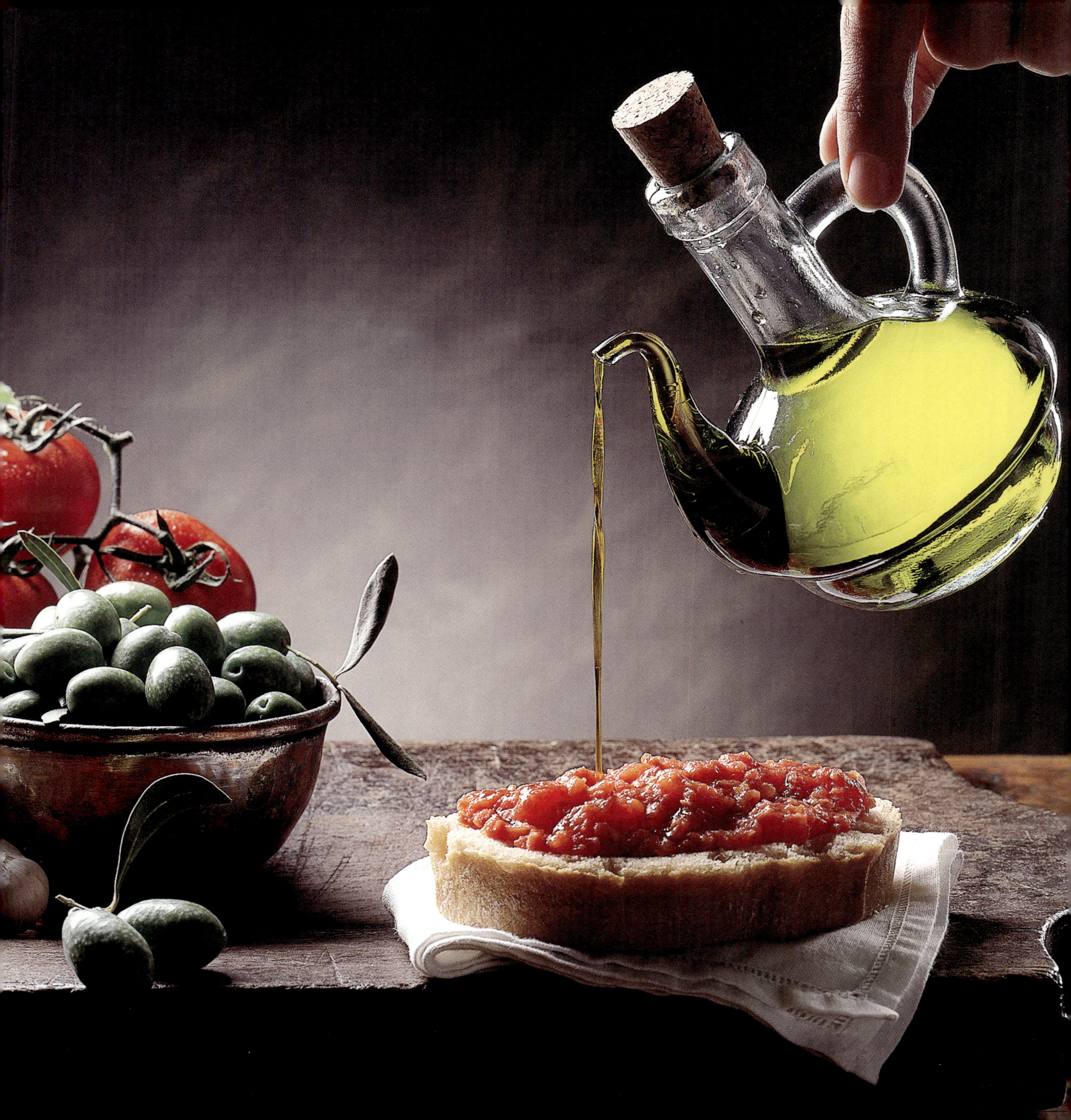

Snacks

During formal dinners or important receptions, several courses are served, and these are preceded by the hors d'oeuvres. This starts the proceedings and precedes the first course. In Italy, the antipasti can be based on meat; a variety of cold cuts; cooked or raw fish; cooked or raw vegetables; or simply a selection of snacks, savory crackers, and the like.

In this chapter, we will take a look at the snacks that accompany the aperitifs and that should stimulate the appetite, priming it for the alcoholic and nonalcoholic drinks. The most common snacks are chips, olives, salted almonds or peanuts, and a variety of pickles.

There are many other ways for enhancing the enjoyment and pleasure of this moment, for example, thin breadsticks wrapped with a slice of Parma ham, sticks of smoked ham, diced mortadella, small pieces of pizza or olive oil bread (focaccia), slices of cheese (Parmesan or other), every variety of cracker, whole olives, or olive paste spread on toasted bread.

To be even more original, and particularly to avoid an excessive consumption of food that is salty or high in calories that could easily unbalance the daily diet or the dinner, the choice could fall on something more natural such as the "crudités": some vegetables such as cucumber, carrots, zucchini, artichokes, radishes, mushrooms, and the like can be used in the preparation of wonderful and tasty hors d'oeuvres.

These are delicious for nibbling, while waiting for lunch or dinner to be served, washed-down by a glass of good wine or a fruit-based, low-alcohol aperitif, on the rocks, or a cocktail based on fruit juice and a dry spumante or champagne.

Imagination is extremely important in the preparation of snacks. It is possible to create a number of combinations with a variety of tastes, colors, and aromas that will satisfy every palate.

These snacks can also be the solution for a quick meal and the ideal solution for lunch or dinner when guests arrive unexpectedly. Even if there are only a handful of ingredients available, a good wholesome meal can be presented without too much work involved.

What follows are just some indicative ideas but, with a touch of imagination and taste, we can do a whole lot more.

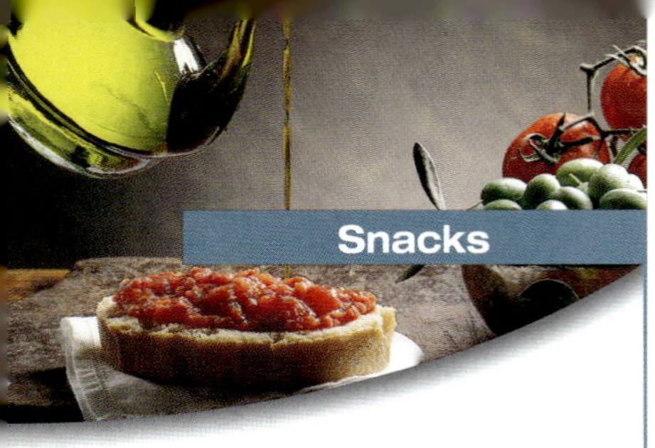

Simple bruschetta

(pronounced brusketta)

Bromatological evaluation per portion

Kcal	183
Protein (%)	8.8
Fats (%)	25.7
Carbohydrates (%)	65.5
Fiber (g)	1.9
Cholesterol (mg)	0

Valuable contents for the eye: ★

The more wholesome the **bread**, the richer it is in vitamins and fibers.

Olive oil is an excellent source of unsaturated fatty acids.

Garlic contains selenium, zinc, and aliine, a substance responsible for the taste and penetrating, persistent smell of garlic. Aliine transforms into allicine, which has antibacterial, cholesterol-lowering, and blood pressure-lowering properties.

Ingredients and amounts for 4 people

- ✓ 4 slices of homemade or farmhouse bread
- ✓ 2 cloves of garlic, cut in half
- ✓ 2 tablespoons extra virgin olive oil
- ✓ salt and pepper to taste

Preparation

Toast the bread on the grill or in the oven.
Rub the half cloves of garlic onto one side of the bread.
Season with oil, salt, and pepper.
This simple bruschetta can be enriched with a variety of ingredients; unquestionably, the most popular is the tomato.

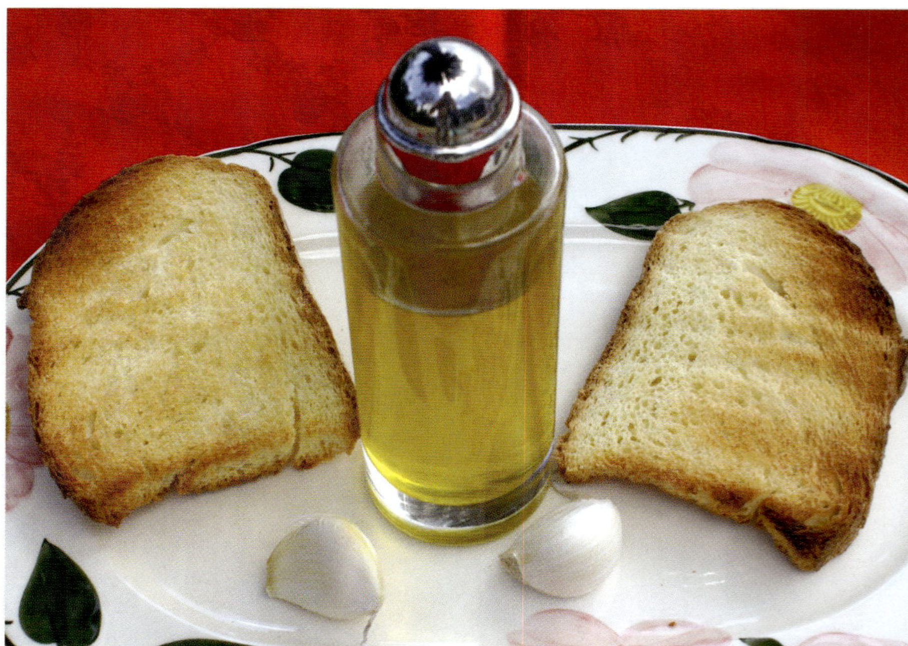

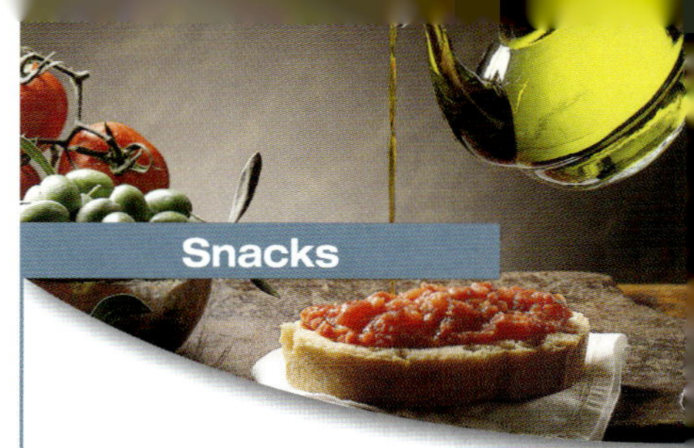

Bruschetta with tomato

Ingredients and amounts for 4 people

✓ 4 slices of farmhouse bread
✓ 4 ripe tomatoes with firm flesh
✓ 2 cloves of garlic
✓ 8 basil leaves
✓ 4 tablespoons extra virgin olive oil
✓ salt and pepper to taste

Preparation

Scald the tomatoes for a few seconds in boiling water and peel; cut into small pieces, remove the seeds, add salt, and allow the water to drain; place in a bowl.
Wash and dry the basil leaves, add to the bowl containing the tomatoes.
Add 1 teaspoon of salt and some black pepper. Mix and let sit for 30 to 40 minutes.
Toast the bread and rub the garlic cloves over each slice.
Spoon the tomato mixture onto the bread and drizzle each slice with good quality extra virgin olive oil.

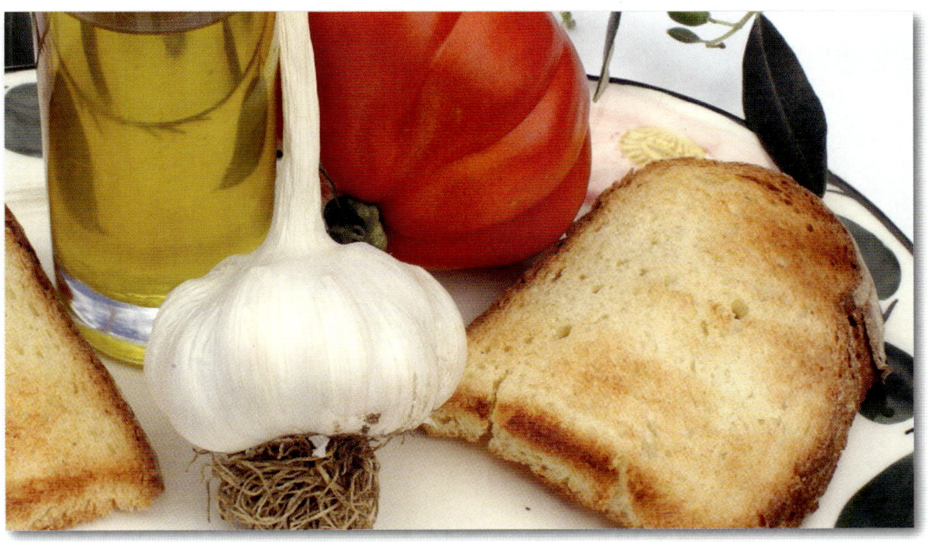

Bromatological evaluation per portion

Kcal	201
Protein (%)	10
Fats (%)	12.3
Carbohydrates (%)	77.7
Fiber (g)	2.7
Cholesterol (mg)	0

Valuable contents for the eye: ★

Tomatoes are rich in vitamins and oligoelements; they contain carotenoids and are an important source of lycopene.
The more wholesome the **bread**, the richer it is in vitamins and fibers.
Olive oil is an excellent source of unsaturated fatty acids.
Basil owes its aroma to the numerous essential oils it contains, which can stimulate salivary and gastric secretion.

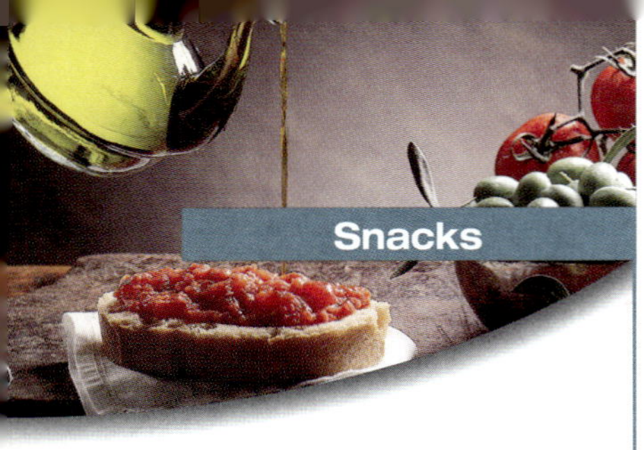

Rich bruschetta

Bromatological evaluation per portion

Kcal	226
Protein (%)	8.7
Fats (%)	36
Carbohydrates (%)	55.3
Fiber (g)	2.6
Cholesterol (mg)	0

Valuable contents for the eye: ★

Tomatoes are rich in vitamins and oligoelements; they contain carotenoids and are an important source of lycopene.
Capers contain vitamins A, C, and E and also a large quantity of sodium.
Basil owes its aroma to the numerous essential oils it contains, which can stimulate salivary and gastric secretion.
The more wholesome the **bread**, the richer it is in vitamins and fibers.

Ingredients and amounts for 4 people

- ✓ 4 slices of homemade or farmhouse bread
- ✓ 4 mature, firm tomatoes
- ✓ 8 basil leaves
- ✓ 2 tablespoons extra virgin olive oil
- ✓ 1 tablespoon desalted capers
- ✓ 8 stoned olives
- ✓ 1 teaspoon dried oregano
- ✓ salt and pepper to taste

Preparation

Drop tomatoes into boiling water for 10 to 15 seconds. Peel and cut into strips. Remove the seeds, and allow to drain.
Mix together some of the tomatoes, olives, and basil leaves.
Add the strips of tomato to the bread, and dust with dried oregano.
Add some capers, a sliced olive, the chopped tomato, olive, and basil.
Season with salt, pepper, and oil.

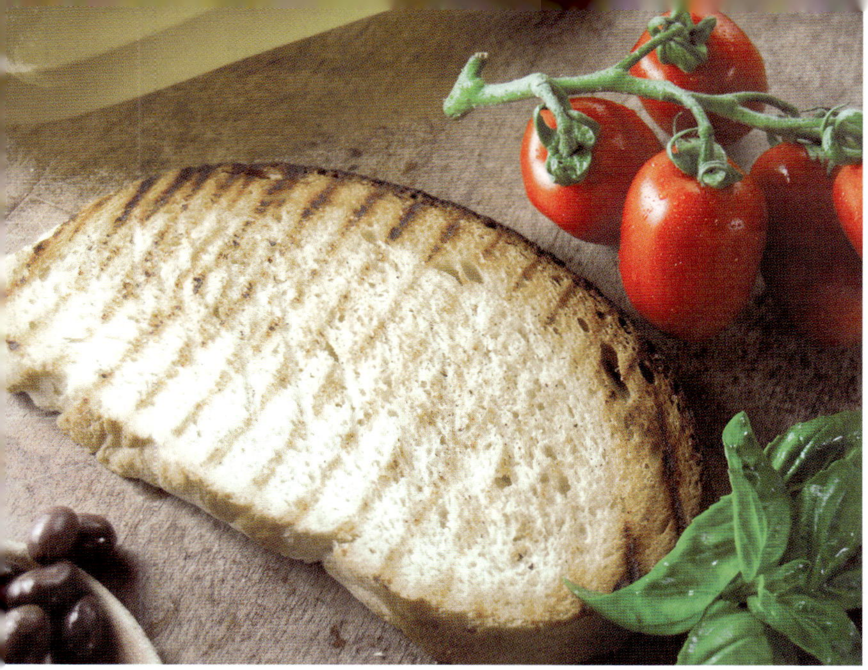
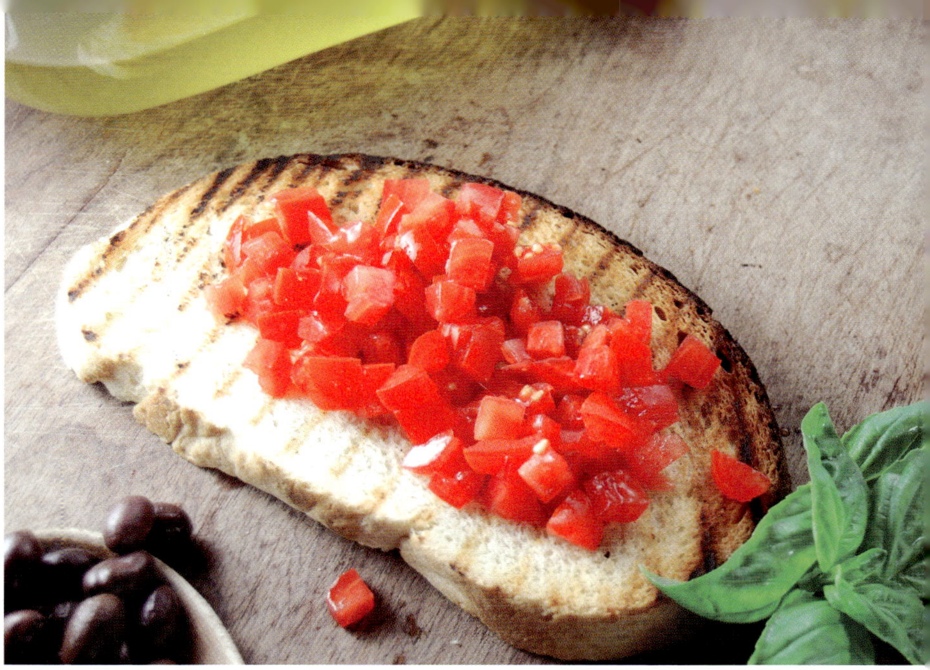
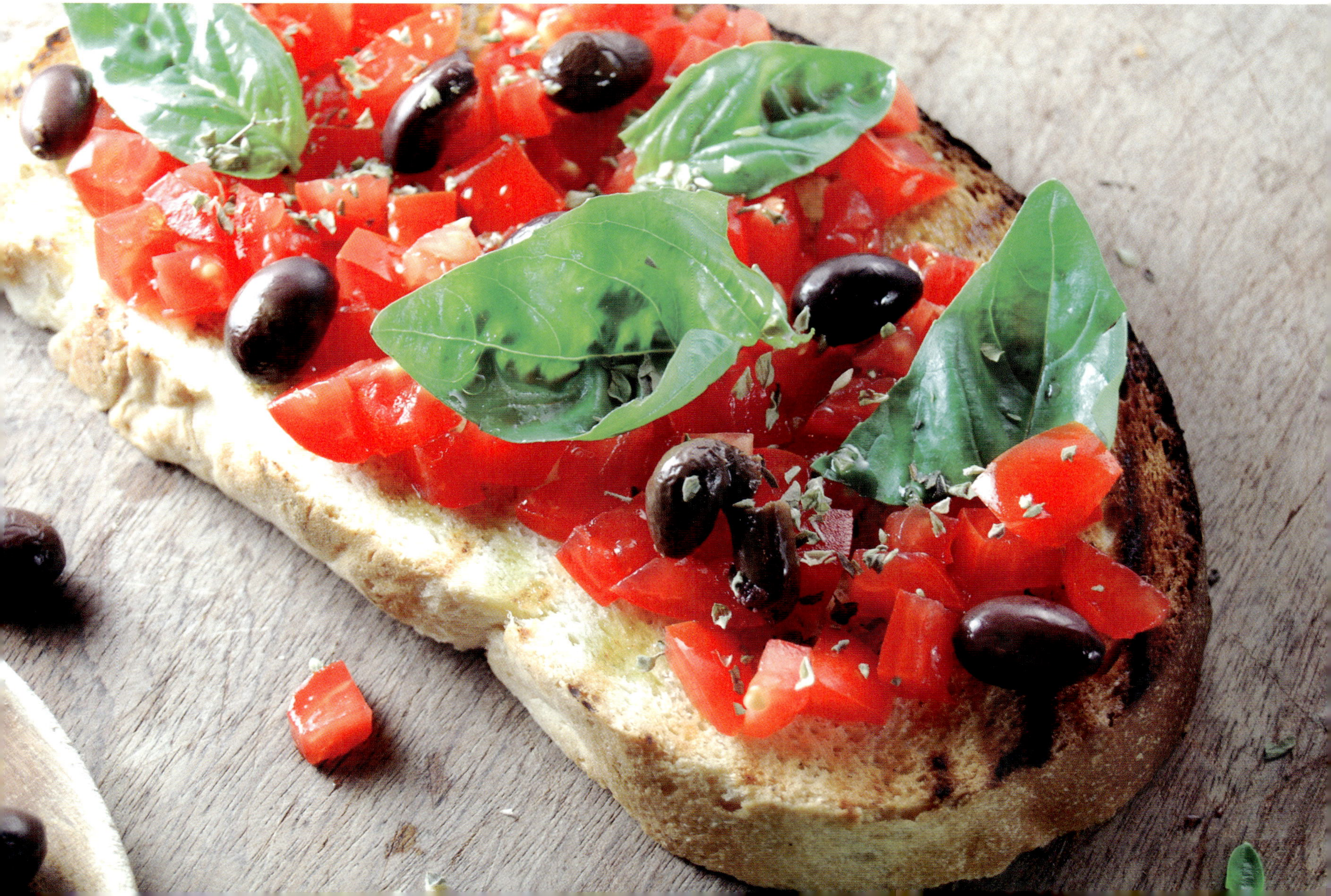

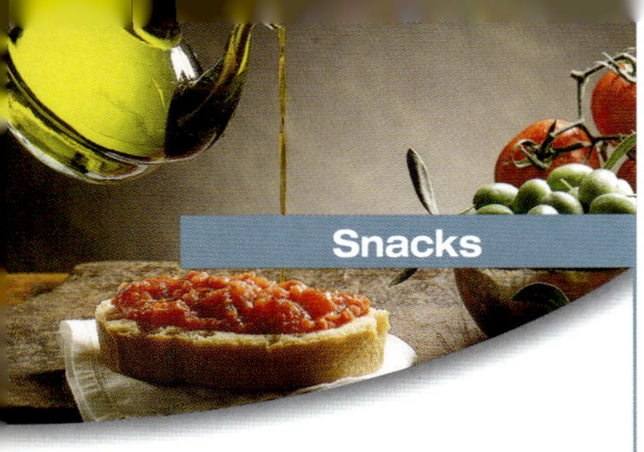

Bruschetta with parmigiano reggiano and balsamic vinegar

Bromatological evaluation per portion

Kcal	221
Protein (%)	13.8
Fats (%)	32.7
Carbohydrates (%)	53.5
Fiber (g)	1.9
Cholesterol (mg)	9.1

Valuable contents for the eye: ★

The more wholesome the **bread**, the richer it is in vitamins and fibers.

Parmesan cheese is rich in easily digestible proteins; it has a low fat content, and contains vitamin A and some vitamins of the B-group.

Olive oil is an excellent source of unsaturated fatty acids.

Balsamic vinegar is low in calories but has a very strong taste.

Ingredients and amounts for 4 people

- ✓ 4 slices of Tuscan bread (salt-free)
- ✓ 1.8 oz (3½ tablespoons) of parmigiano reggiano (Parmesan cheese)
- ✓ 1 tablespoon balsamic vinegar
- ✓ 2 tablespoons extra virgin olive oil
- ✓ salt and pepper to taste

Preparation

Blend the cheese with the olive oil, balsamic vinegar, salt, and pepper until creamy.

Toast the slices of Tuscan bread and spread the cream onto the warm slices.

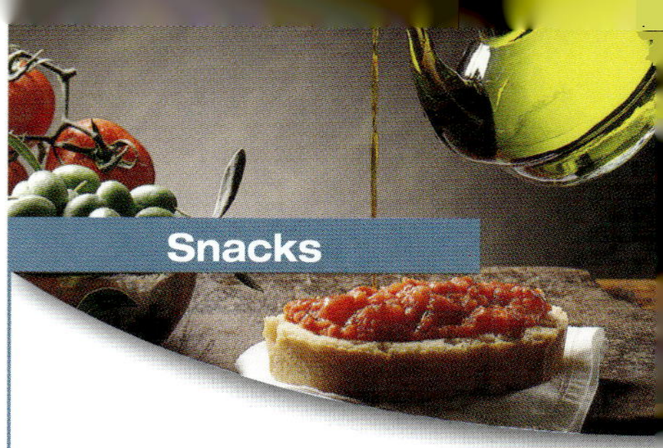

Bruschetta with anchovies

Ingredients and amounts for 4 people

- ✓ 4 slices of toast
- ✓ 8 anchovy fillets in oil
- ✓ 2 tablespoons butter

Preparation

Cut the slices of toast in half.
Spread a thin layer of butter onto the bread.
Place an anchovy fillet on each piece of bread.

Bromatological evaluation per portion

Kcal	311
Protein (%)	7.7
Fats (%)	83.7
Carbohydrates (%)	8.6
Fiber (g)	5.3
Cholesterol (mg)	0

Valuable contents for the eye: ★★

The more wholesome the **bread**, the richer it is in vitamins and fibers.
Anchovies are low in fat and contain omega-3 fatty acids.
Butter is made from milk and contains high quantities of saturated fatty acids.

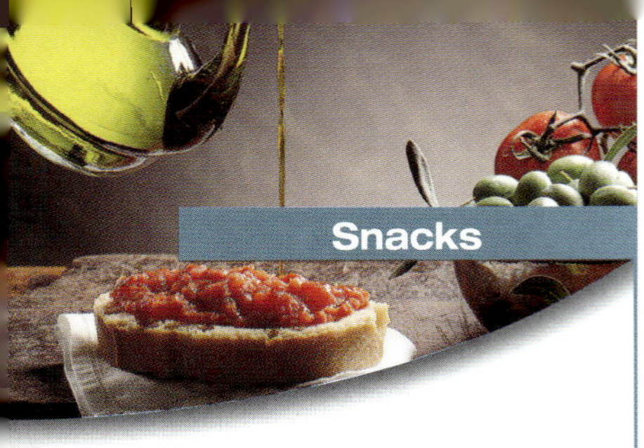

Greek cheese with **olives** and **basil**

Bromatological evaluation per portion

Kcal	270
Protein (%)	19.2
Fats (%)	78.5
Carbohydrates (%)	2.3
Fiber (g)	0
Cholesterol (mg)	54.4

Valuable contents for the eye: ★

Greek cheese (feta), made from cow's and sheep's milk, is tasty and not high in fat.

Olives are rich in monounsaturated fats, vitamin E, and potassium.

Basil owes its aroma to the numerous essential oils it contains, which can stimulate salivary and gastric secretion.

Ingredients and amounts for 4 people

✓ 16 cubes of Greek cheese or fresh sheep's milk cheese

✓ 16 basil leaves

✓ 16 stoned Taggiasche olives (small, tasty black olives)

Preparation

Place a leaf of basil on top of each cube of cheese, add an olive, and use a toothpick to keep the ingredients together.

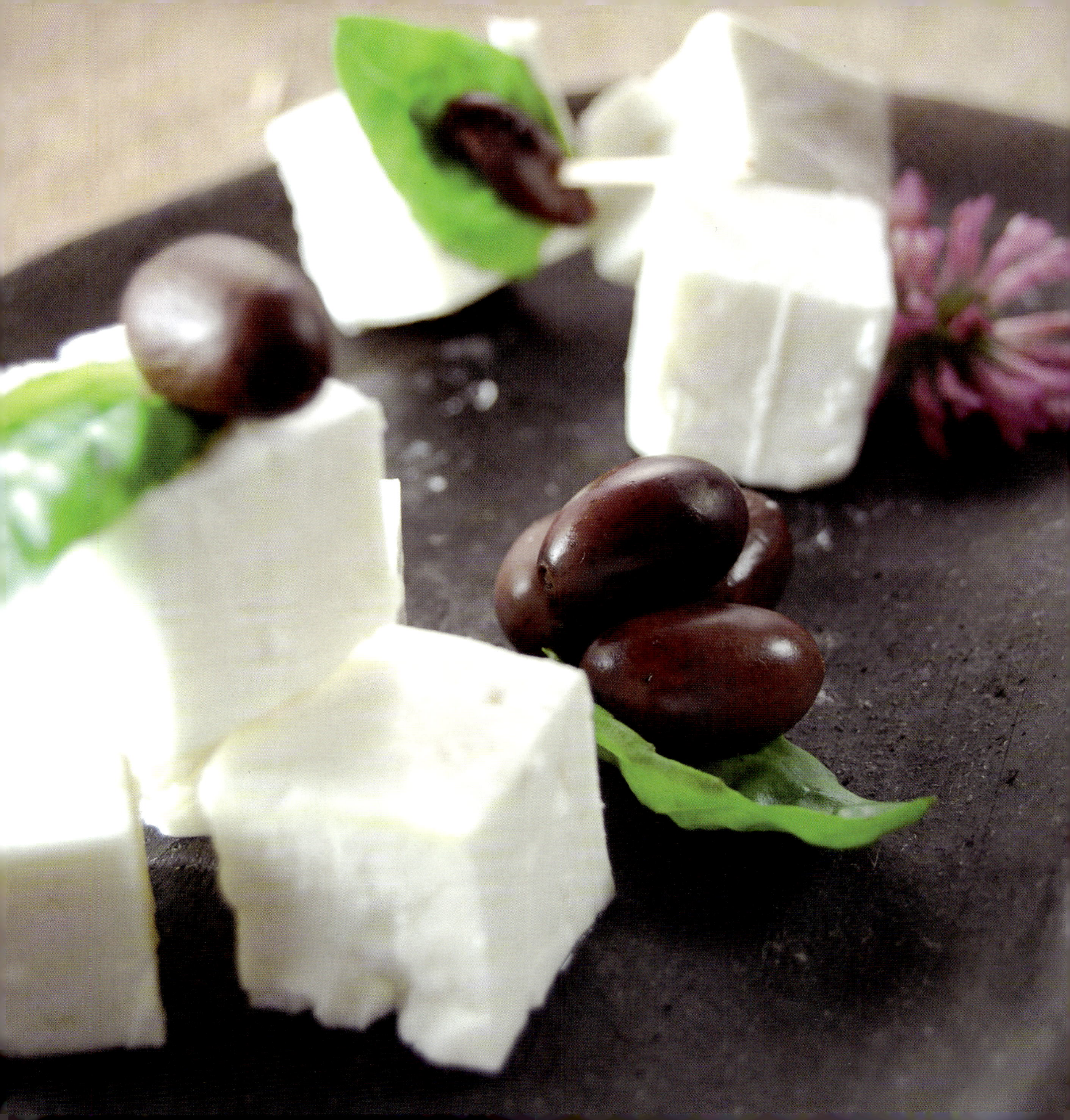

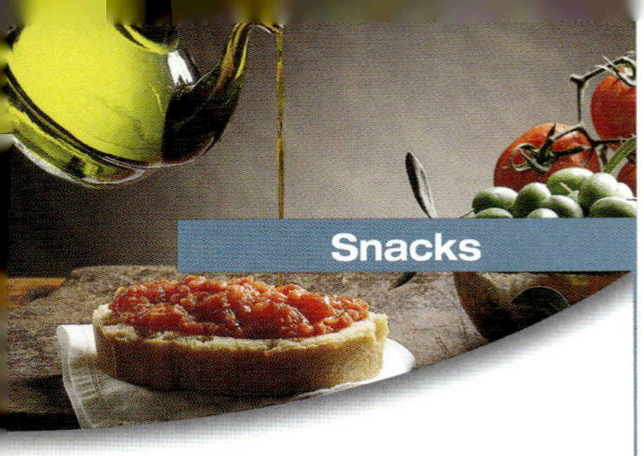

Bromatological evaluation per portion

Kcal	182
Protein (%)	22.1
Fats (%)	73.3
Carbohydrates (%)	4.6
Fiber (g)	0
Cholesterol (mg)	23

Valuable contents for the eye: ★ ★

Tomatoes are rich in vitamins and oligoelements; they contain carotenoids and are an important source of lycopene.
Mozzarella cheese contains easily digestible protein and calcium.
Basil owes its aroma to the numerous essential oils it contains, which can stimulate salivary and gastric secretion.
In addition, **basil pesto** contains **olive oil,** small amounts of **basil**, **pine-nuts**, **Parmesan cheese**, **goat's milk cheese,** and **garlic**.

Cherry tomatoes with **mozzarella cheese** and (basil) **pesto**

Ingredients and amounts for 4 people

- ✓ 8 cherry tomatoes
- ✓ 1 mozzarella cheese, cut into cubes
- ✓ 1 tablespoon (basil) pesto

Preparation

Dip the cherry tomatoes for approximately 10 seconds in boiling water, cool them under running water, and peel.
Top and tail the tomatoes, remove the seeds, and add salt.
Fill each tomato with one or more cubes of mozzarella cheese and add some fresh basil pesto.

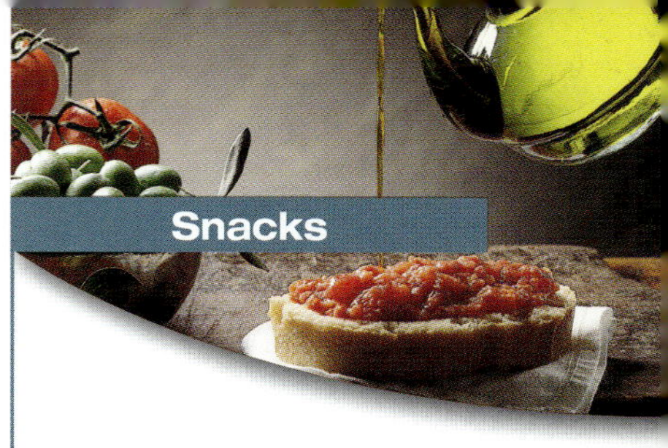

Cherry tomatoes with ricotta cheese

Ingredients and amounts for 4 people

- ✓ 1 cup fresh ricotta cheese
- ✓ 16 small plum or Piccadilly tomatoes
- ✓ 16 basil leaves
- ✓ 1 clove of garlic, cut into 4 to 6 pieces
- ✓ 1 tablespoon extra virgin olive oil
- ✓ salt and pepper to taste

Preparation

Wash and dry the tomatoes, cut the tops off, and remove the flesh.
Turn upside down and drain for approximately 15 minutes.
Put the oil, garlic, salt, pepper, ricotta, and the tomato flesh into a bowl.
Mix to produce a smooth, thick cream (the ricotta and the tomatoes must produce a sauce that is not liquid).
Remove the pieces of garlic, fill the tomatoes with the cream, and place the basil leaf over the top.
Cool in the fridge for 20 to 30 minutes and then serve.

Bromatological evaluation per portion

Kcal	160
Protein (%)	17.3
Fats (%)	72
Carbohydrates (%)	10.7
Fiber (g)	0.9
Cholesterol (mg)	39.9

Valuable contents for the eye: ★ ★

Ricotta is a milk product that is light and tasty. It is high in calcium and contains a modest quantity of vitamins.

Tomatoes are rich in vitamins and oligoelements; they contain carotenoids and are an important source of lycopene.

Olive oil is an excellent source of unsaturated fatty acids.

Basil owes its aroma to the numerous essential oils it contains, which can stimulate salivary and gastric secretion.

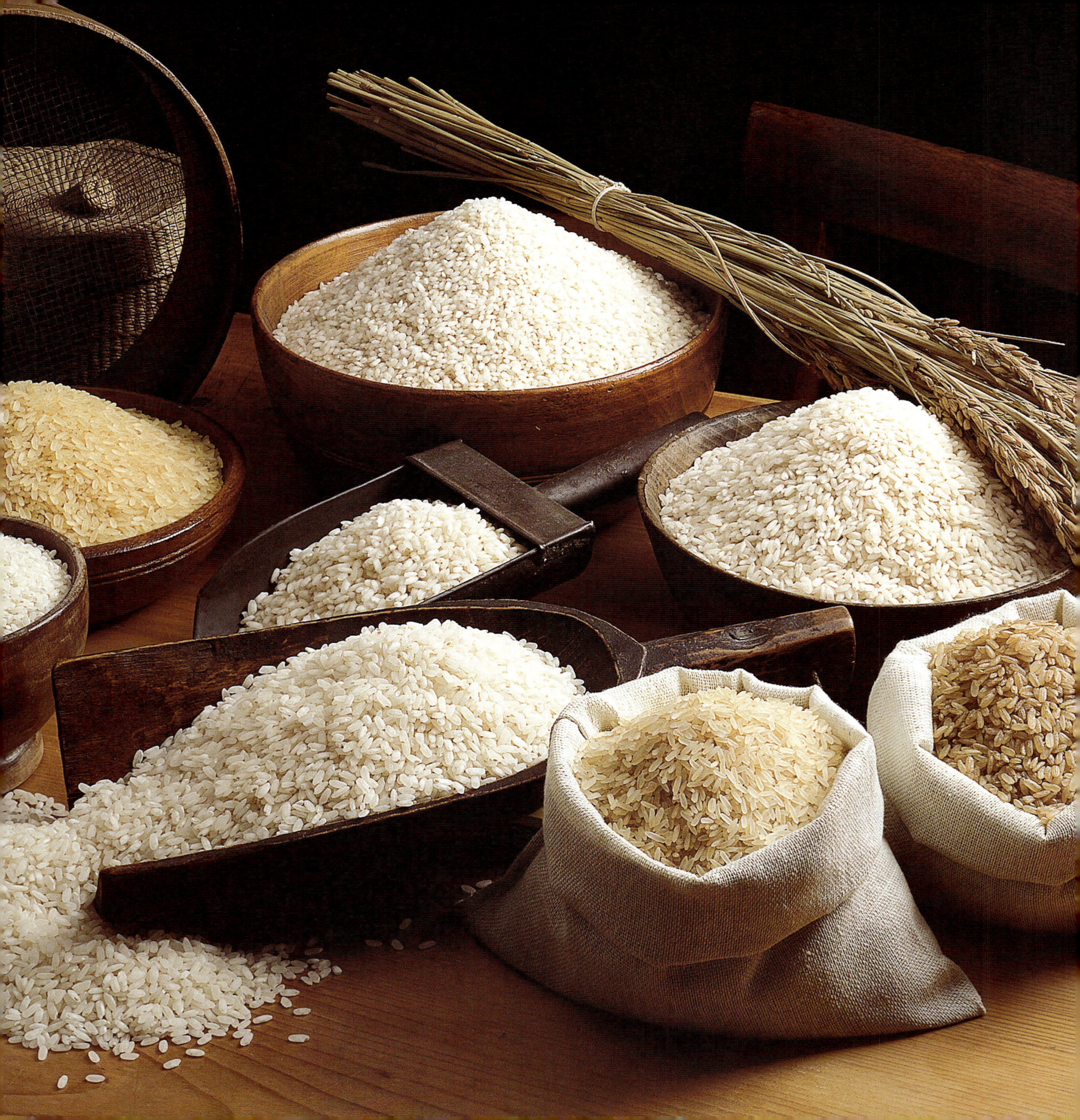

Risotto

For Italians, pasta is the queen of the table, but for at least half of the world's population (Asia at the top of the list), rice has this place of honor.
For more than 6000 years, rice has been cultivated in India and China. At the time of publication, Asia accounts for 90% of the world's rice consumption. However, Italy is the major rice producer in the European Union.
Even though rice only appeared in Europe around 1000 AD, the Italians rapidly included it in the cuisine with risottos, regional soups, timbales, and even in some desserts.
Rice loses some of its vitamins (thiamine) during polishing; however, it has the great advantage of being very easy to digest thanks to the absence of fibers and the quality of the starch, in particular amylase, which is much more digestible than the amylopectins that predominate in corn starch. This characteristic legitimates the dietary "prescription" of rice in forms of colitis or in episodes of diarrhea; nevertheless, the energy levels of rice from its carbohydrate content is similar to pasta. Across the different varieties of rice, this content oscillates at around 78%.
There is one slight dietary defect associated with the carbohydrates of rice and that is the "glycemic index"; the final product of its digestion (glucose) will enter the blood more rapidly, with the need for a rapid insulin response. Consequently, it is not indicated for people who are obese or diabetic. This problem can be overcome by using parboiled rice, which has a better glycemic index and a larger quantity of thiamine, thanks to the industrial processing method that reiterates the age-old procedure used by the Asian populations of soaking unrefined rice in water. The rice was then boiled for a few minutes and left to dry in the sun. This procedure improved the storage time.
Rice contains approximately 3 to 4 g less protein than pasta; however, the combination of its amino acids is better in biological terms (ie, it is closer to the completeness of animal proteins). Lastly, rice is gluten free, making it an essential ingredient in the diet of people suffering from celiac disease. It can be consumed as a main course, as a side dish to accompany proteins, or in desserts.

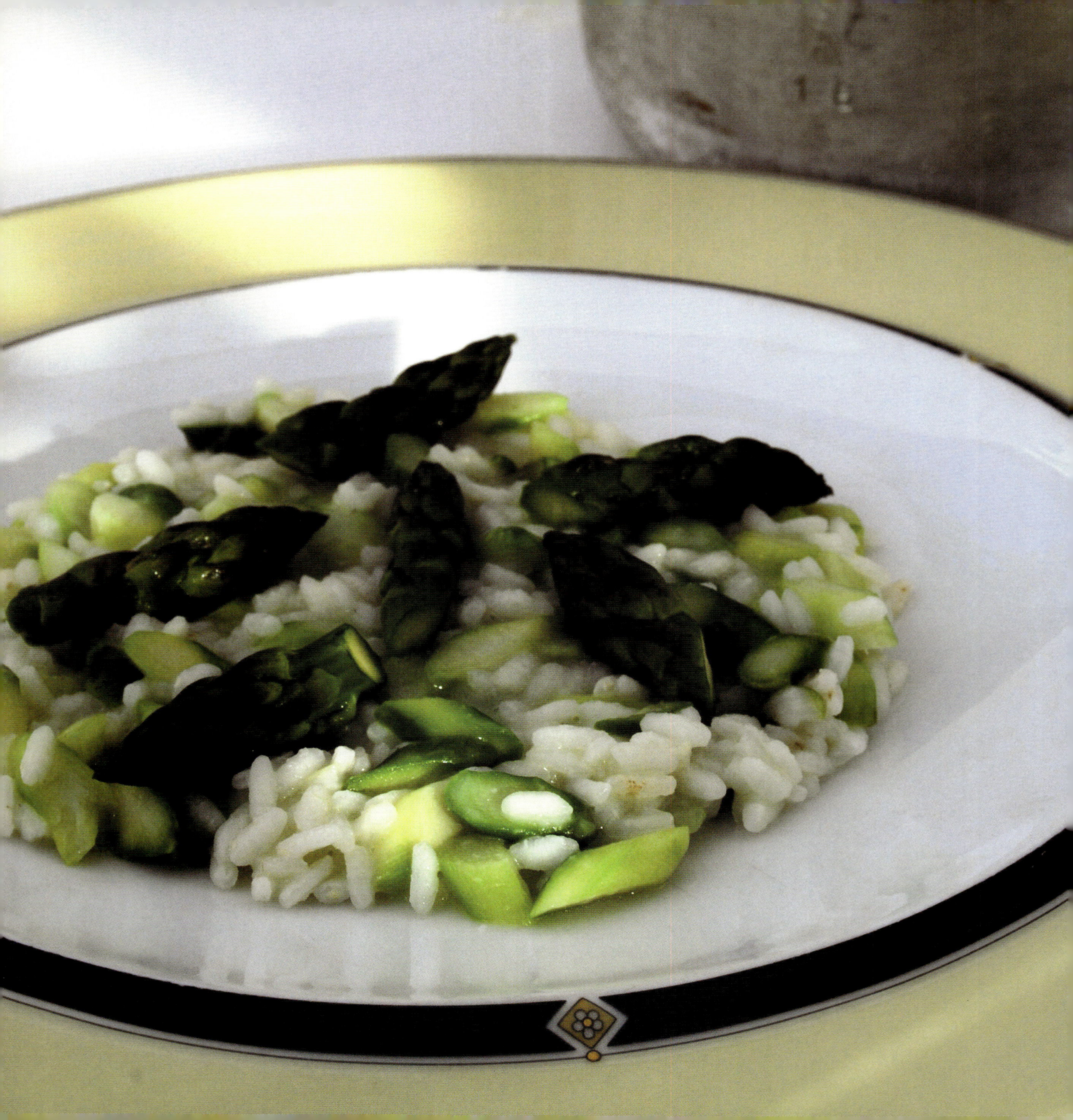

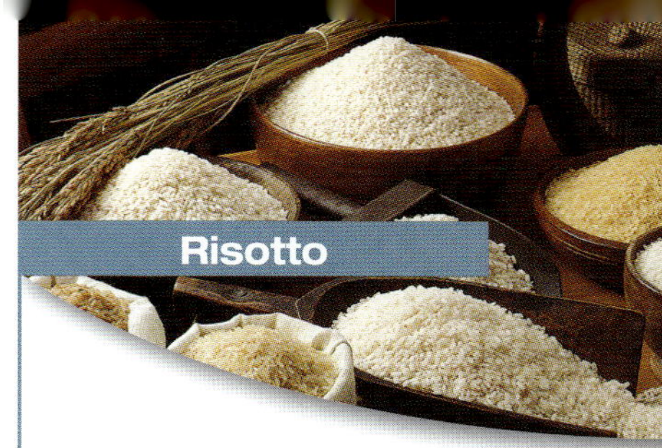

Risotto with **asparagus**

Ingredients and amounts for 4 people

- ✓ 10½ oz (1⅓ cups) Arborio rice
- ✓ 1 bunch of green asparagus (washed)
- ✓ 1/4 onion
- ✓ 1 liter (33.8 oz) vegetable stock
- ✓ 4 tablespoons butter
- ✓ 4 tablespoons grated Parmesan cheese
- ✓ 4 tablespoons extra virgin olive oil
- ✓ fresh parsley
- ✓ salt and pepper to taste

Preparation

Place the onion and oil in a pan and heat the onion until soft.
Season with a pinch of salt and pepper.
Add the rice and heat thoroughly.
Add a couple ladlefuls of boiling vegetable stock; cook the rice, stirring occasionally.
Add more broth when needed until the rice is almost cooked. Increase the heat.
In the meantime, peel the asparagus and remove the tough woody parts; slice the tip and the stalk into thin disks; add to the risotto about 5 minutes after it has started to cook.
When the rice is almost ready, add the butter and Parmesan cheese and mix until smooth.
Let sit for a couple of minutes and serve with a finely chopped parsley garnish.

Bromatological evaluation per portion

Kcal	579
Protein (%)	10.4
Fats (%)	46.5
Carbohydrates (%)	43.1
Fiber (g)	2.9
Cholesterol (mg)	60

Valuable contents for the eye: ★

Asparagus is rich in fiber; it contains vitamins B6 and C, folic acid, carotenoids, and flavonoids.
Parmesan cheese is rich in easily digestible protein, is low in fat, and contains vitamin A and some vitamins of the B group.
Butter is made from milk and contains high quantities of saturated fatty acids.
Onion contains vitamin C and a good quantity of flavonoids (quercetin).

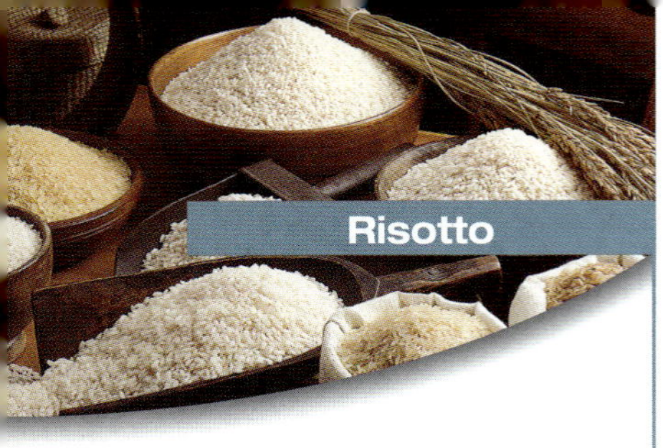

Risotto with bream

Bromatological evaluation per portion

Kcal	766
Protein (%)	20.6
Fats (%)	44.6
Carbohydrates (%)	34.8
Fiber (g)	0.9
Cholesterol (mg)	150

Valuable contents for the eye: ★★

Bream is a lean easily digested fish, rich in protein and omega-3 fatty acid.
Olive oil is an excellent source of unsaturated fatty acids.
Parmesan cheese is rich in easily digestible protein, is low in fat, and contains vitamin A and some vitamins of the B group.
Butter is made from milk and contains high quantities of saturated fatty acids.
Wine contains small amounts of flavonoids.
Like onion, **shallots** also contain flavonoids.

Ingredients and amounts for 4 people

- ✓ 10½ oz (1⅓ cup) Arborio rice
- ✓ 17½ oz fillet of bream (boned)
- ✓ 4 tablespoons extra virgin olive oil
- ✓ 1 shallot
- ✓ 1 glass of dry white wine
- ✓ 7 tablespoons grated Parmesan cheese
- ✓ 4 tablespoons butter
- ✓ 1 liter (33.8 oz) fish stock
- ✓ salt and pepper to taste

Preparation

Fry the finely sliced shallot in the oil in a pan until soft.
Add the pieces of boned fish.
Cook for 1 to 2 minutes, and then add salt and pepper.
Add the rice, and stir frequently; pour in the wine, and allow to evaporate.
Add the boiling fish stock, one ladleful at a time, adding when the previous has been absorbed.
When the rice is almost ready, add the butter and Parmesan cheese and mix until smooth.
Serve hot.

Risotto with artichokes

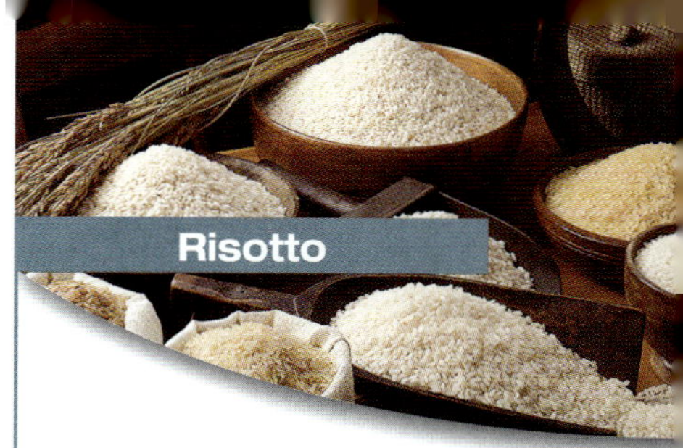

Ingredients and amounts for 4 people

- ✓ 10½ oz (1⅓ cups) Arborio rice
- ✓ 4 artichokes
- ✓ juice of ½ lemon
- ✓ 1/8 onion
- ✓ 1 liter (33.8 oz) vegetable stock (homemade or with a stock cube dissolved in boiling water)
- ✓ 4 tablespoons butter
- ✓ 4 tablespoons grated Parmesan cheese
- ✓ 4 tablespoons extra virgin olive oil
- ✓ salt and pepper to taste

Preparation of the artichokes

Remove the tougher outer leaves; cut 2/3 off the top, and divide the remainder into quarters, removing any sharp pieces and the tufts. Cut into thin slices and soak in water and lemon juice.

Preparation of the risotto

In a pan, fry the onion in the oil over low heat.
Add the artichokes, and cook for 7 to 8 minutes.
Season with a pinch of salt and pepper.
Add the rice and heat gently.
Add a couple ladlefuls of boiling stock and cook the rice, stirring occasionally; add stock when needed until the rice is almost cooked.
When the rice is almost ready, add the butter and Parmesan cheese and mix until smooth.
Let sit for a couple of minutes and serve with a finely chopped parsley garnish.

Bromatological evaluation per portion

Kcal	579
Protein (%)	10.4
Fats (%)	46.5
Carbohydrates (%)	43.1
Fiber (g)	3.2
Cholesterol (mg)	60

Valuable contents for the eye: ★★

In addition to high quantities of fiber and mineral salts, **artichokes** are also high in folic acid.
Parmesan cheese is rich in easily digestible protein, is low in fat, and contains vitamin A and some vitamins of the B group.
Butter is made from milk and contains high quantities of saturated fatty acids.
Lemon contains high quantities of vitamin C and β-carotene. It also contains flavonoids (particularly in the pith or albedo, which is underneath the peel).
Onion contains vitamin C and a good quantity of flavonoids (quercetin).

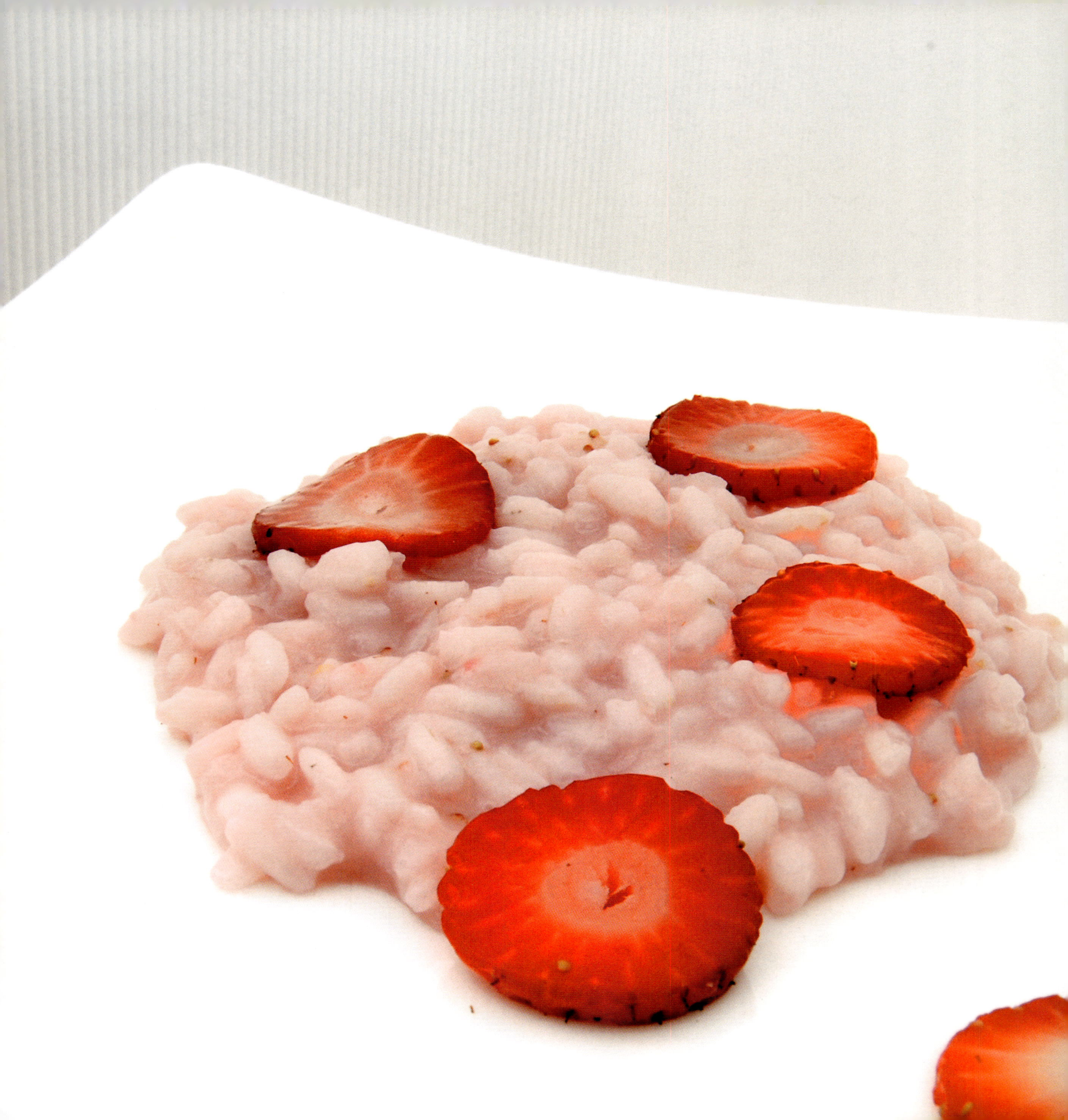

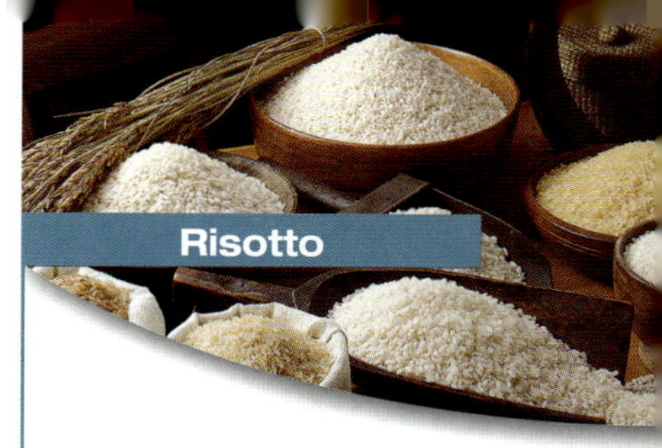

Risotto with strawberries

Ingredients and amounts for 4 people

- ✓ 10½ oz (1⅓ cups) rice
- ✓ 7 oz strawberries
- ✓ ½ glass dry white wine
- ✓ 1 liter (33.8 oz) vegetable stock
- ✓ 1 shallot
- ✓ 2 tablespoons butter
- ✓ 2 tablespoons extra virgin olive oil
- ✓ 2 tablespoons Parmesan cheese

Preparation

Cook the chopped shallot very slowly in a small amount of oil and butter.
Add the rice and cook for a couple of minutes.
Add the wine and cook until it has evaporated.
Continue cooking the rice, adding one ladleful of boiling stock each time all the liquid has been absorbed.
When the rice is almost completely cooked, add the chopped strawberries.
Then add the butter and Parmesan cheese and mix until smooth.
Decorate with strawberries cut in half and serve.
For a greater contrast in flavor, the risotto can be served garnished with shavings of Parmesan cheese.

Bromatological evaluation per portion

Kcal	503
Protein (%)	11.4
Fats (%)	35.8
Carbohydrates (%)	52.8
Fiber (g)	1.7
Cholesterol (mg)	60.2

Valuable contents for the eye: ★ ★

Strawberries are a good source of vitamin C and anthocyanosides.
Butter is made from milk and contains high quantities of saturated fatty acids.
Parmesan cheese is rich in easily digestible protein, is low in fat, and contains vitamin A and some vitamins of the B group.
Wine contains small amounts of flavonoids.
Like onion, **shallots** also contain flavonoids.

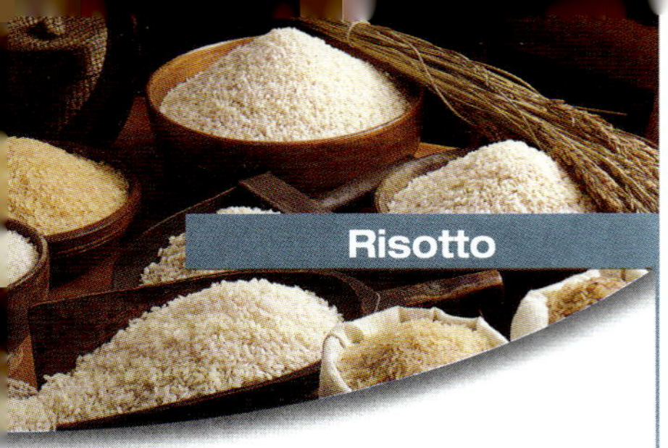

Risotto with red radicchio

Bromatological evaluation per portion

Kcal	588
Protein (%)	10.8
Fats (%)	45.7
Carbohydrates (%)	43.5
Fiber (g)	2.6
Cholesterol (mg)	60

Valuable contents for the eye: ★ ★

Radicchio is rich in flavonoids and vitamins A, B, and C.

Parmesan cheese is rich in easily digestible protein, is low in fat, and contains vitamin A and some vitamins of the B group.

Onion contains vitamin C and a good quantity of flavonoids (quercetin).

Olive oil is an excellent source of unsaturated fatty acids.

Red wine contains resveratrol and flavonoids.

Ingredients and amounts for 4 people

✓ 10½ oz (1⅓ cups) Vialone Nano rice
✓ 1¾ cups red radicchio
✓ 4 tablespoons butter
✓ 3 tablespoons extra virgin olive oil
✓ 1 onion
✓ ½ glass red wine
✓ 1 liter (33.8 oz) meat stock
✓ 4 tablespoons grated Parmesan cheese
✓ salt and pepper to taste

Preparation

Wash, dry, and cut the radicchio into pieces. Leave aside the hearts, which have been cut into segments.
Soften the onion in the oil, add the radicchio, and cook for 2 to 3 minutes.
Add the red wine and allow it to evaporate.
Add the rice and mix; add boiling broth, one ladleful at a time.
Cook the radicchio hearts in butter and when they are still quite crunchy, add to the rice and finish cooking.
Last, add the Parmesan cheese and a pinch of salt and pepper; mix well and serve piping hot.

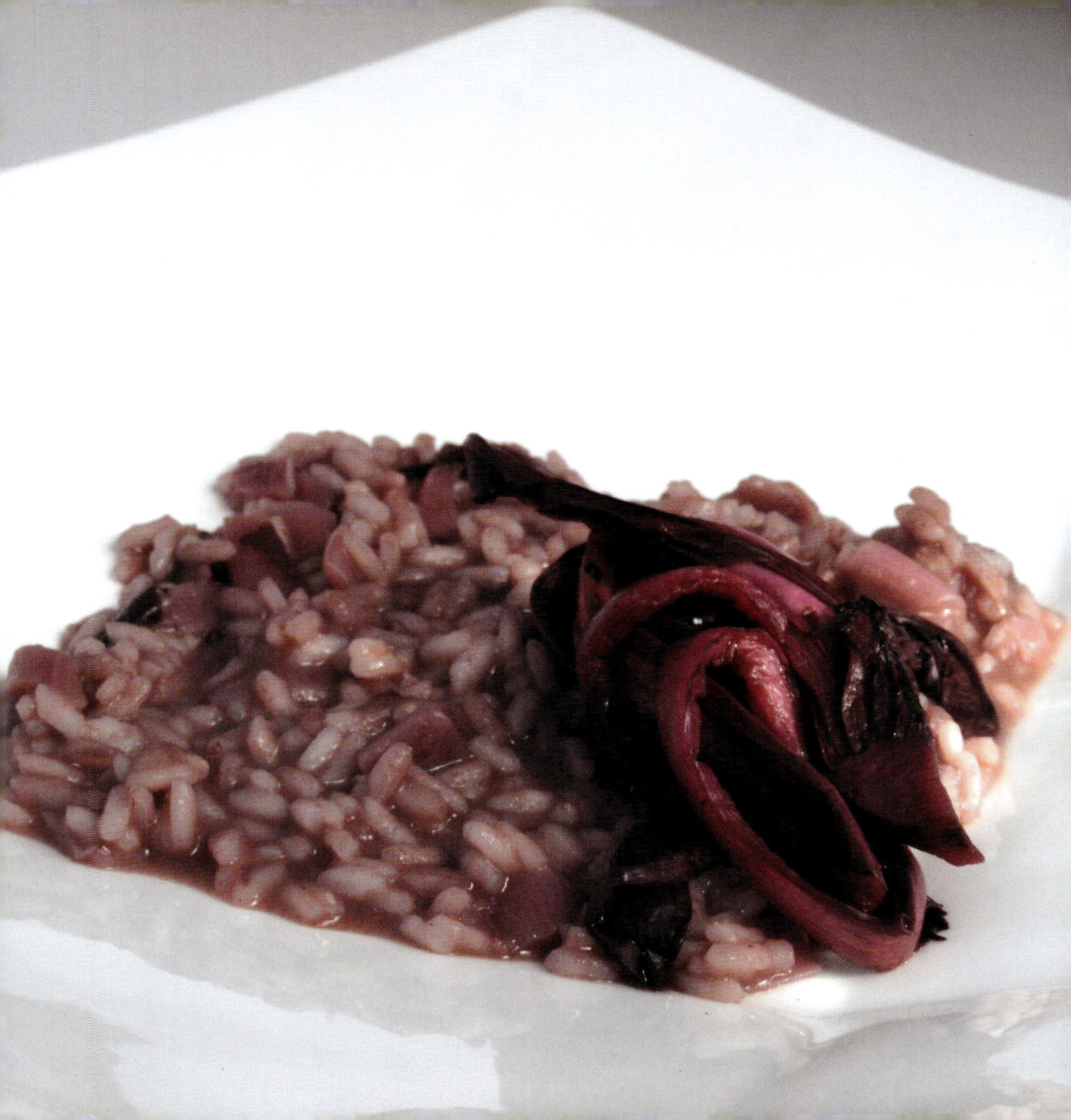

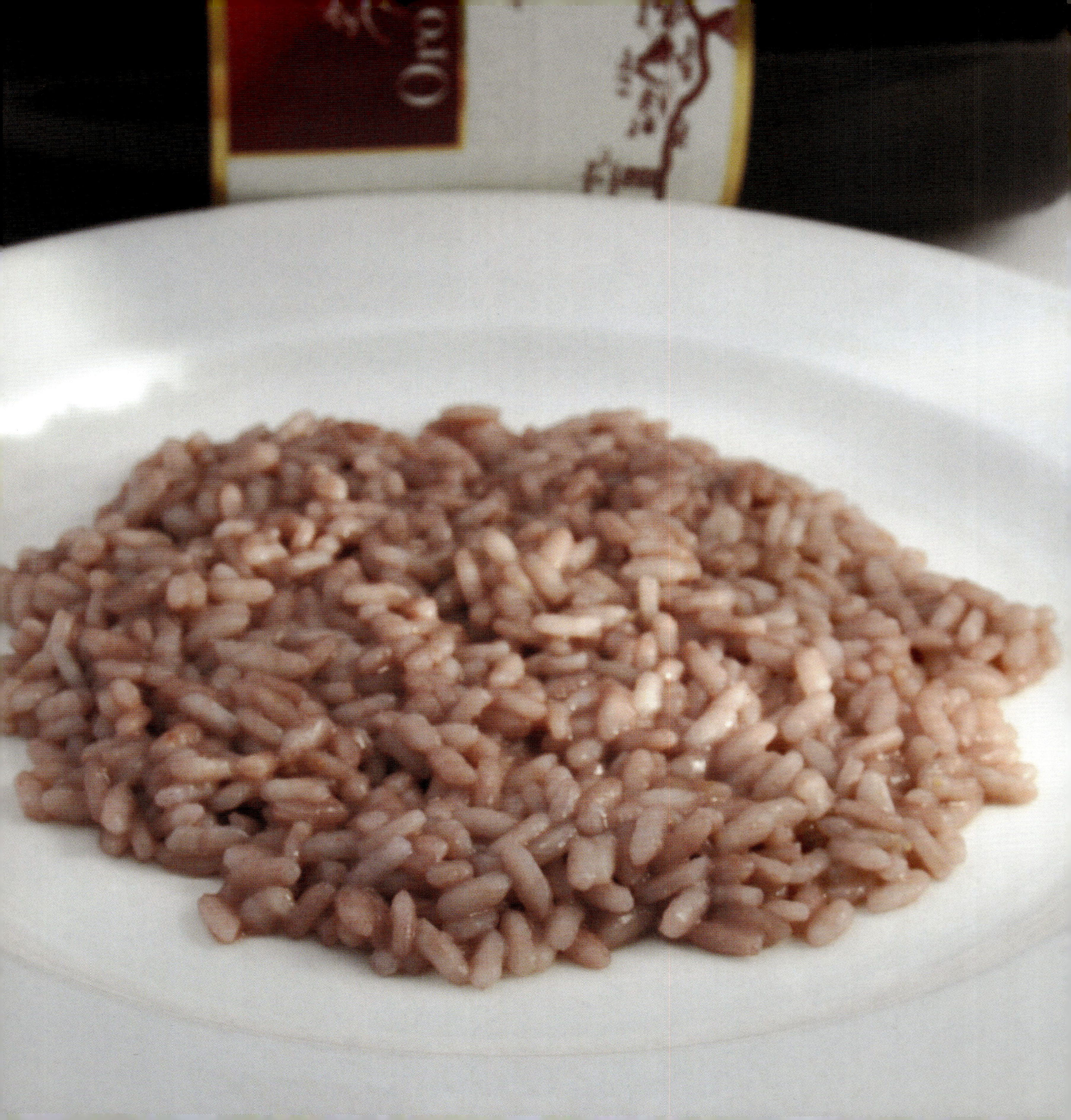
Oro

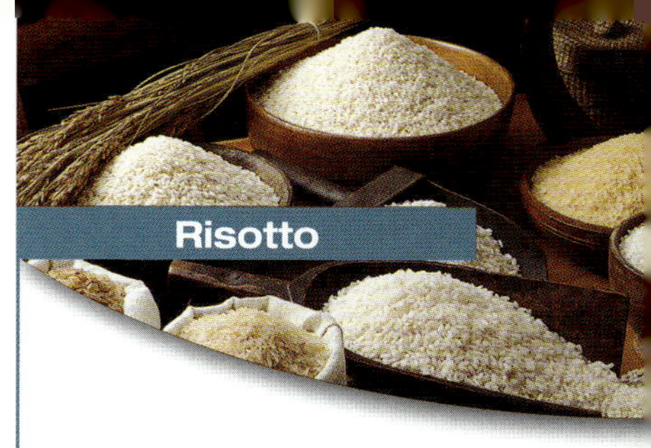

Risotto with **red wine**

Ingredients and amounts for 4 people

- ✓ 10½ oz (1⅓ cups) Carnaroli rice
- ✓ 2 glasses red wine (Amarone, Barolo, or Barbera preferred)
- ✓ 4 tablespoons extra virgin olive oil
- ✓ ⅛ onion, finely sliced
- ✓ ¼ carrot, finely sliced
- ✓ 1 stalk of celery, finely sliced
- ✓ 1 liter (33.8 oz) meat stock
- ✓ 4 tablespoons Parmesan cheese
- ✓ 4 tablespoons butter
- ✓ salt and pepper to taste

Preparation

Soften the onion, carrot, and celery in the hot oil.
Add the rice and coat with the oil.
Add the wine and allow to evaporate.
Add the boiling meat stock, one ladleful at a time, adding when the liquid has evaporated. Add the salt and pepper.
When the rice is almost cooked, add the butter and Parmesan cheese and mix until smooth.

Bromatological evaluation per portion

Kcal	678
Protein (%)	8.7
Fats (%)	39.7
Carbohydrates (%)	51.6
Fiber (g)	2.2
Cholesterol (mg)	60.1

Valuable contents for the eye: ★★

Red wine contains resveratrol and flavonoids.
Butter is made from milk and contains high quantities of saturated fatty acids.
Parmesan cheese is rich in easily digestible protein, is low in fat, and contains vitamin A and some vitamins of the B group.
Celery is a diuretic and also an aphrodisiac. It contains minerals, water-soluble vitamins, and flavonoids.
Carrots are an excellent source of β-carotene; they stimulate diuresis and intestinal motility.
Onion contains vitamin C and a good quantity of flavonoids (quercetin).
Olive oil is an excellent source of unsaturated fatty acids.

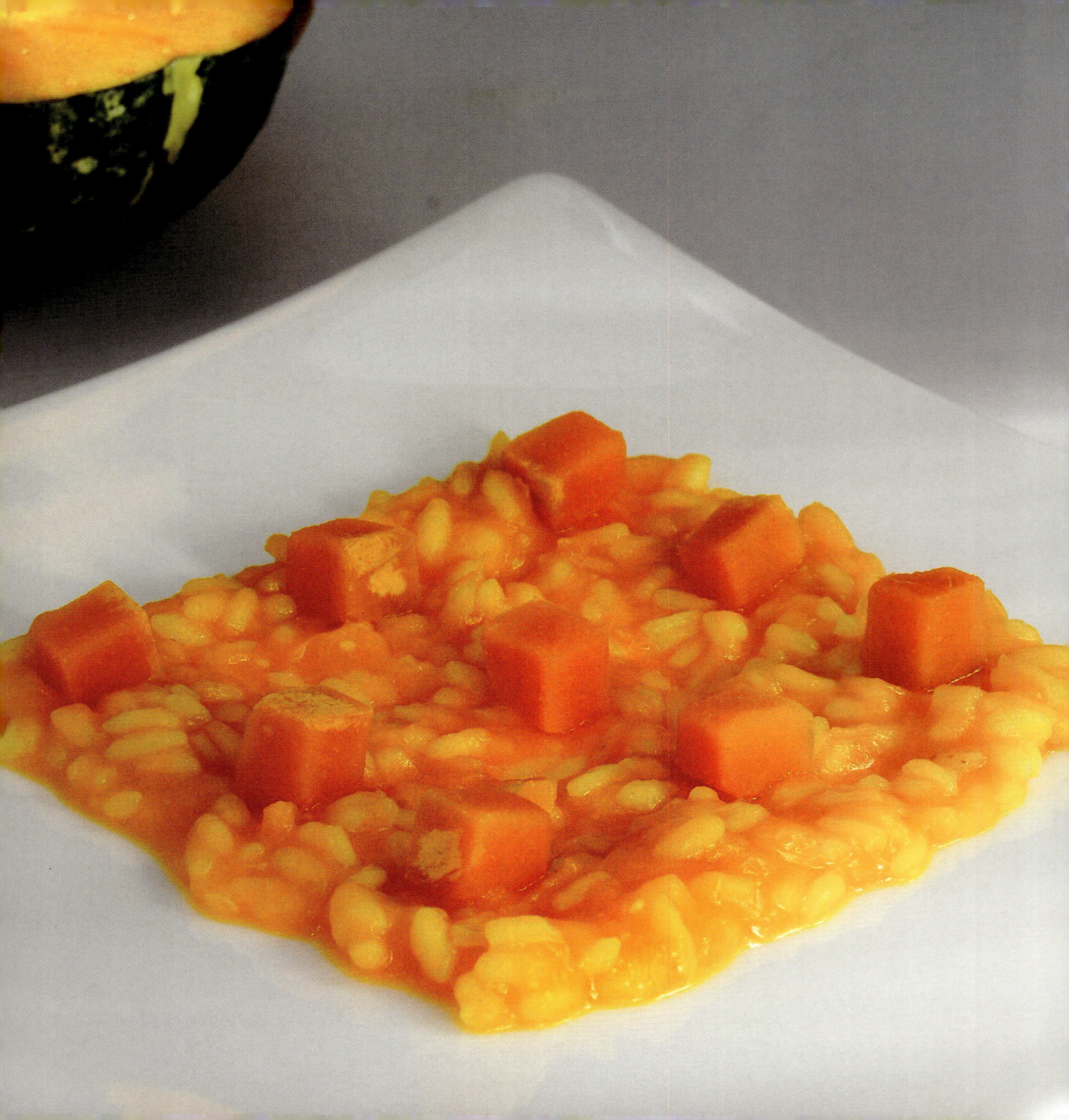

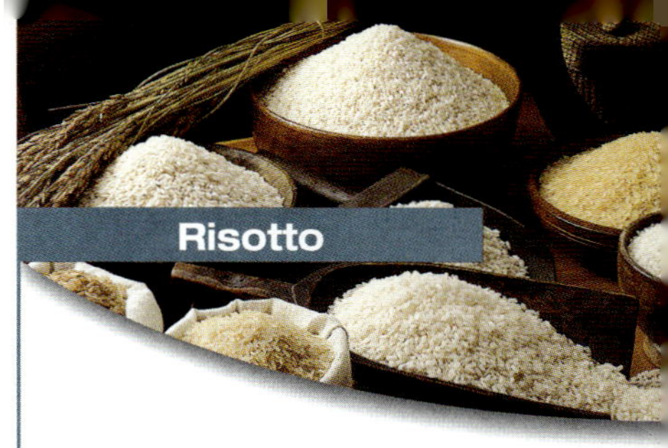

Risotto with **pumpkin**

Ingredients and amounts for 4 people

- ✓ 10½ oz (1⅓ cups) Carnaroli rice
- ✓ 28 oz (3½ cups) diced pumpkin pulp
- ✓ 4 tablespoons extra virgin olive oil
- ✓ ½ onion
- ✓ 1 liter (33.8 oz) vegetable stock
- ✓ 4 tablespoons butter
- ✓ 4 tablespoons Parmesan cheese
- ✓ salt and black pepper
- ✓ ½ glass dry white wine (optional)

Preparation

Heat the oil in a casserole, and cook the onion until soft.
Add the diced pumpkin and cook for approximately 10 minutes or longer until soft.
Add the rice and mix well; add salt and pepper to taste.
If wine is being used, add to the mixture at this point.
Add ladlefuls of boiling stock as the liquid is absorbed.
When the rice is almost cooked, add the butter and the Parmesan cheese and mix until smooth.

Bromatological evaluation per portion

Kcal	599
Protein (%)	10.5
Fats (%)	45
Carbohydrates (%)	44.5
Fiber (g)	0.9
Cholesterol (mg)	60.2

Valuable contents for the eye: ★ ★

Pumpkin is an excellent source of carotenoids, vitamin C, and vitamins of the B group.
Butter is made from milk and contains high quantities of saturated fatty acids.
Parmesan cheese is rich in easily digestible protein, is low in fat, and contains vitamin A and some vitamins of the B group.
Olive oil is an excellent source of unsaturated fatty acids.

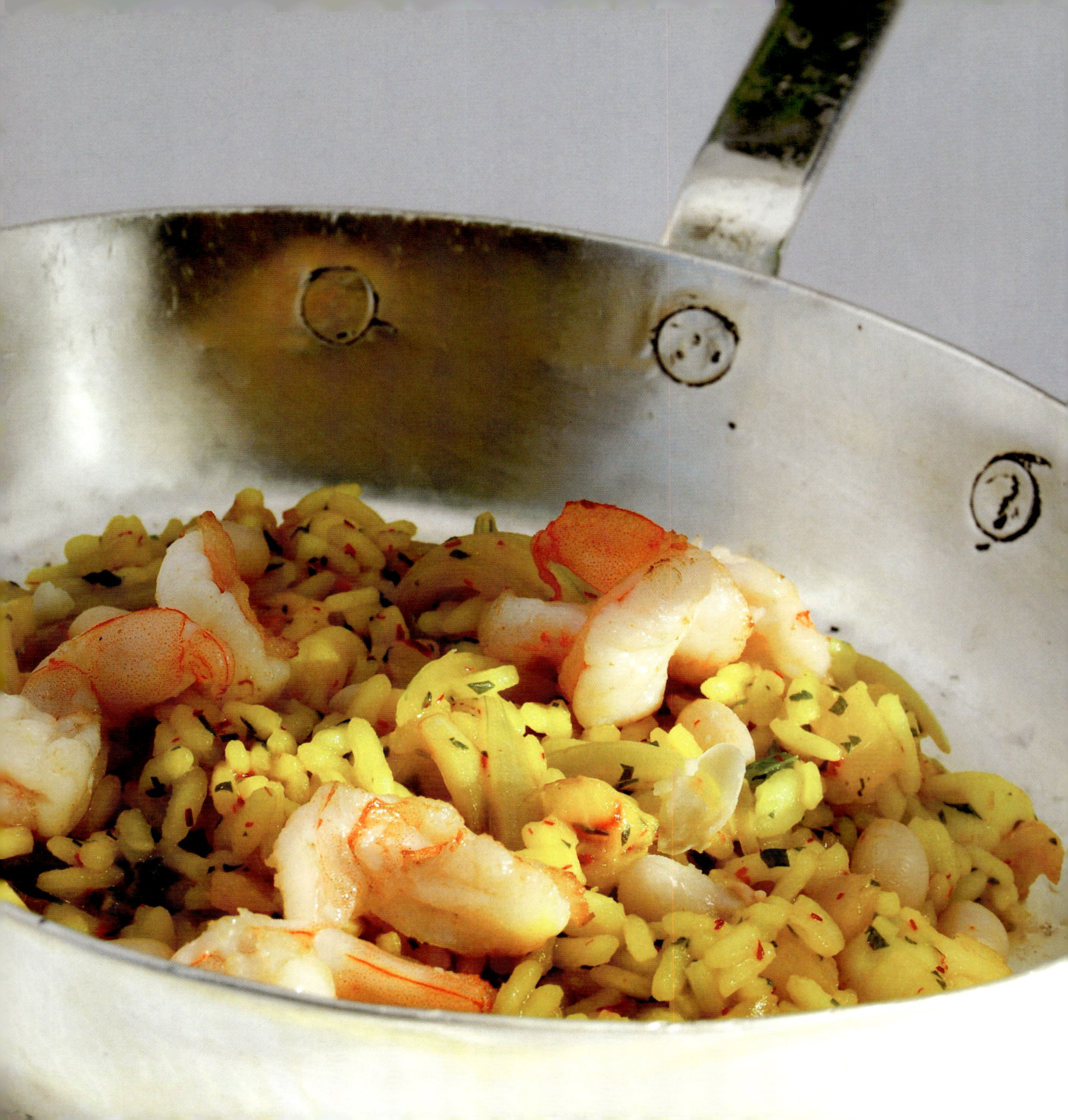

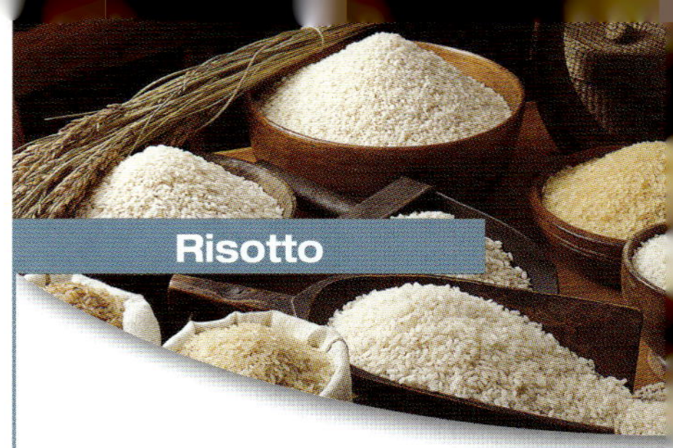

Caribbean-style paella

Ingredients and amounts for 4 people

- ✓ 10½ oz (1⅓ cups) Arborio or Vialone Nano rice
- ✓ 3 sweet green peppers
- ✓ 7 oz kidney beans (boiled)
- ✓ 16 shelled prawns
- ✓ 3 or 4 unshelled prawns
- ✓ 2 large onions
- ✓ 1 clove of garlic
- ✓ 4 sachets of saffron powder
- ✓ 1 pineapple
- ✓ 1 liter (33.8 oz) vegetable stock
- ✓ 1 bunch of parsley, chopped finely
- ✓ 6 tablespoons extra virgin olive oil
- ✓ salt and pepper to taste

Preparation

Heat the oil in a large pan with 2 handles; cook the prawns gently.
Remove the prawns and keep to one side.
Add the whole garlic clove and the onions cut into segments; then, add the peeled peppers, cut into thin circles.
Add the rice, mix, and cook for a few minutes; remove the garlic.
Add the shelled prawns to the rice-vegetable mixture.
Add salt and pepper to taste.
Peel and core the pineapple; remove all the other inedible parts and cut into pieces.
Add the pieces of pineapple and a large helping of chopped parsley to the mixture; cook for a few moments.
Mix well and add the saffron diluted in a small amount of warm water.
Add the beans and the warm vegetable stock and heat over low heat for 20 to 25 minutes until the rice has cooked and all the liquid has been absorbed.
Garnish the dish with 3 or 4 unshelled prawns.

Bromatological evaluation per portion

Kcal	610
Protein (%)	18.1
Fats (%)	25.6
Carbohydrates (%)	56.3
Fiber (g)	5.1
Cholesterol (mg)	0

Valuable contents for the eye: ★★★

Sweet peppers are a good source of carotenoids, particularly luteine.
Saffron contains an extremely high percentage of luteine, some vitamins of the B group, and substances that activate digestion.
Beans contain protein and fiber and are a good source of carotenoids and flavonoids.
Onion contains vitamin C and a good quantity of flavonoids (quercetin).
Pineapple is sweet and replenishing; it is rich in potassium and β-carotene; it contains bromeline, an anti-inflammatory.
Prawns are rich in omega-3 and oligominerals, particularly astaxanthin, which they obtain from the algae they eat.

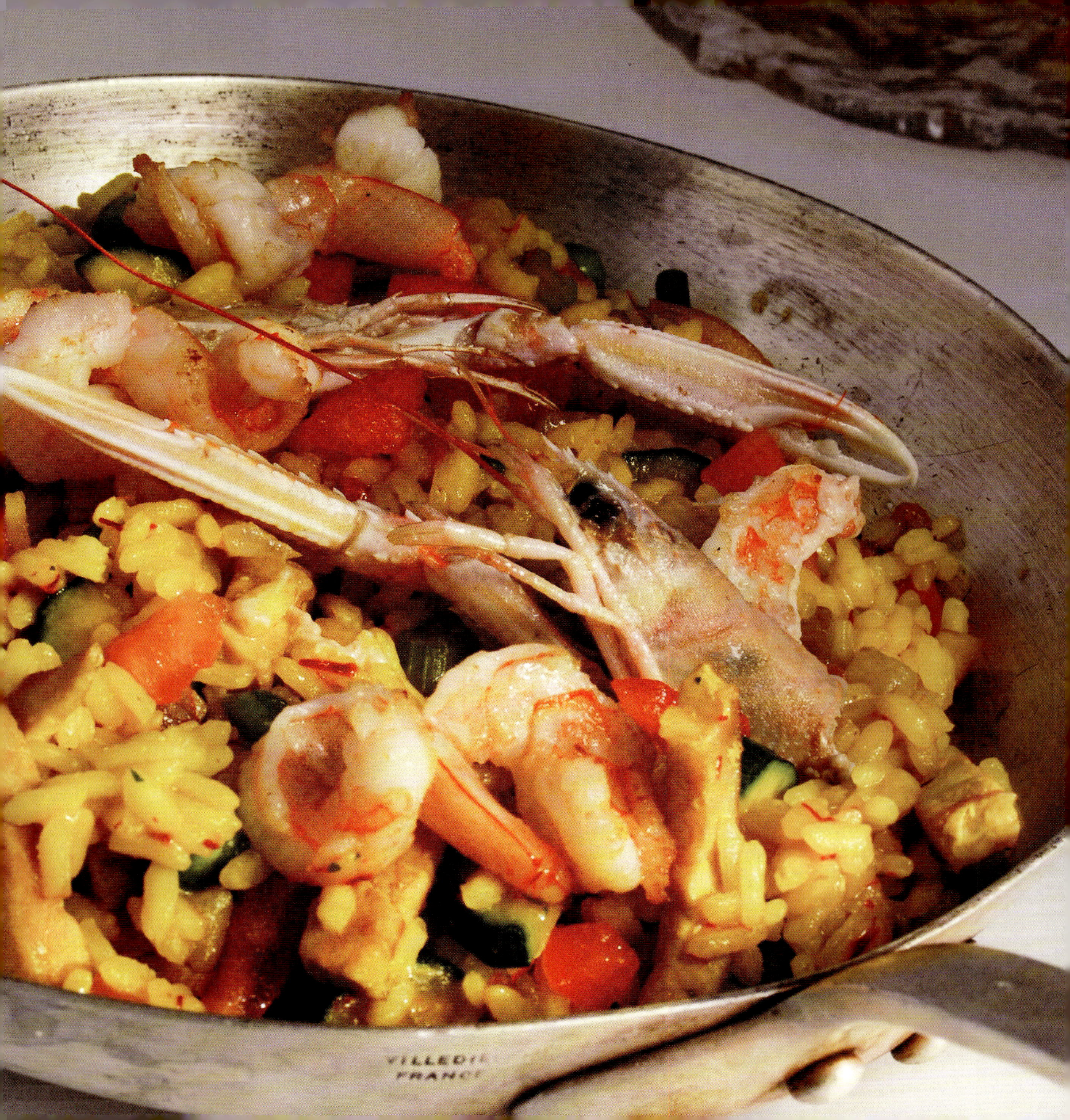
VILLEDI
FRANCE

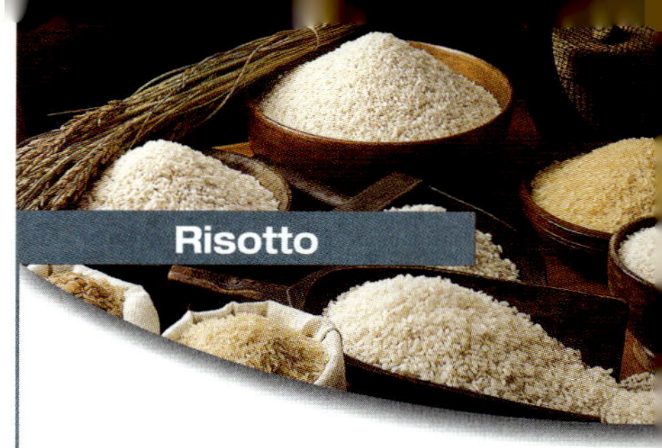

Paella

Ingredients and amounts for 4 people

- ✓ 1¾ cups rice
- ✓ 2 cloves of garlic
- ✓ 1 onion
- ✓ 7 oz skinless, boneless chicken, cut into pieces
- ✓ 7 oz boned rabbit, cleaned and cut into pieces
- ✓ 4 ripe tomatoes, peeled
- ✓ 4 zucchine trombetta (little trumpet zucchini)
- ✓ 3½ oz fresh or frozen peas (or broad beans)
- ✓ 2 red and green sweet peppers
- ✓ 3½ oz diced cooked ham, bacon, or sausage
- ✓ 4 sachets of saffron
- ✓ 6¾ oz shrimp or prawn stock
- ✓ 8 prawns
- ✓ 8 shrimp
- ✓ 4 tablespoons extra virgin olive oil
- ✓ salt and pepper to taste
- ✓ optional: 7 oz diced swordfish or other fish fillet cut into pieces

Preparation

Place the sweet peppers in the oven for approximately 10 minutes.
Wrap them in newspaper for 3 to 4 minutes, then peel, clean, and cut them into pieces.
Fry the cloves of garlic in the oil and then remove them.
Add the chopped onion and the pieces of chicken and rabbit and brown for a few minutes in the oil.
Add the peeled tomatoes, chopped zucchini, peas or broad beans, and peppers.
Add the diced cooked ham, bacon, or sausage; add salt and pepper to taste; and cook for approximately 15 minutes.
Add the rice.
Optional: add diced swordfish or other fish fillet.
Mix all the ingredients together and add the saffron, which was diluted in warm water; stop stirring the rice at this point.
Add 3 to 4 tablespoons boiling stock of shrimp or prawn and start cooking (the pan can be placed in the oven at 350°F for 20 minutes or over low heat, adding broth when necessary).
When almost cooked, add the shelled prawns and shrimp; last, decorate with prawns or shrimp (2 to 3 per person) that have been fried in another pan. (Cut the prawns in half lengthwise, leaving the head and the shell).
For optimal cooking of the paella and to present it properly at the table, a special electrical appliance called a *paelliera* can be used. It allows perfect adjustment of the temperature and time of cooking.

Stock: In a saucepan, boil the prawn heads in at least 1 liter (33.8 oz) of water, remove the heads, and use this liquid to cook the rice.

Bromatological evaluation per portion

Kcal	836
Protein (%)	28.5
Fats (%)	32.6
Carbohydrates (%)	38.9
Fiber (g)	3.3
Cholesterol (mg)	98.2

Valuable contents for the eye: ★★★

Zucchini is low in calories and rich in carotenoids and vitamin C and E.
Sweet peppers are a good source of carotenoids, particularly luteine.
Peas are rich in vitamin C and carotenoids; they also contain phytosterols (which lower the cholesterol levels).
Chicken contains digestible proteins and has a good ratio of saturated and unsaturated fatty acids.
Rabbit is a lean white meat.
Crustaceans are rich in omega-3 and oligominerals, particularly astaxanthin, which they obtain from the algae they eat.
Saffron contains an extremely high percentage of luteine, some vitamins of the B group, and substances that activate the digestion.

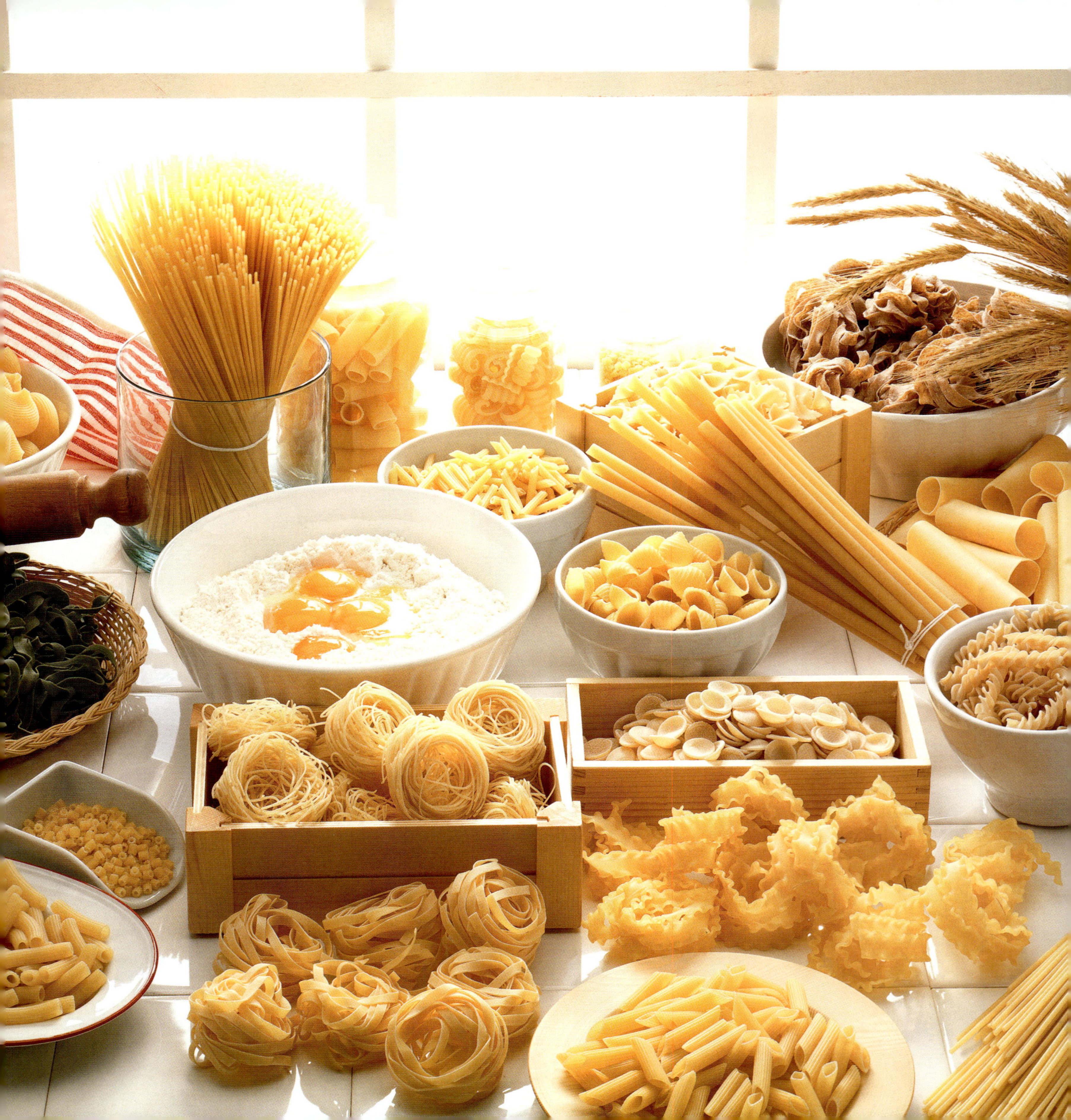

Pasta

Studies in the 1950s and 1960s that focused on the dietary benefits of the "Mediterranean diet" projected pasta into the international limelight and legitimized its gastronomic success, exalting the dietetic benefits that in the past were misunderstood or undervalued by nutritionists.

The rediscovery of the importance of complex carbohydrates in the diet of an omnivore, such as man, has revaluated not just the dietary model of Southern Italy, based on pasta, legumes, vegetables, and oil, but has actually become a prototype to be imitated.

With regards to pasta, there is the widespread promotion of this diet by the scientific community in the wake of backing from the epidemiological observations of the relationship between diet and ischemic cardiopathies and following the definition of the dietary guidelines, all in favor of slow-burning carbohydrates with a low "glycemic index."

Apart from anything else, there is no truth to the rumor that pasta causes weight gain! There is no need for a degree in medicine to know that no food on its own "causes weight gain." Obesity develops only when the total amount of energy introduced with food exceeds the total amount of energy expenditure. As a result, pasta can be a part of low-calorie diets and high-calorie diets; it is just a question of quantity and the sauce! If the ration of pasta is interpreted as more than 3.5 oz of spaghetti, with a lot of condiment—cream, butter, and cheese as part of a daily diet of soda and French fries—then there is a lack of common sense, and the pasta cannot be blamed for any weight increase.

Pasta could be accused of not being a complete and well-balanced food because there is no fat and because its proteins lack 2 important amino acids (lysine and threonine). However, no one eats pasta that is completely free from sauce! Just a few teaspoons of cheese or meat sauce are needed to transform it into a one-course meal.

Nevertheless, it is advisable that the people who live sedentary lifestyles opt for more simple sauce (tomato, basil, chili pepper, etc) and avoid the unnecessary second course (which can be eaten at another meal). They can satisfy the appetite with side dishes of vegetables (unlimited in terms of choice and quantity) and a portion of seasonal fruit.

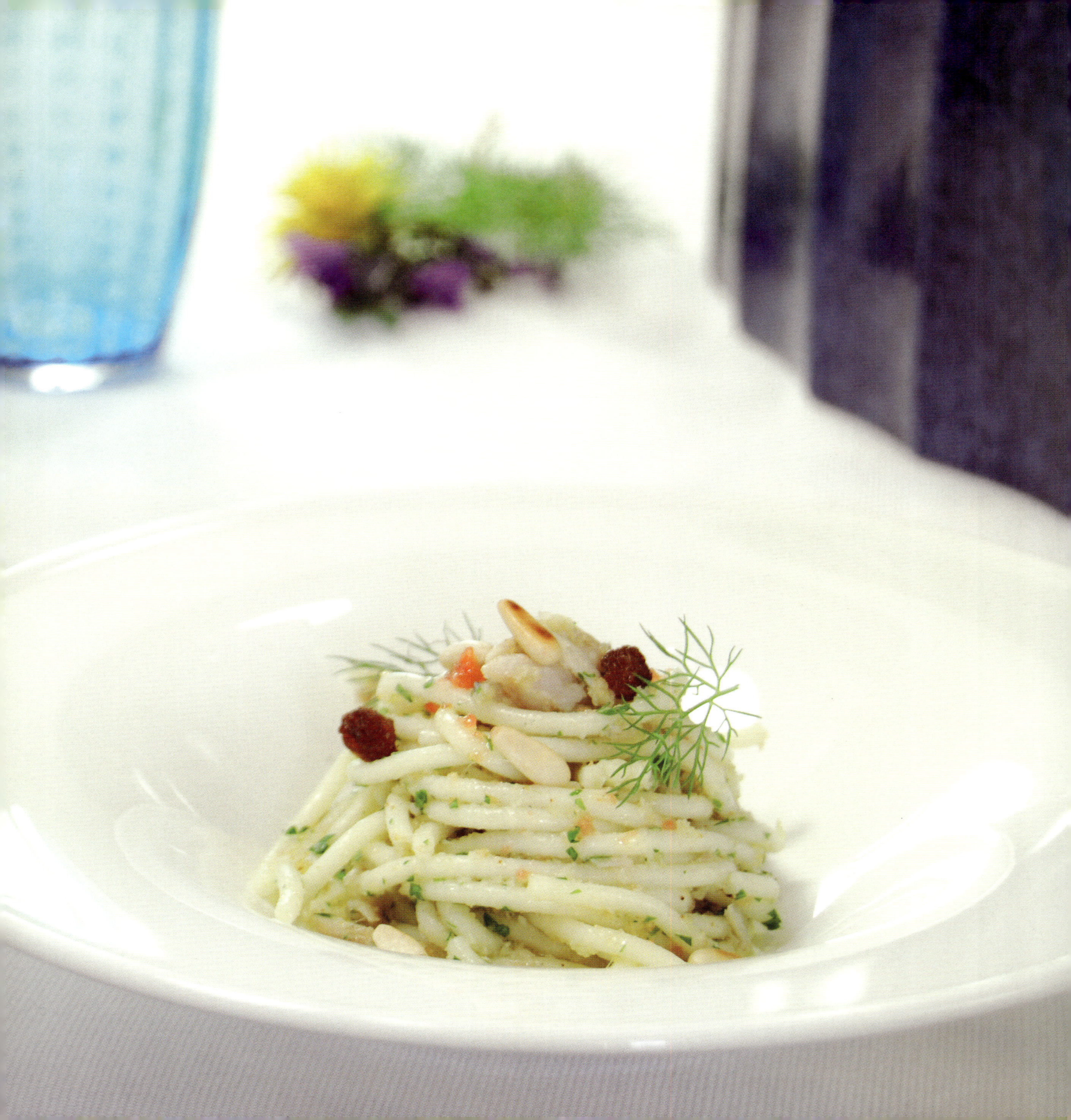

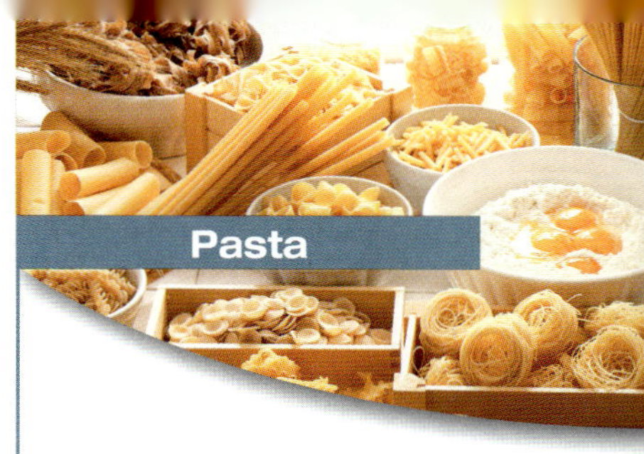

Bucatini with sardines

Ingredients and amounts for 4 people

- ✓ 10½ oz (1⅓ cups) bucatini pasta
- ✓ 1¾ cups sardines
- ✓ 1 bunch of wild fennel leaves
- ✓ 1¾ cups tomatoes, cut into pieces
- ✓ 1 teaspoon pine nuts
- ✓ 1 teaspoon raisins
- ✓ 1 onion
- ✓ 4 tablespoons extra virgin olive oil
- ✓ salt and pepper to taste

Preparation

Clean the fresh sardines, and remove the heads and the scales.
Cut them in half, wash in salty water, and dry.
Soak the raisins in water for 10 to 15 minutes to soften them.
In a pan, cook the onion in the oil over low heat for a fairly long time; then add the sardines and the raisins until they are browned. Then, add the tomatoes.
Add salt and pepper and cook for 10 minutes more.
In the meantime, cook the bucatini, drain, and add the sauce, adding the pine nuts and wild fennel leaves, which have been chopped finely and blanched in the water used to cook the pasta.

Bromatological evaluation per portion

Kcal	485
Protein (%)	20.8
Fats (%)	27.8
Carbohydrates (%)	51.4
Fiber (g)	2.9
Cholesterol (mg)	0

Valuable contents for the eye: ★ ★

Sardines are rich in omega-3 fatty acid.
Tomatoes are rich in vitamins and oligominerals, but particularly they contain carotenoids and are the most important source of lycopene.
Pine nuts are very small but rich in flavonoids and omega-6 fatty acid.
Raisins are dried grapes that are rich in sugars, potassium, calcium, and iron.
Onions contain vitamin C and a good quantity of flavonoids (quercetin).
Olive oil is an excellent source of unsaturated fatty acids.
Fennel leaves contain essential oils and flavonoids.

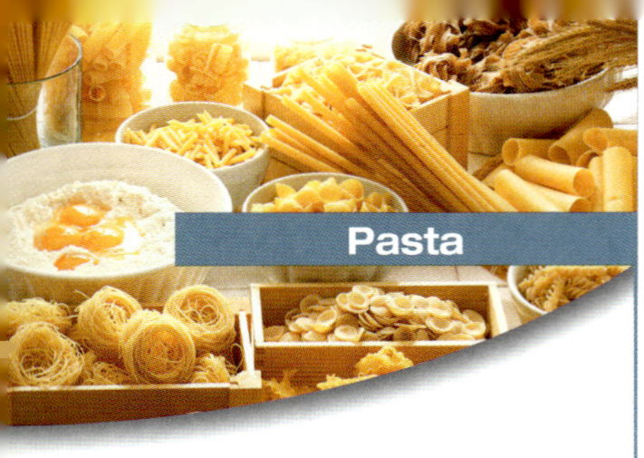

Pasta shells with pumpkin

Bromatological evaluation per portion

Kcal	492
Protein (%)	14
Fats (%)	36.4
Carbohydrates (%)	49.6
Fiber (g)	2.3
Cholesterol (mg)	45.6

Valuable contents for the eye: ★ ★

Pumpkin is an excellent source of carotenoids, vitamins C, and vitamins of the B group.
Ricotta is a milk-based product that is tasty and light; it contains a large quantity of calcium and a modest quantity of vitamins.
Onions contain vitamin C and a good quantity of flavonoids (quercetin).
Olive oil is an excellent source of unsaturated fatty acids.
Nutmeg contains essential oils and has digestive properties.
Once washed well, the skin of the **orange** can be used, the flavedo, as it contains essential oils and carotenoids.

Ingredients and amounts for 4 people

- ✓ 10½ oz (1⅓ cups) pasta shells
- ✓ 21 oz peeled pumpkin, seeds and filaments removed
- ✓ 10½ oz (1⅓ cups) ricotta cheese
- ✓ 1 white onion, chopped
- ✓ 4 tablespoons extra virgin olive oil
- ✓ pinch of grated nutmeg
- ✓ pinch of orange zest
- ✓ salt and black pepper to taste

Preparation

Pour the oil into a pan and heat, add the onion and cook until soft. Add the pumpkin, and cook until it is soft, adding water where necessary. Add salt and pepper to taste.
Place the ricotta in a preheated dish with a couple of tablespoons of hot water and add salt and pepper and grated nutmeg. Mix until a smooth cream is obtained.
Cook the pasta shells and pour them while still hot into the dish containing the ricotta cheese. Add the pumpkin and mix together. Add a pinch of grated orange zest and serve.

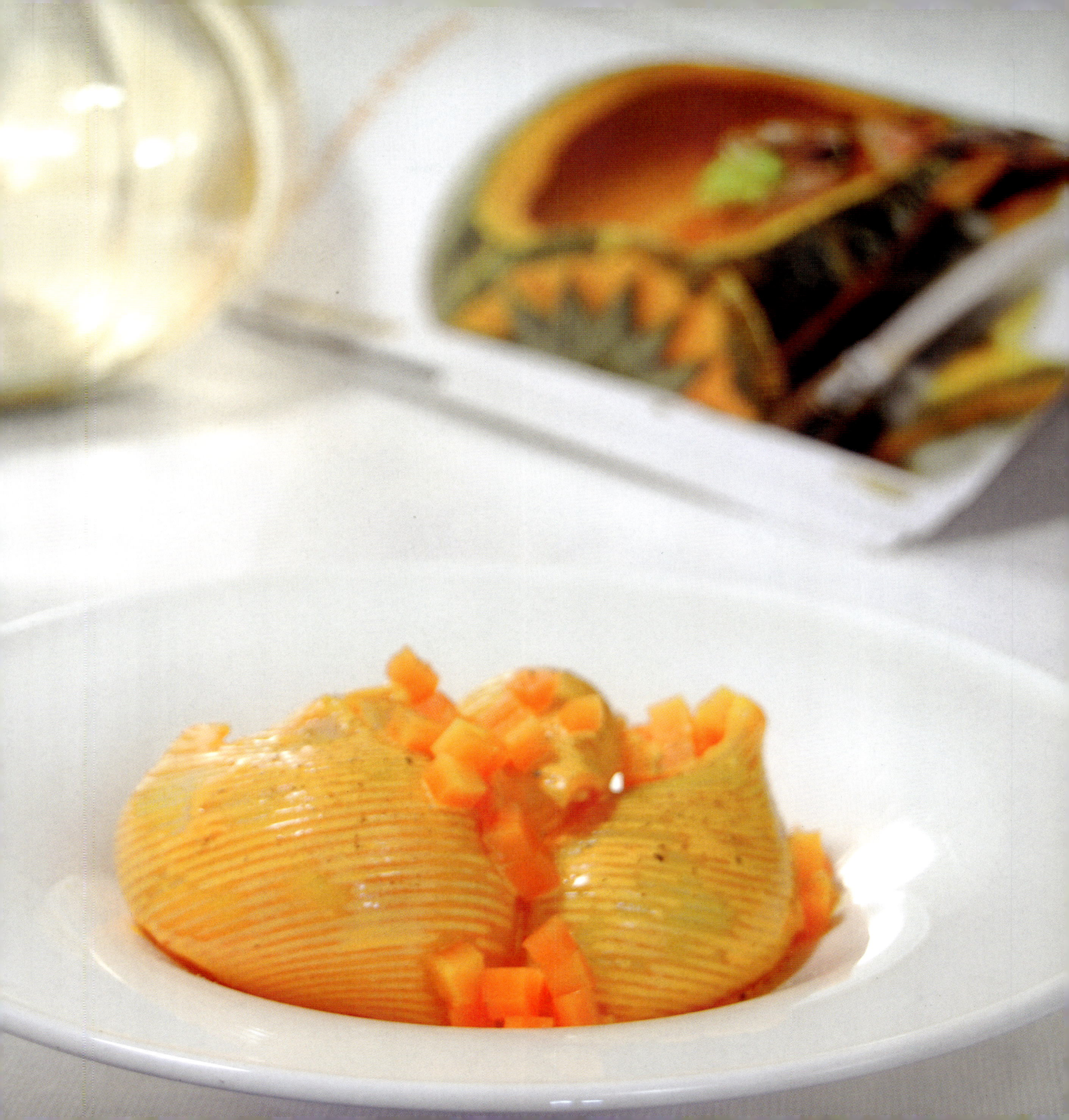

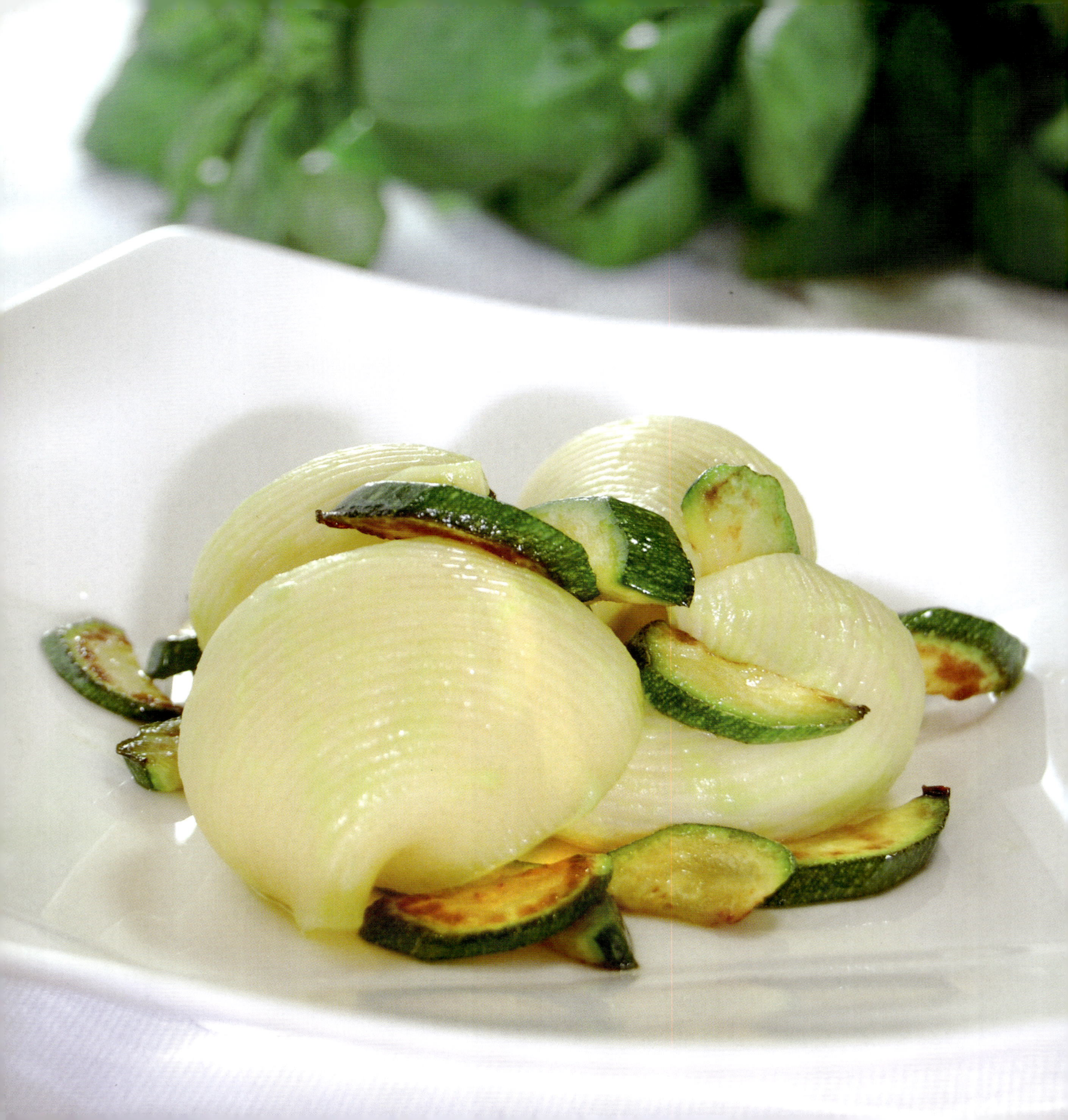

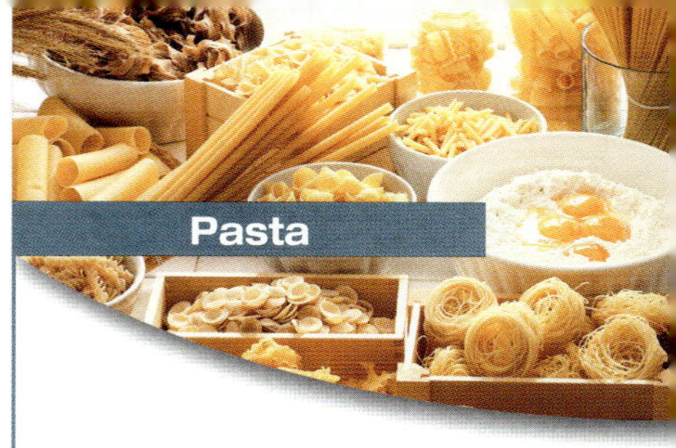

Pasta shells with **zucchini**

Ingredients and amounts for 4 people

- ✓ 10½ oz (1⅓ cups) pasta shells
- ✓ 6 small zucchinis
- ✓ 4 tablespoons extra virgin olive oil
- ✓ ½ onion, chopped
- ✓ salt and pepper to taste

Preparation

Soften the onion very slowly in the oil; add the zucchinis, which have been cut into disks; and cook them in the oil for a few minutes.

Boil the pasta shells in abundant salty water, cook till al dente, and drain.

In a large bowl, mix the pasta shells and the zucchinis; season with a small amount of olive oil, salt, and pepper.

Bromatological evaluation per portion

Kcal	363
Protein (%)	11
Fats (%)	27.7
Carbohydrates (%)	61.3
Fiber (g)	3.4
Cholesterol (mg)	0

Valuable contents for the eye: ★★

Zucchinis are low in calories and very rich in carotenoids and vitamins C and E.

Onions contain vitamin C and a good quantity of flavonoids (quercetin).

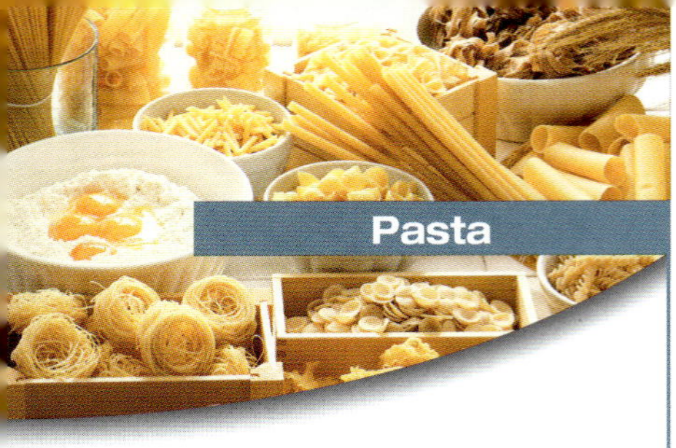

Linguine with **fish sauce**

Bromatological evaluation per portion

Kcal	578
Protein (%)	29
Fats (%)	32.1
Carbohydrates (%)	38.9
Fiber (g)	2.7
Cholesterol (mg)	76

Valuable contents for the eye: ★★

Fish in general is rich in omega-3.

Tomatoes are rich in vitamins and oligominerals, but particularly they contain carotenoids and are the most important source of lycopene.

Garlic contains selenium, zinc, and alline, which is responsible for the taste and the penetrating, persistent odor of garlic. When alline is transformed into allicine, it has an antibacterial action, and it lowers cholesterol and blood pressure levels.

Olive oil is an excellent source of unsaturated fatty acids.

Ingredients and amounts for 4 people

- ✓ 10½ oz (1⅓ cups) linguine pasta
- ✓ 1 scorpion fish (10 to 14 oz)
- ✓ 7 oz mixed fish (anchovies, mackerel, grouper, gurnard, cod)
- ✓ 1 clove of garlic
- ✓ 3½ oz tomato pulp or 4 small Pachino cherry tomatoes cut into quarters
- ✓ 4 tablespoons extra virgin olive oil
- ✓ salt and pepper to taste

Preparation

Clean the fish carefully; remove the scales, the skin, the insides, and the bones. Cut into fillets or pieces.
Brown the fish in the olive oil and add the garlic.
Add the tomato pulp or 4 small Pachino cherry tomatoes and some water and allow the fish to cook.
Add salt and pepper to taste.
Cook for 10 to 15 minutes, allowing it to dry.
At the same time, cook the linguine in salted water, cook till al dente, and drain.
Add the pasta to the sauce, mix, and cook for another 1 to 2 minutes.
The quality of the sauce depends on the freshness and type of fish and on the sweetness of the tomatoes.
Optional: Add the flavors typical of the Mediterranean to taste: oregano, basil, and capers.

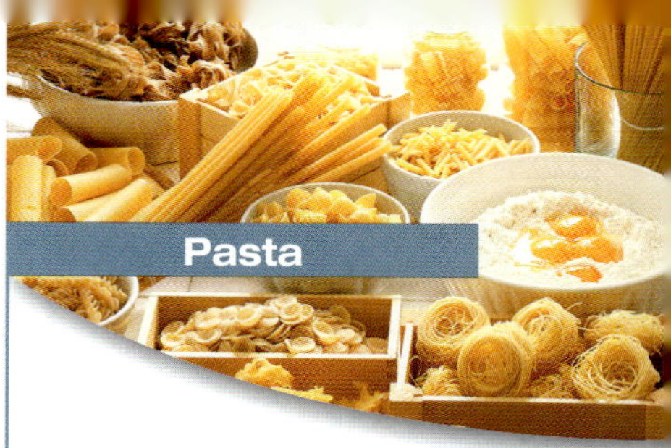

Orecchiette pasta (Pugliese style)

Ingredients and amounts for 4 people

✓ 10½ oz (1⅓ cups) orecchiette pasta
✓ 1¾ cups turnip tops
✓ 1 clove of garlic
✓ 1 teaspoon currants
✓ 1 teaspoon pine nuts
✓ 2 anchovy fillets in oil, cut into small pieces
✓ ½ chili pepper, chopped
✓ 6 tablespoons extra virgin olive oil
✓ salt and pepper to taste

Preparation

Wash the turnip tops, and cut them at the base of each flower.
Boil in abundant salted water.
After 5 minutes, add the orecchiette.
When they are cooked but still slightly al dente, drain them along with the turnip tops, pour into a bowl, add a couple of tablespoons of oil, and season with salt and pepper.
In the meantime, pour 4 tablespoons of oil into a pan, and heat the crushed garlic without allowing it to change color; add the anchovies, chili pepper, currants, and pine nuts and then add the pasta with the turnip tops.
Allow to cook for a few minutes, mixing before serving.

Bromatological evaluation per portion

Kcal	427
Protein (%)	13.5
Fats (%)	29.1
Carbohydrates (%)	57.4
Fiber (g)	4.8
Cholesterol (mg)	0

Valuable contents for the eye: ★★★

Turnip tops are rich in carotenoids and vitamin C.
Currants are dried grapes and are rich in sugars, potassium, calcium, and iron.
Pine nuts are very small but rich in flavonoids and omega-6.
Anchovies are low in calories and contain omega-3 fatty acids.
Chili peppers contain capsaicin, which makes them spicy; they also contain carotenoids and flavonoids.
Olive oil is an excellent source of unsaturated fatty acids.
Garlic contains selenium, zinc, and alline, which is responsible for the taste and the penetrating, persistent odor of garlic. When alline is transformed into allicine, it has an antibacterial action, and it lowers cholesterol and blood pressure levels.

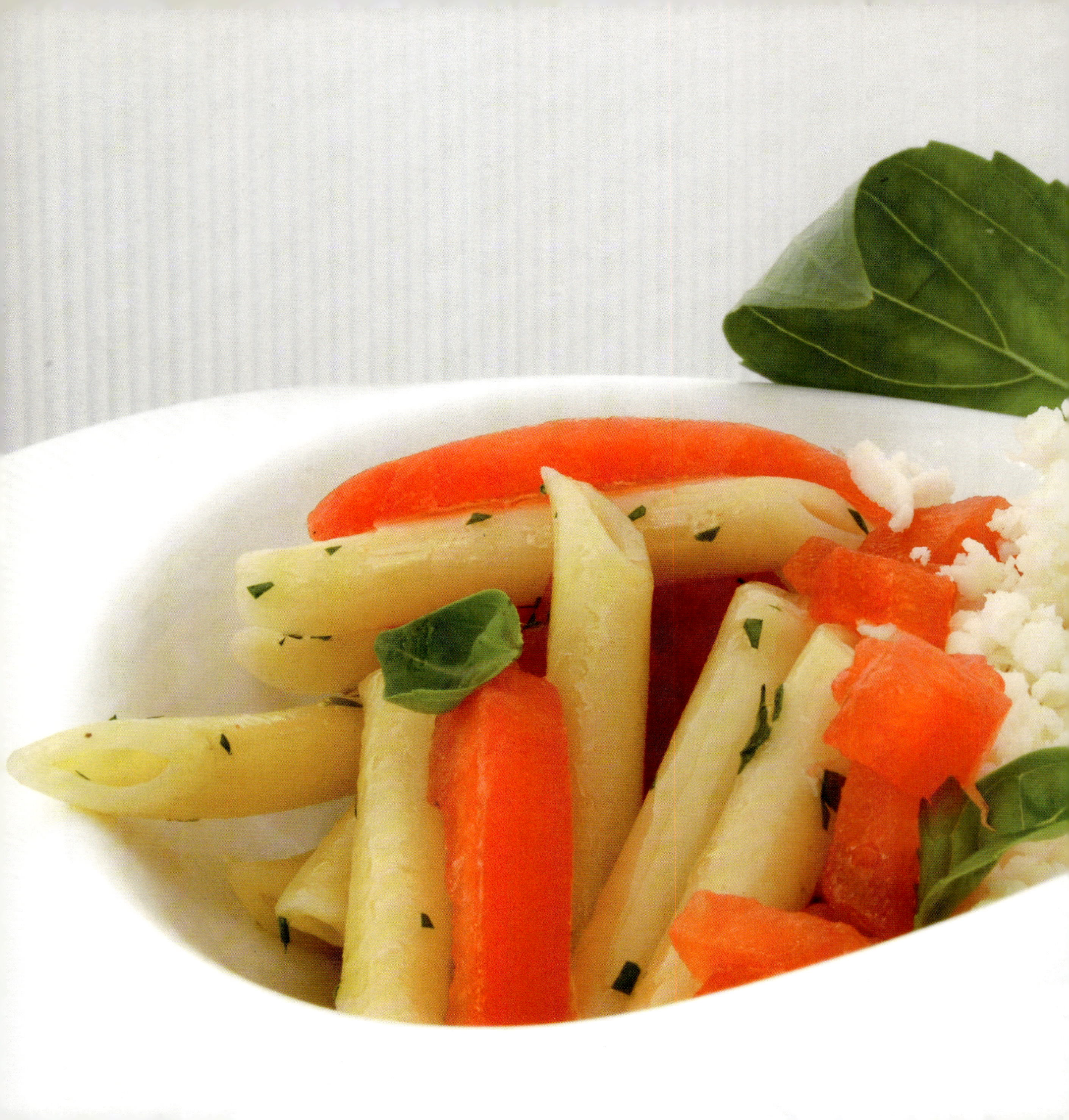

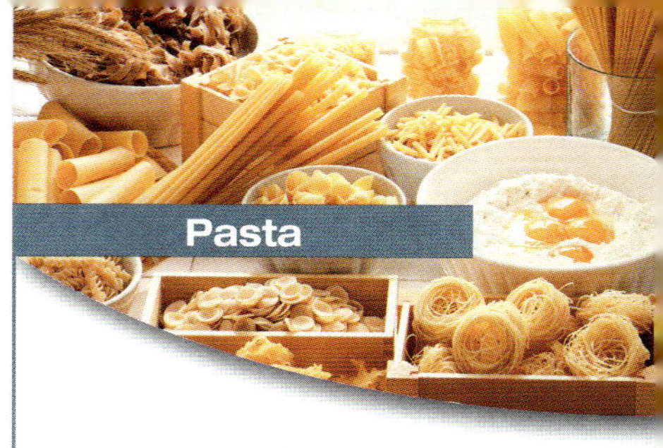

Maccheroncini pasta (Caprese style)

Ingredients and amounts for 4 people

- ✓ 10½ oz (1⅓ cups) maccheroncini pasta
- ✓ 4 ripe tomatoes
- ✓ 1⅓ cups mozzarella
- ✓ 1 oz stoned Taggiasche olives (small tasty black olives)
- ✓ 2 tablespoons desalted capers
- ✓ ½ teaspoon oregano
- ✓ 6 basil leaves
- ✓ 4 tablespoons extra virgin olive oil
- ✓ salt to taste

Preparation

Peel and cut the tomatoes; remove the seeds, and let the water drain.
Cut the mozzarella into pieces and the olives into disks.
Cook and drain the pasta and let it cool . Add a tablespoon of oil, and stir to prevent it from sticking; place in a dish.
Add the tomatoes, mozzarella, olives, capers, oil, salt, oregano, and basil and stir well.

Bromatological evaluation per portion

Kcal	589
Protein (%)	16.8
Fats (%)	43.9
Carbohydrates (%)	39.3
Fiber (g)	4.1
Cholesterol (mg)	36.8

Valuable contents for the eye: ★

Tomatoes are rich in vitamins and oligominerals, but particularly they contain carotenoids and are the most important source of lycopene.
Mozzarella contains easily digested protein and calcium.
Olives are rich in monounsaturated fats, vitamin E, and potassium.
Olive oil is an excellent source of unsaturated fatty acids.
Capers contain vitamins A, C, and E but also a large quantity of sodium.
Oregano is rich in essential oils.
Basil owes its aroma to the numerous essential oils it contains; these stimulate salivary and gastric secretions.

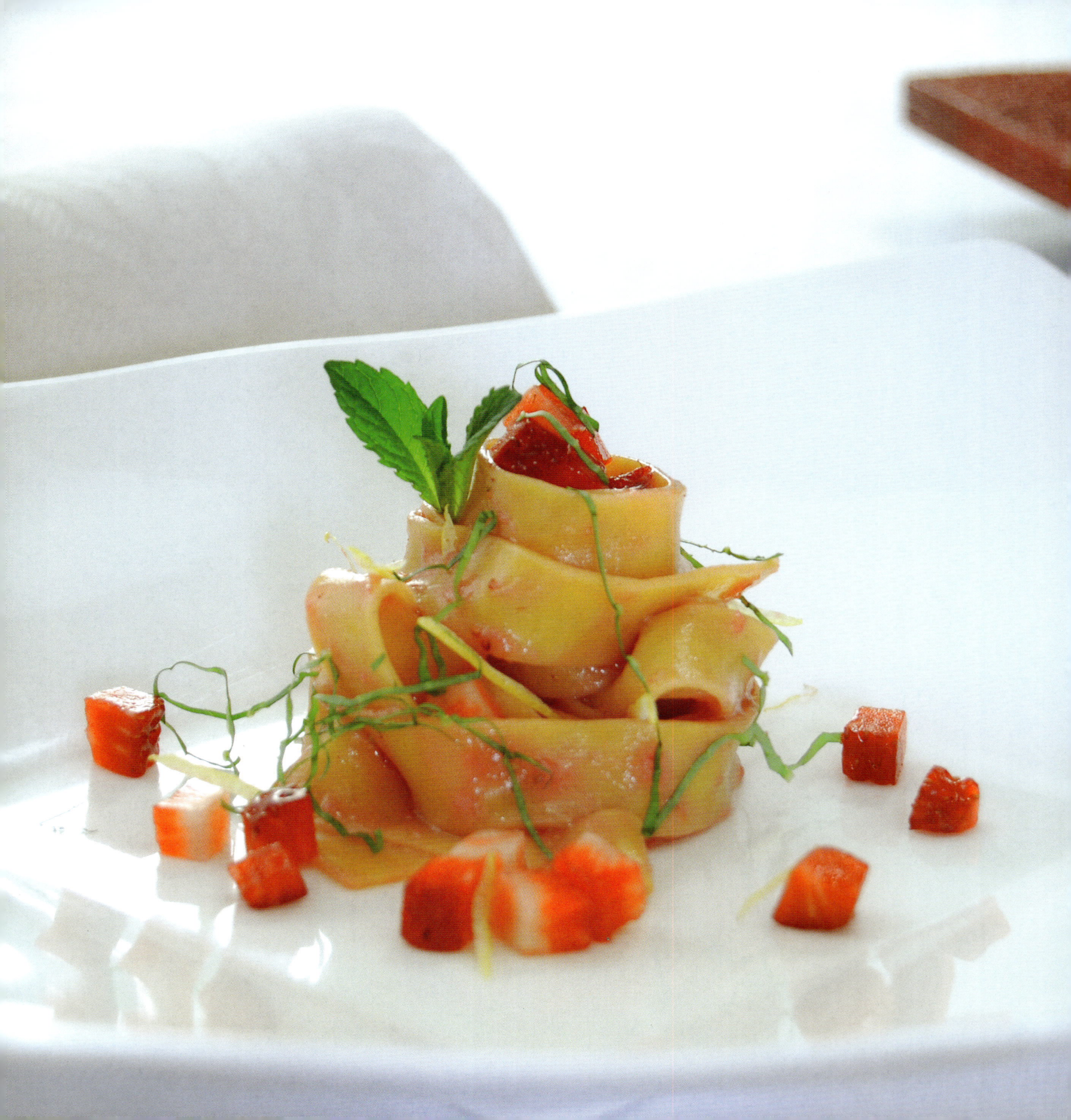

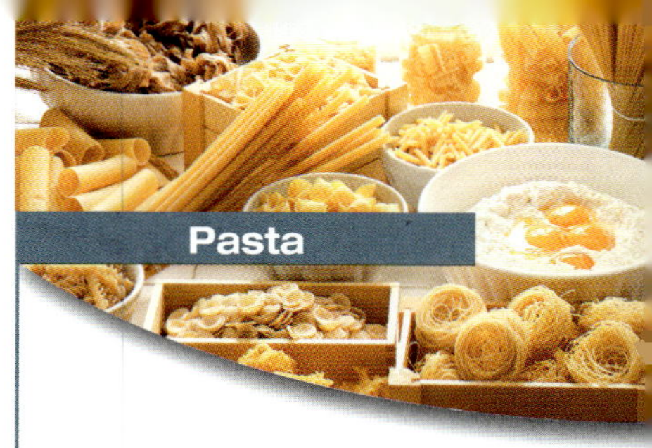

Pappardelle with strawberries

Ingredients and amounts for 4 people

- ✓ 10½ oz (1⅓ cups) egg pappardelle pasta or broad tagliatelle
- ✓ 10½ oz (1⅓ cups) small, ripe strawberries
- ✓ 7 tablespoons natural white yogurt
- ✓ 1.8 oz sheep's milk ricotta
- ✓ 2 tablespoons extra virgin olive oil
- ✓ yellow peel of ½ a lemon
- ✓ 4 mint leaves, chopped fine
- ✓ 6 basil leaves

Preparation

Put half the quantity of strawberries, yogurt, and ricotta in a blender. Blend well.

Cook the pasta in salted water and drain.

Pour some oil into a pan. Add the basil leaves and the pasta, and mix for a few seconds.

Turn off the heat and pour in the strawberry cream, mixing well.

Add the mint leaves and the lemon peel and mix. Finally, garnish with the remaining strawberries cut into large pieces, mix, and serve.

Bromatological evaluation per portion

Kcal	445
Protein (%)	12.5
Fats (%)	30.2
Carbohydrates (%)	57.3
Fiber (g)	3.6
Cholesterol (mg)	85.6

Valuable contents for the eye: ★★

Yogurt has a high repletion index; in addition to the live milk enzymes, it contains vitamins of the B group and folic acid.

Ricotta is a milk-based product that is tasty and light; it contains a large quantity of calcium and a modest quantity of vitamins.

Olive oil is an excellent source of unsaturated fatty acids.

Mint leaves contain flavonoids, and its essential oil has an antispastic effect.

Basil owes its aroma to the numerous essential oils it contains; these stimulate salivary and gastric secretions.

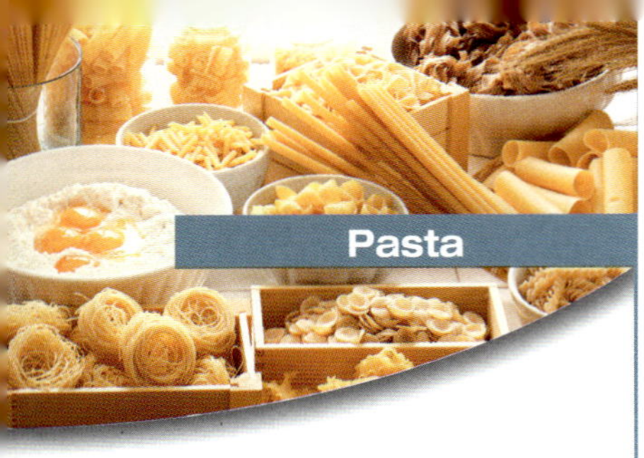

Bromatological evaluation per portion

Kcal	405
Protein (%)	10.3
Fats (%)	25.3
Carbohydrates (%)	64.4
Fiber (g)	5.4
Cholesterol (mg)	0

Valuable contents for the eye: ★ ★ ★

Zucchinis are low in calories and rich in carotenoids and vitamins C and E.

The **apple** is rich in fructose. It contains flavonoids (quercetin) and oligoelements such as zinc and selenium.

Sweet peppers are a good source of carotenoids, particularly luteine.

Tomatoes are rich in vitamins and oligominerals, but particularly they contain carotenoids and are the most important source of lycopene.

Onion contains vitamin C and a good quantity of flavonoids (quercetin).

Olive oil is an excellent source of unsaturated fatty acids.

Cold and colored penne pasta

Ingredients and amounts for 4 people

✓ 10½ oz (1⅓ cups) penne pasta
✓ 3 zucchinis
✓ 1 onion, sliced
✓ 2 tomatoes
✓ 2 red apples
✓ ½ sweet pepper
✓ 4 tablespoons extra virgin olive oil
✓ 8 basil leaves
✓ 1 tablespoon parsley, chopped
✓ salt and pepper to taste

Preparation

Wash and clean the vegetables (zucchinis, apples, peppers, and tomatoes) and cut them into strips.

Put onion and olive oil in a pan, and heat until the onion starts to fry. Remove from the heat and cool.

Drain the oil (discarding the onion) into a blender; add all the sliced vegetables; blend until a creamy mixture is obtained.

Add salt to taste, then add pepper, basil, and parsley.

Cook the pasta in abundant salted water; drain but do not rinse as this would remove the salt used for cooking; spread onto a tray to allow to cool. Add a small quantity of oil to prevent the pasta from sticking together.

Mix the pasta and the blended cream together in a dish and mix well.

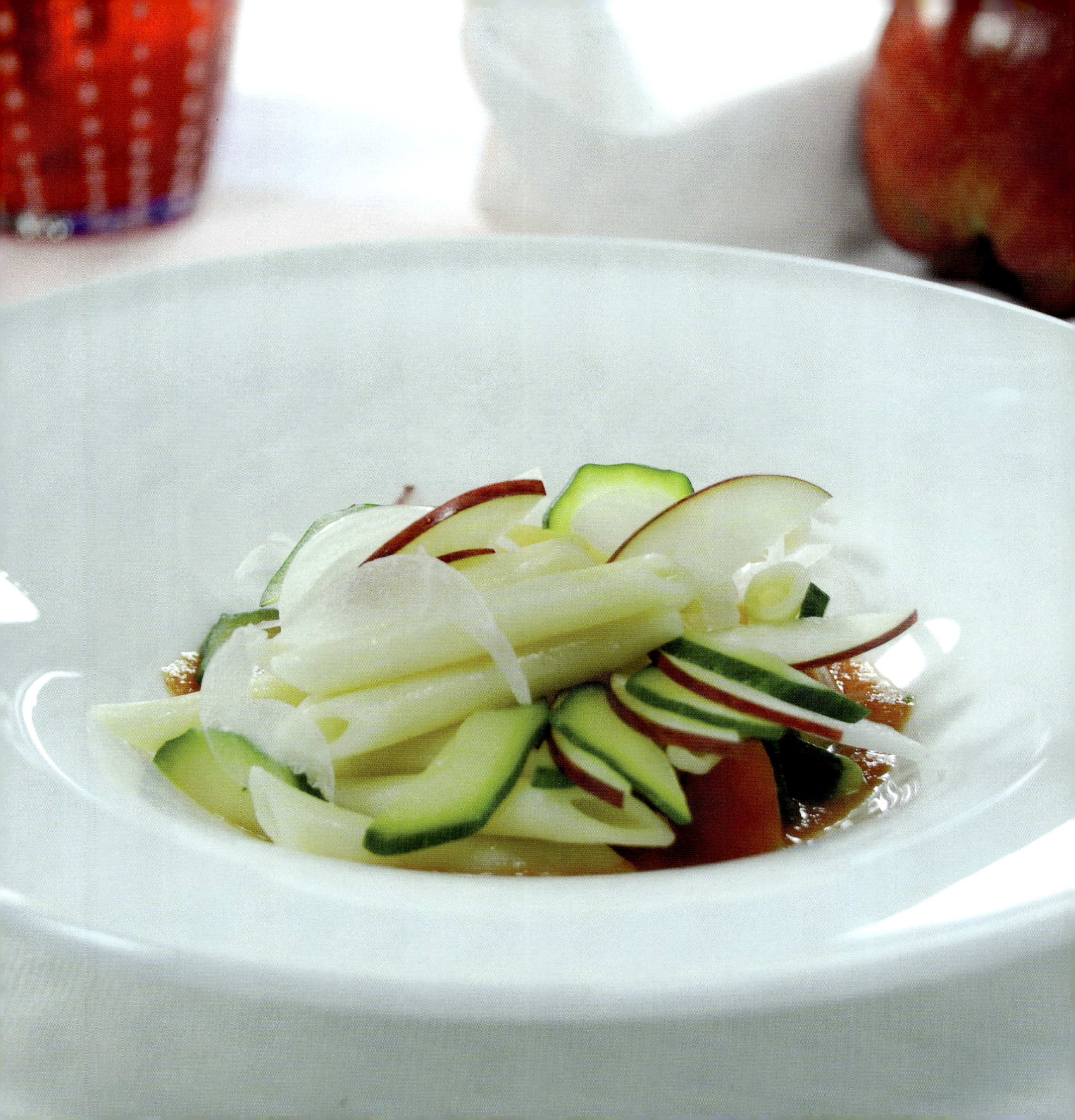

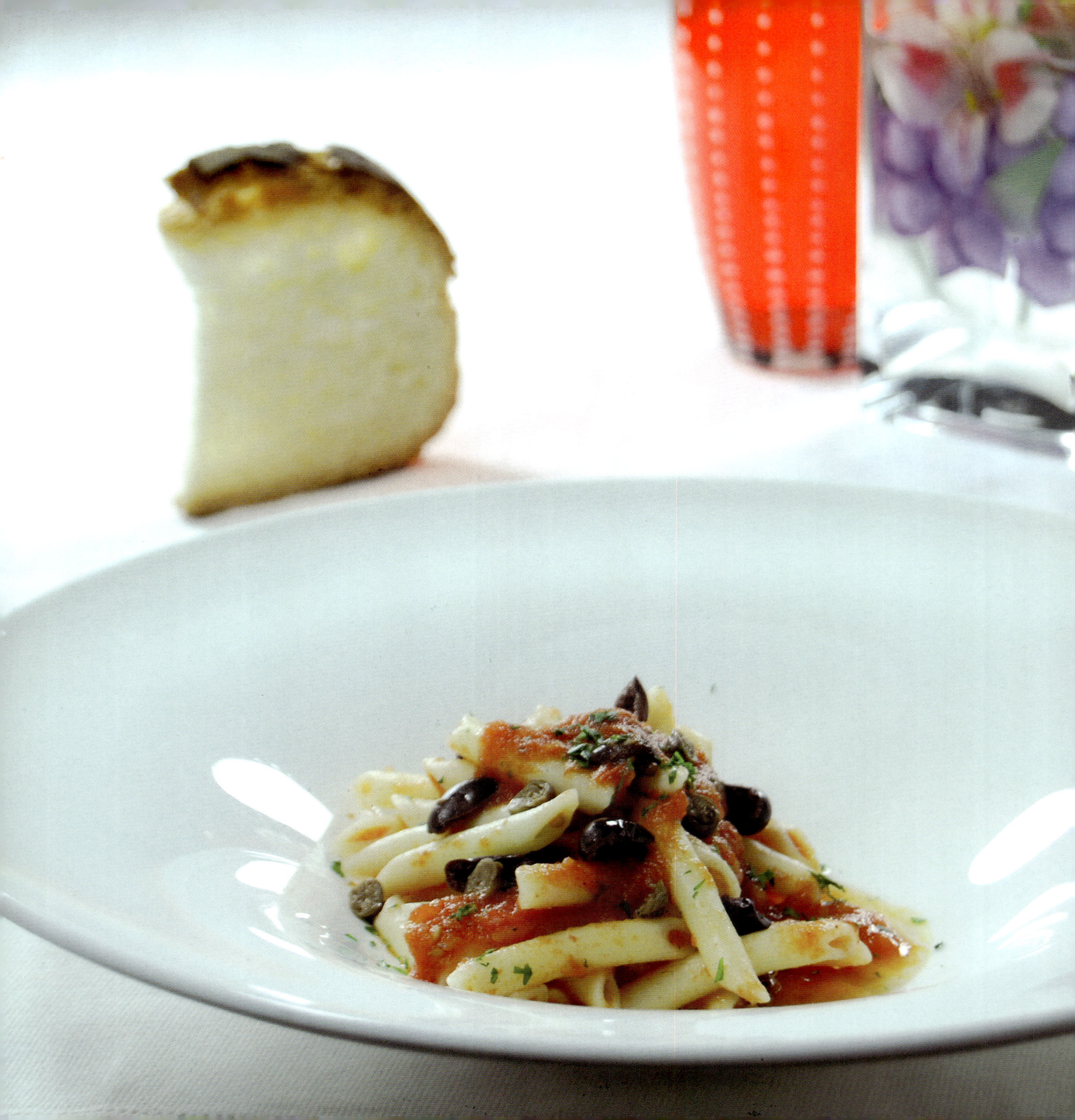

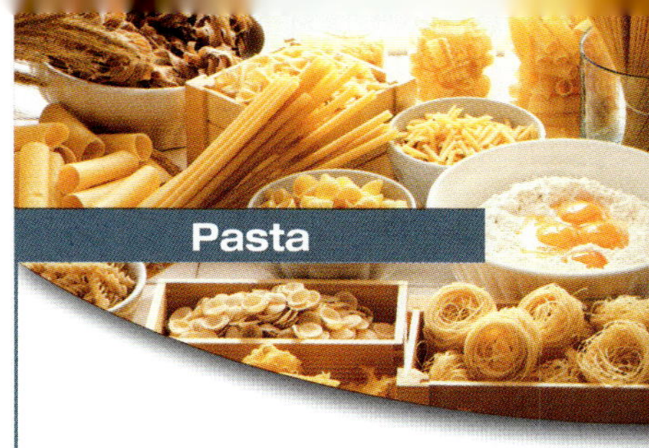

Penne pasta or spaghetti all'arrabbiata

Ingredients and amounts for 4 people

- ✓ 10½ oz (1⅓ cups) penne pasta or spaghetti
- ✓ 1¾ cups fresh tomato pulp
- ✓ 1 oz onion, chopped
- ✓ 1 oz stoned Taggiasche olives (small, tasty black olives)
- ✓ 1 teaspoon salted capers
- ✓ 1 whole chili pepper
- ✓ 1 sprig of basil
- ✓ 3 tablespoons extra virgin olive oil

Preparation

In a large casserole, heat the oil, and slowly cook the onion.
Crush and add the chili peppers, olives, and capers.
Add the tomato, and cook the mixture for approximately 5 minutes.
Cook the pasta, drain, and mix with the sauce in the casserole dish; garnish with fresh basil and serve.

Bromatological evaluation per portion

Kcal	393
Protein (%)	10.5
Fats (%)	30.2
Carbohydrates (%)	59.3
Fiber (g)	4.4
Cholesterol (mg)	0

Valuable contents for the eye: ★

Tomatoes are rich in vitamins and oligominerals, but particularly they contain carotenoids and are the most important source of lycopene.
Chili peppers contain capsaicin, which makes them spicy; they also contain carotenoids and flavonoids.
Olives are rich in monounsaturated fats, vitamin E, and potassium.
Capers contain vitamins A, C, and E, but also a large quantity of sodium.

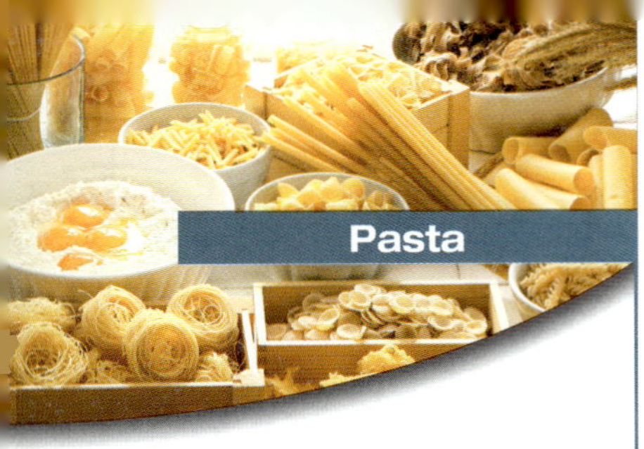

Penne pasta with tomato and basil sauce

Bromatological evaluation per portion

Kcal	447
Protein (%)	14.7
Fats (%)	34.1
Carbohydrates (%)	51.2
Fiber (g)	4.1
Cholesterol (mg)	18.2

Valuable contents for the eye: ★

Tomatoes are rich in vitamins and oligominerals, but particularly they contain carotenoids and are the most important source of lycopene.

Basil owes its aroma to the numerous essential oils it contains; these stimulate salivary and gastric secretions.

Parmesan cheese is rich in easily digestible protein, is low in fat, and contains vitamin A and some vitamins of the B group.

Olive oil is an excellent source of unsaturated fatty acids.

Ingredients and amounts for 4 people

✓ 10½ oz (1⅓ cups) penne pasta

✓ 4 very ripe tomatoes

✓ 6 tablespoons extra virgin olive oil

✓ 16 basil leaves

✓ 8 tablespoons freshly grated Parmesan cheese

Preparation

Thirty minutes before the meal, peel the tomatoes, remove the seeds, cut tomatoes into pieces, add salt, and drain. Remove the water extracted from the tomatoes, add the oil and the basil, and mix well. Let sit for 20 to 30 minutes.

Cook the pasta till al dente and drain.

Drain off any water formed in the dish containing the tomato, oil, and basil. Add the pasta, and mix well.

Sprinkle the Parmesan cheese over the pasta and sauce before serving.

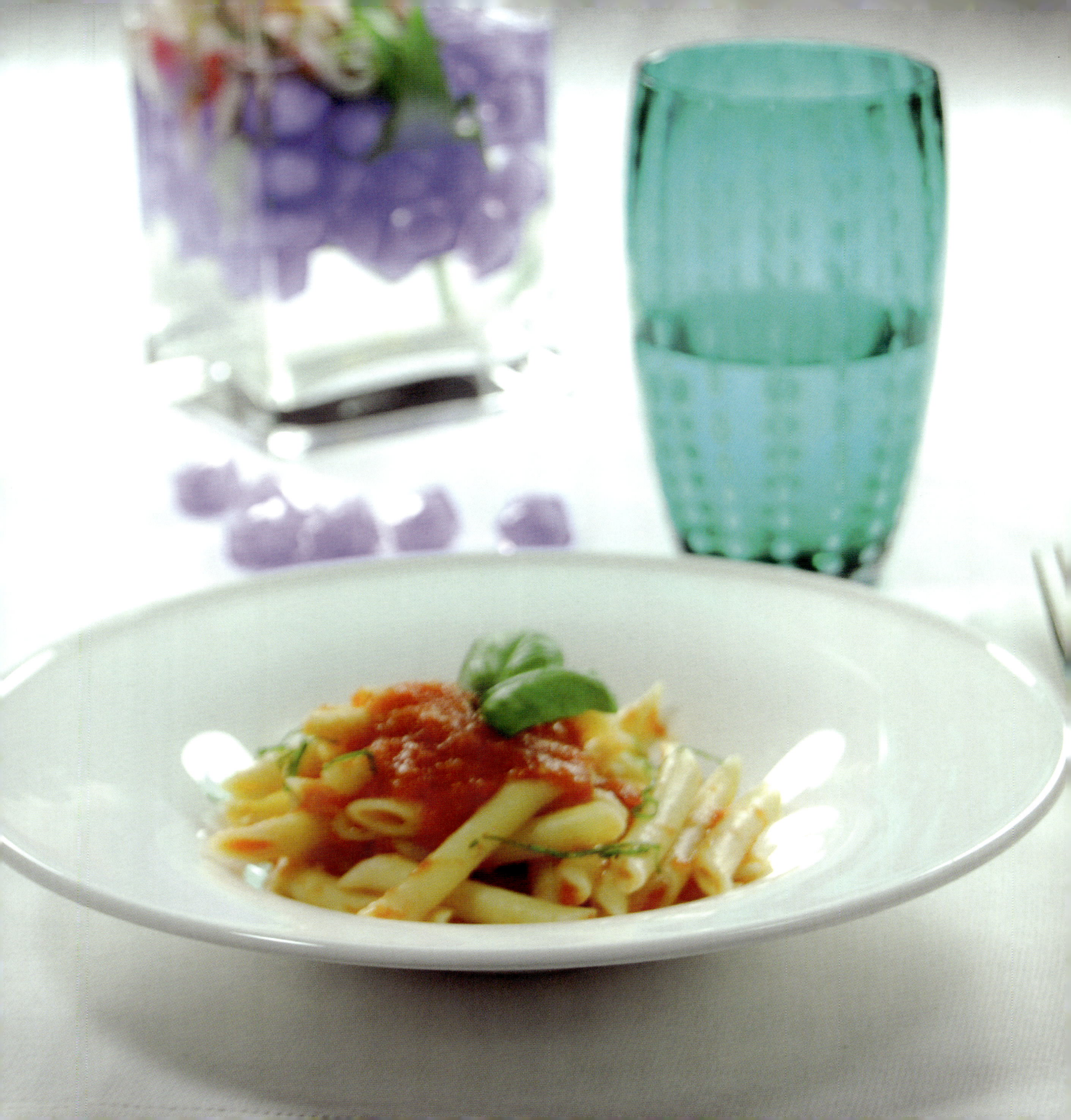

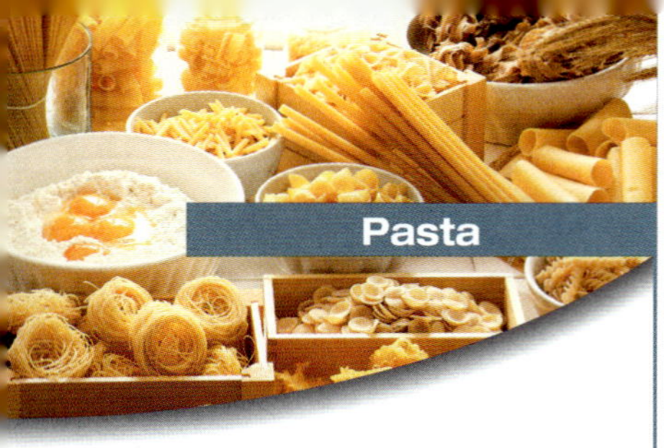

Bromatological evaluation per portion

Kcal	573
Protein (%)	17.2
Fats (%)	42.2
Carbohydrates (%)	40.6
Fiber (g)	4.2
Cholesterol (mg)	36.8

Valuable contents for the eye: ★

Tomatoes are rich in vitamins and oligominerals, but particularly they contain carotenoids and are the most important source of lycopene.
Mozzarella contains easily digested protein and calcium.
Olive oil is an excellent source of unsaturated fatty acids.
Basil owes its aroma to the numerous essential oils it contains; these stimulate salivary and gastric secretions.
Parsley contains flavonoids and is also an apiol, an antispastic, and an antipyretic. It also stimulates uterine contractions.

Cold penne pasta with **mozzarella** and **tomatoes**

Ingredients and amounts for 4 people

✓ $10\frac{1}{2}$ oz ($1\frac{1}{3}$ cups) penne pasta
✓ 1 large mozzarella, finely sliced
✓ 4 very ripe tomatoes
✓ 1 clove of garlic
✓ 1 bunch of parsley
✓ 1 bunch of basil
✓ 4 tablespoons extra virgin olive oil
✓ salt and black pepper to taste

Preparation

Add the tomatoes to the boiling water that will be used to cook the pasta. Blanch for about 10 seconds, remove, and cool in a bowl of cold water. Skin the tomatoes and cut into 2 pieces, remove the seeds, and cut into small pieces; allow the water to drain.
Place the tomatoes in a large salad bowl and marinate with salt, pepper, garlic, parsley, basil, and olive oil.
Cook the pasta in abundant salted water, drain, and dry well with a cloth; this will allow it to fully maintain the flavor.
Add the pasta to the salad bowl, and mix with the other ingredients.
Add the finely sliced mozzarella.

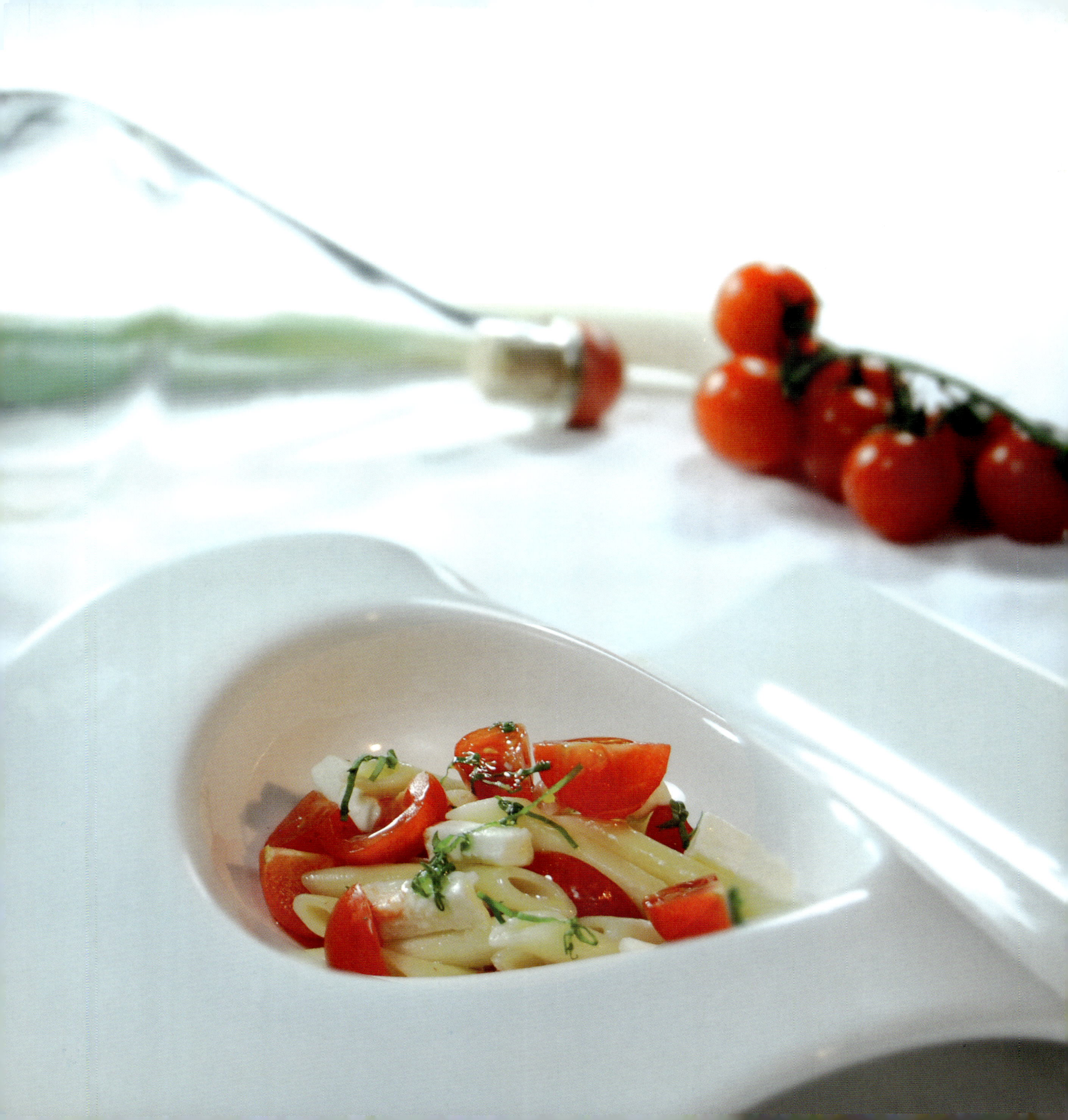

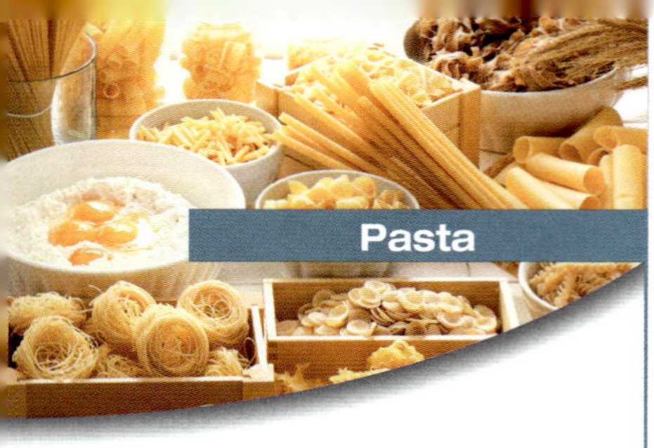

Penne pasta with ricotta cheese

Bromatological evaluation per portion

Kcal	341
Protein (%)	15.5
Fats (%)	14
Carbohydrates (%)	70.5
Fiber (g)	2.1
Cholesterol (mg)	16.1

Valuable contents for the eye: ★

Milk (particularly whole milk) has a good balance of sugars, fats, and proteins; it contains high quantities of calcium and phosphorous, but particularly fat-soluble anti-oxidant vitamins and water-soluble vitamins.
Ricotta is a milk-based product that is tasty and light; it contains a large quantity of calcium and a modest quantity of vitamins.
Cinnamon is highly aromatic and is also an aphrodisiac; it stimulates the digestion, reduces the blood cholesterol and triglyceride levels, and enhances the action of insulin.
Marjoram is rich in essential oils.

Ingredients and amounts for 4 people

✓ 10½ oz (1⅓ cups) penne pasta
✓ 7 oz milk, heated
✓ 7 tablespoons ricotta cheese
✓ 1 teaspoon sugar
✓ 1 teaspoon ground cinnamon
✓ 1 teaspoon marjoram
✓ salt and pepper to taste

Preparation

While the pasta is cooking in abundant salted water, place the ricotta cheese in a large salad bowl with the milk, sugar, cinnamon, salt, pepper, and marjoram. Mix these ingredients with a fork to produce a soft, smooth cream.
Drain the pasta well, and add the ricotta cream; mix well and serve.

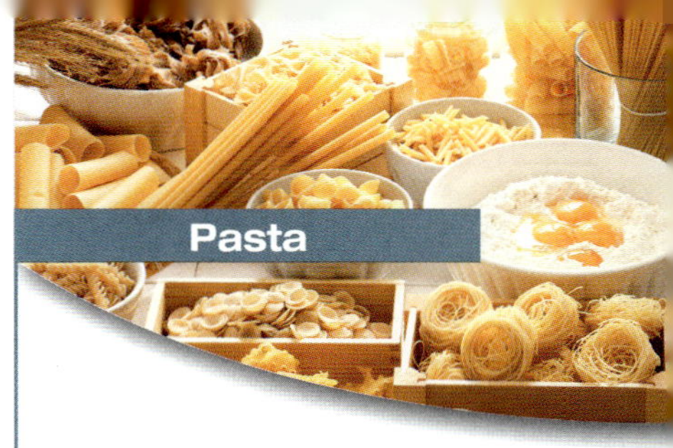

Penne pasta with Mediterranean garden vegetables (served hot or cold)

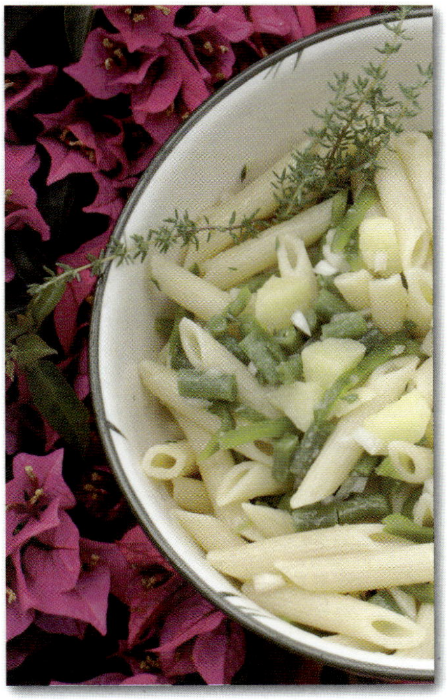

Ingredients and amounts for 4 people

- ✓ 10½ oz (1⅓ cups) penne pasta
- ✓ ⅔ cup potatoes, finely sliced
- ✓ 3½ oz fresh tender runner beans
- ✓ 1 sweet pepper
- ✓ 1 sprig of thyme
- ✓ 1 spring onion
- ✓ 4 to 6 tablespoons extra virgin olive oil
- ✓ salt

Preparation

Heat the sweet pepper in the oven for a few minutes. Remove the skin and seeds and cut into strips.
Clean and thinly slice the onion.
Cook the pasta, potatoes, and runner beans together in abundant salted water.
Rinse under cold water to stop the cooking process; drain all the ingredients together.
Add the peppers, olive oil, a handful of salt, and thyme.
Mix and serve.

Bromatological evaluation per portion

Kcal	411
Protein (%)	10.8
Fats (%)	25.5
Carbohydrates (%)	63.7
Fiber (g)	4.4
Cholesterol (mg)	0

Valuable contents for the eye: ★★

The **potato** is rich in starch, and it contains potassium, vitamin C, and vitamin B5.
Runner beans contain protein and fiber and are a good source of carotenoids and flavonoids.
Sweet peppers are a good source of carotenoids, particularly luteine.
The **spring onion** contains vitamin C and a good quantity of flavonoids (quercerin).
Olive oil is an excellent source of unsaturated fatty acids.
Thyme contains essential oils and flavonoids.

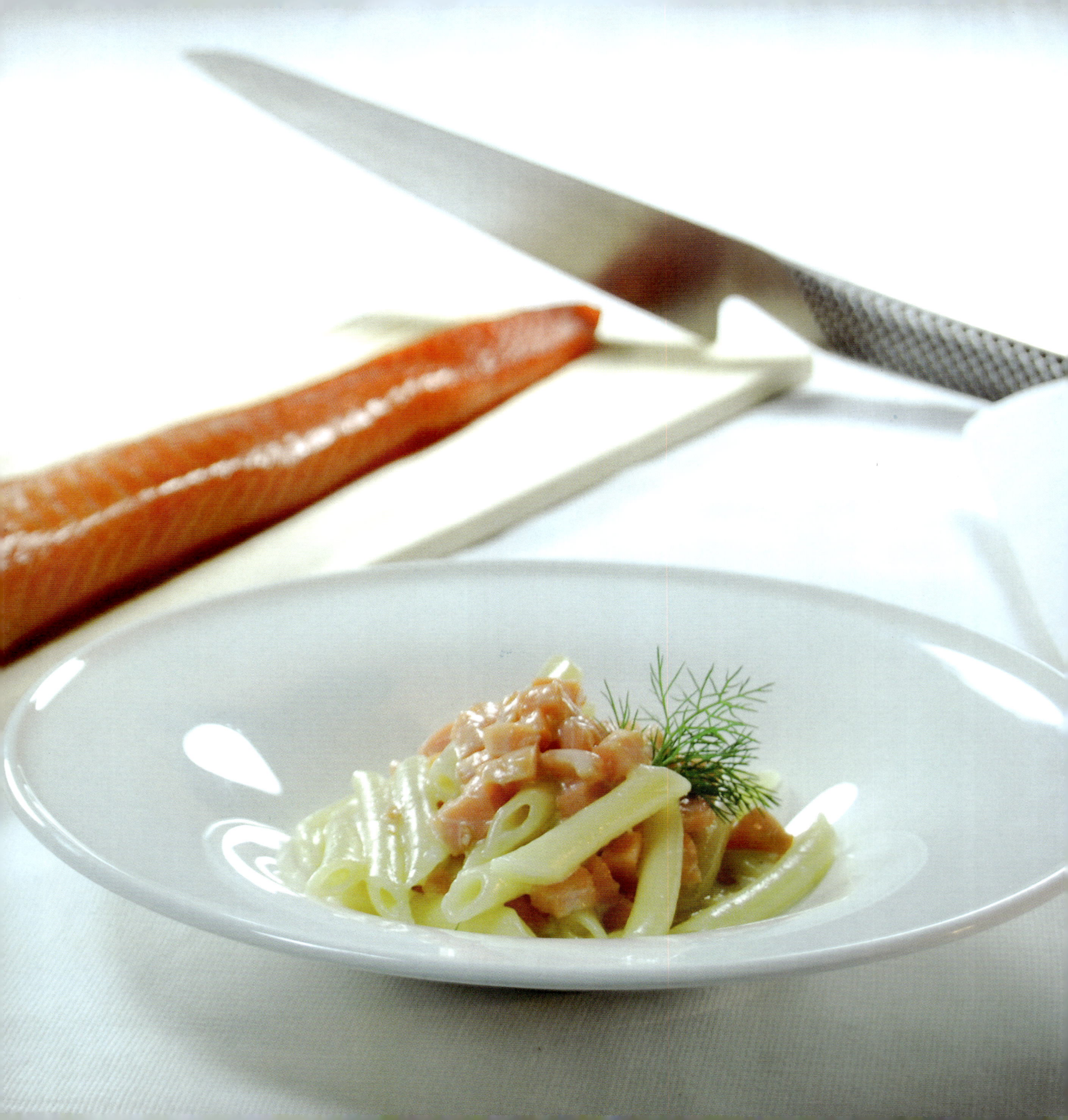

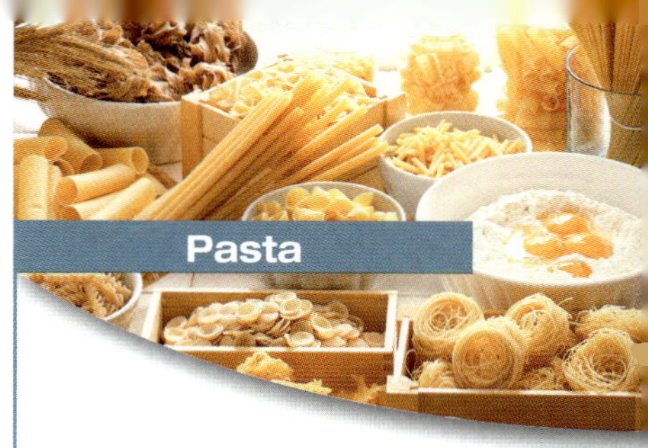

Penne pasta with salmon

Ingredients and amounts for 4 people

- ✓ 10½ oz (1⅓ cups) penne pasta
- ✓ ⅔ cup smoked salmon
- ✓ ⅓ cup heavy cream
- ✓ 1 shot-glass of vodka
- ✓ 4 tablespoons butter
- ✓ 1 sprig of chopped fennel leaves

Preparation

Cut the salmon into thin, small pieces.
Heat the butter in a pan, and cook the salmon slowly over low heat.
Add the vodka, and allow to evaporate.
While cooking the salmon, boil the pasta in abundant salted water, and drain when almost cooked al dente.
When the pasta is almost cooked, mix the salmon with the cream and fennel leaves and cook for 1 to 2 minutes.
Add the salmon sauce to the drained pasta, and serve in a large serving dish.

Bromatological evaluation per portion

Kcal	519
Protein (%)	16.8
Fats (%)	36.6
Carbohydrates (%)	46.6
Fiber (g)	2.1
Cholesterol (mg)	62.5

Valuable contents for the eye: ★★

Salmon is a fish rich in omega-3 and oligominerals, particularly astaxanthin, which it obtains from the crustaceans it eats.
Butter is made from milk and contains high quantities of saturated fatty acids.
Cream has a high fat content but is also extremely delicious.
Fennel leaves contain essential oils and flavonoids.

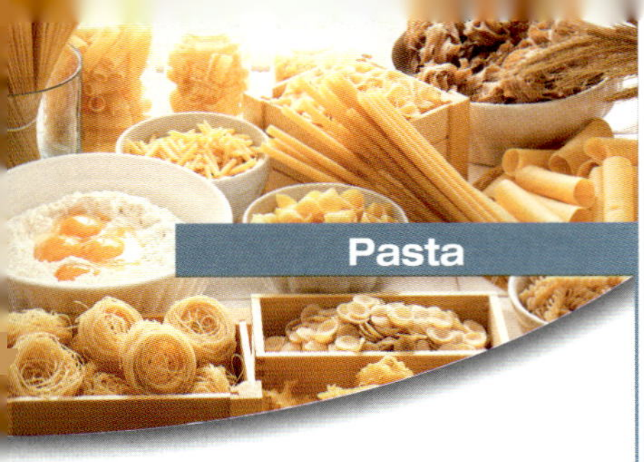

Bromatological evaluation per portion

Kcal	446
Protein (%)	22
Fats (%)	27.3
Carbohydrates (%)	50.7
Fiber (g)	3.9
Cholesterol (mg)	25

Valuable contents for the eye: ★ ★

Asparagus is rich in fiber and contains vitamins C and B6, folic acid, carotenoids, and flavonoids.

Salmon is a fish rich in omega-3 and oligominerals, particularly astaxanthin, which it obtains from the crustaceans it eats.

Wine contains small quantities of flavonoids.

Olive oil is an excellent source of unsaturated fatty acids.

Pink pepper contains essential oils, tannin and flavonoids.

Penne or sedani pasta with asparagus and salmon

Ingredients and amounts for 4 people

- ✓ 10½ oz (1⅓ cups) ridged penne or sedani pasta
- ✓ 10½ oz (1⅓ cups) soft asparagus tips
- ✓ ⅔ cups smoked salmon
- ✓ ½ glass white wine
- ✓ 10 to 12 pink peppercorns
- ✓ 2 tablespoons extra virgin olive oil
- ✓ salt to taste

Preparation

Cook the pasta al dente. Drain, and add a small amount of oil; allow it to cool.

While the pasta is cooking, cut the salmon into strips.

Pour oil into a pan, heat, and add the asparagus tips; pour the white wine into the pan, allow the wine to evaporate, add a ladleful of water, and cook. Blend until the sauce has a creamy consistency.

Pour the asparagus sauce over the pasta and mix; add the salmon and the pink peppercorns.

Mix and serve.

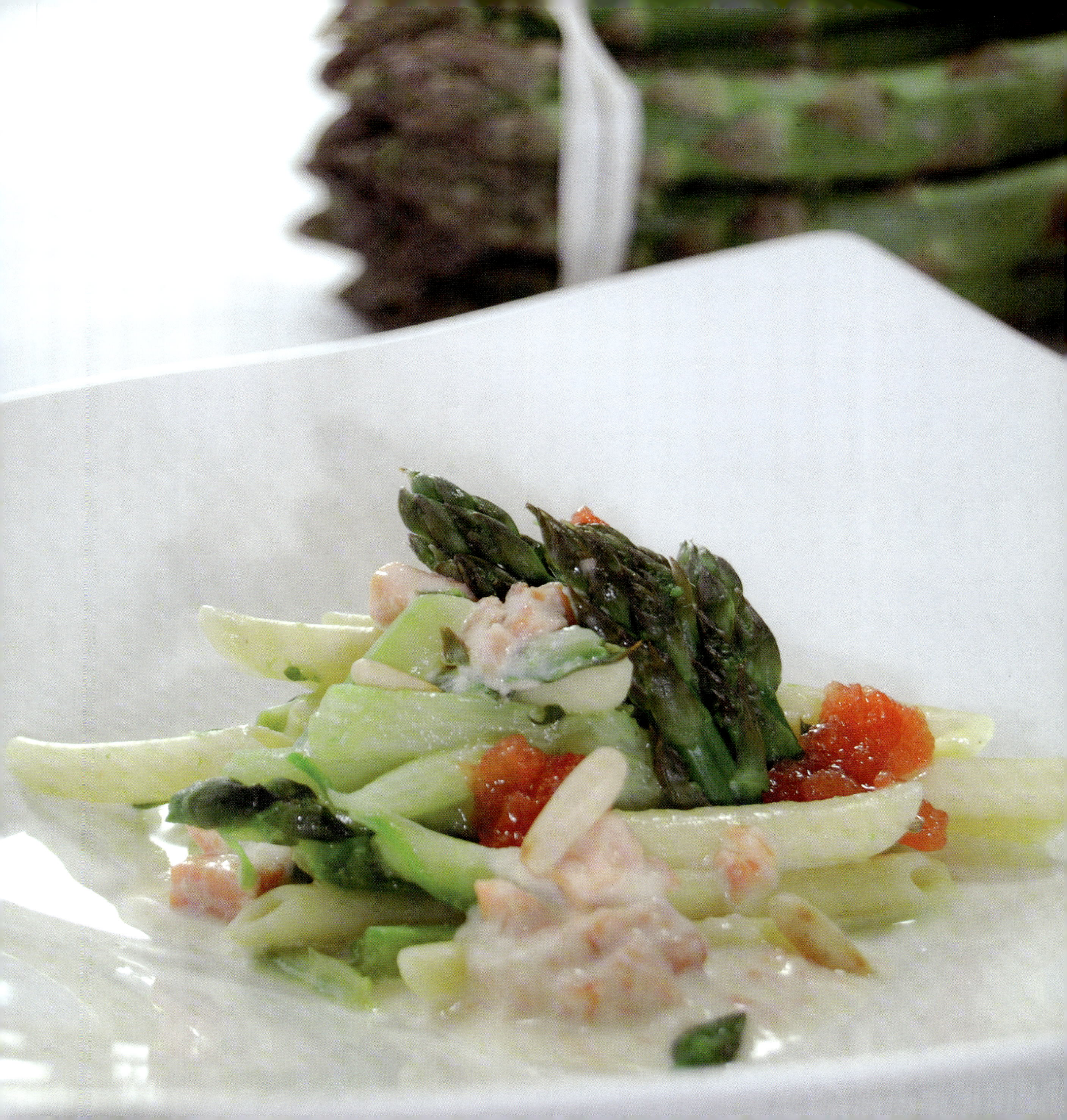

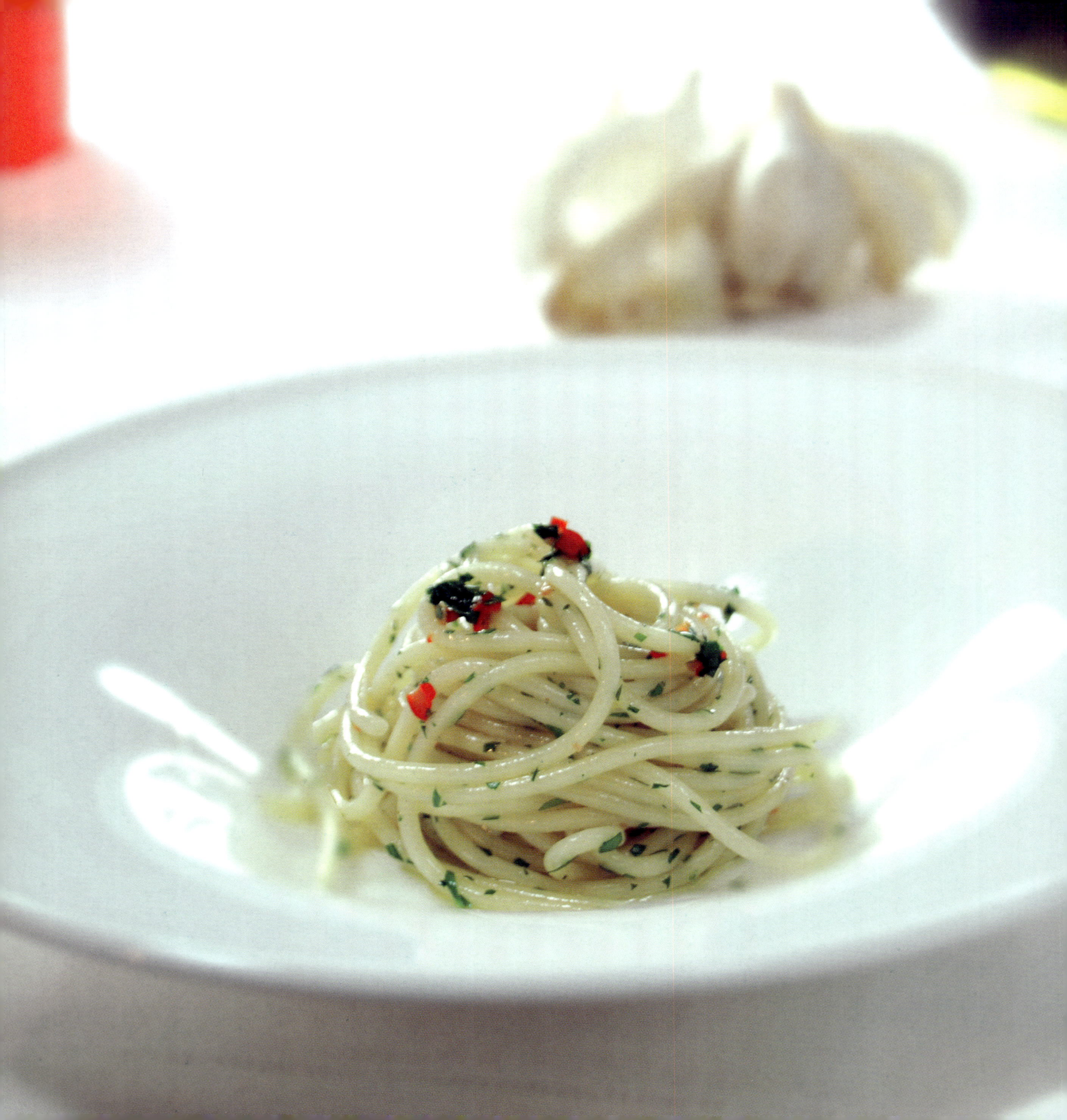

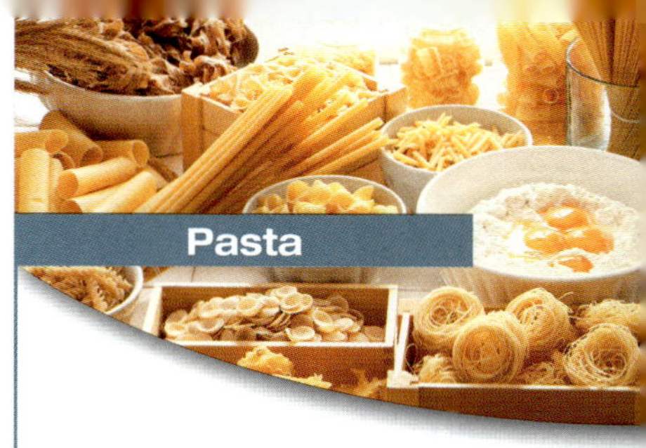

Spaghetti with **garlic, oil,** and **chili pepper**

Ingredients and amounts for 4 people

- ✓ 10½ oz (1⅓ cups) spaghetti
- ✓ 8 tablespoons extra virgin olive oil
- ✓ 2 cloves of garlic
- ✓ 1 fresh red chili pepper
- ✓ 1 sprig of parsley, chopped fine
- ✓ 1 teaspoon white wine
- ✓ salt to taste

Preparation

Pour the oil into a pan; add the garlic and chili pepper.
Heat, and as soon as the garlic shows signs of frying, take off the heat and interrupt the cooking with a dash of white wine.
Add the parsley and a pinch of salt.
Cook the pasta al dente, and drain.
Pour the pasta into the pan, and heat. Mix with the oil, garlic, and chili pepper mixture for approximately 1 minute.
Serve hot.

Bromatological evaluation per portion

Kcal	352
Protein (%)	10.2
Fats (%)	28.5
Carbohydrates (%)	61.3
Fiber (g)	2.6
Cholesterol (mg)	0

Valuable contents for the eye: ★

Garlic contains selenium, zinc, and alline, which is responsible for the taste and the penetrating, persistent odor of garlic. When alline is transformed into allicine, it has an antibacterial action and it lowers cholesterol levels and blood pressure.
Chili peppers contain capsaicin, which makes them spicy; they also contain carotenoids and flavonoids.
Olive oil is an excellent source of unsaturated fatty acids.

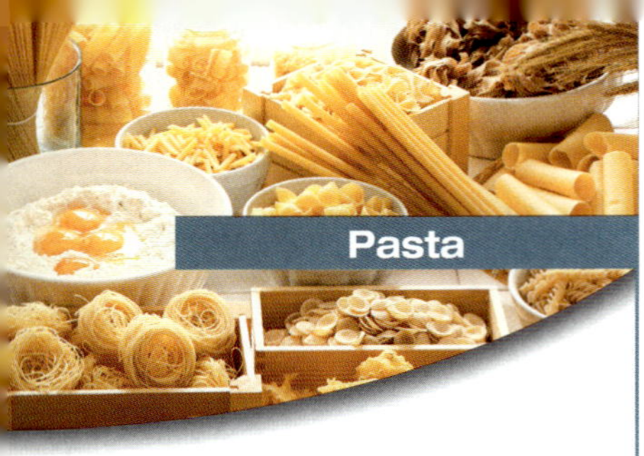

Spaghetti with mullet roe

Bromatological evaluation per portion

Kcal	426
Protein (%)	14.9
Fats (%)	34.3
Carbohydrates (%)	50.8
Fiber (g)	2.2
Cholesterol (mg)	88

Valuable contents for the eye: ★

Mullet roe has a high omega-3 content, but also contains a large quantity of salt and cholesterol.

Olive oil is an excellent source of unsaturated fatty acids.

Lemon contains high quantities of vitamin C, β-carotene, and flavonoids (particularly in the pith or albedo, underneath the peel).

Chili peppers contain capsaicin, which makes them spicy; they also contain carotenoids and flavonoids.

Garlic contains selenium, zinc, and alline, which is responsible for the taste and the penetrating, persistent odor of garlic. When alline is transformed into allicine, it has an antibacterial action, and it lowers cholesterol levels and blood pressure.

Ingredients and amounts for 4 people

- ✓ 10½ oz (1⅓ cups) spaghetti
- ✓ ⅓ cup dried mullet roe
- ✓ ½ clove of garlic, crushed
- ✓ 1 lemon, carefully washed
- ✓ 4 tablespoons extra virgin olive oil
- ✓ salt and pepper to taste
- ✓ 1 dry chili pepper, crushed

Preparation

Grate the mullet roe and the lemon zest into a bowl. Add the garlic to taste and a small amount of chili pepper and high-quality extra virgin oil. Cook the pasta al dente in abundant salted water. While cooking, remove a ladleful of the boiling water and add to the bowl; mix well until the oil and the roe are fully blended.
Drain the pasta, and pour into the bowl.
Mix well and serve.

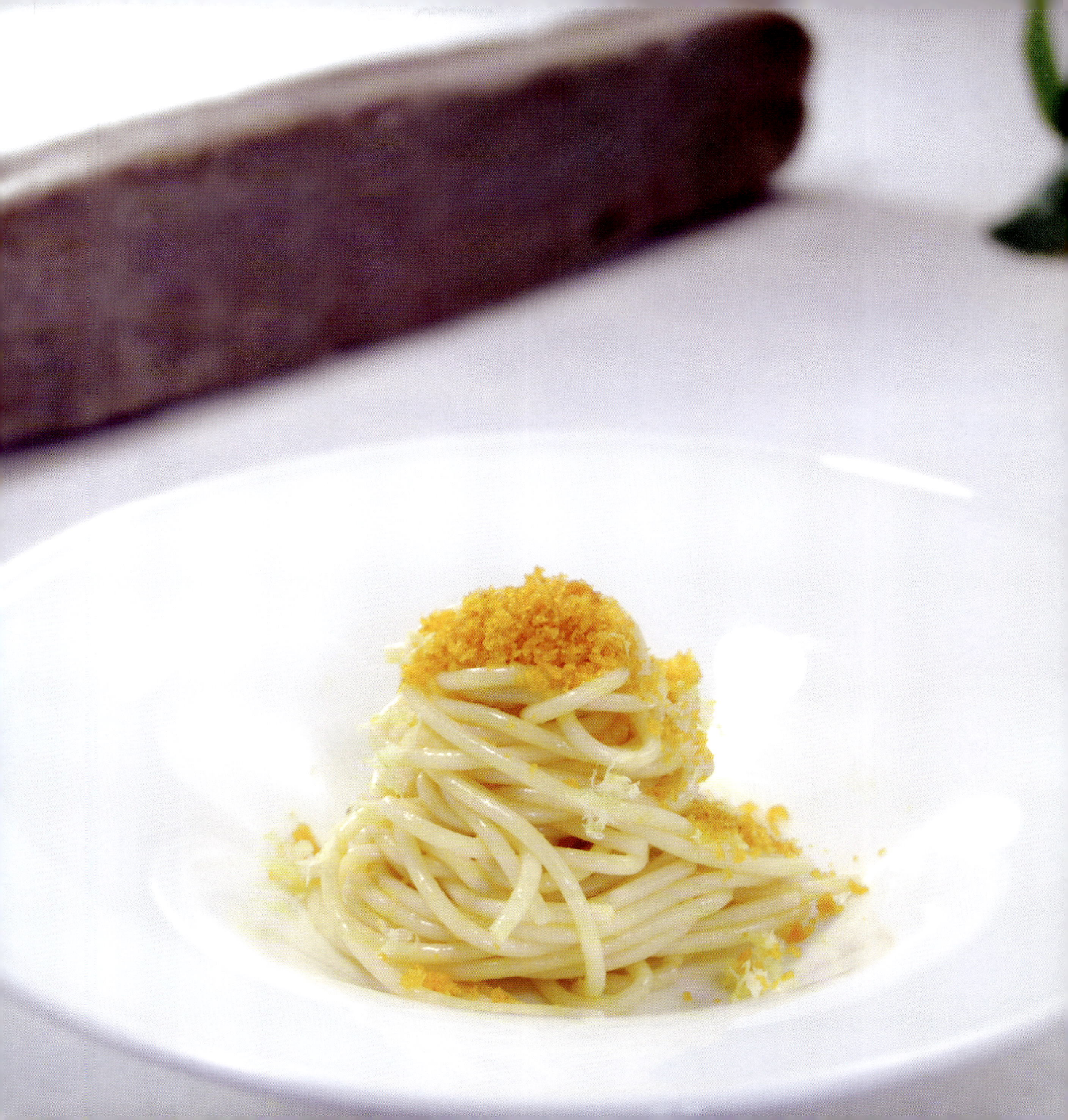

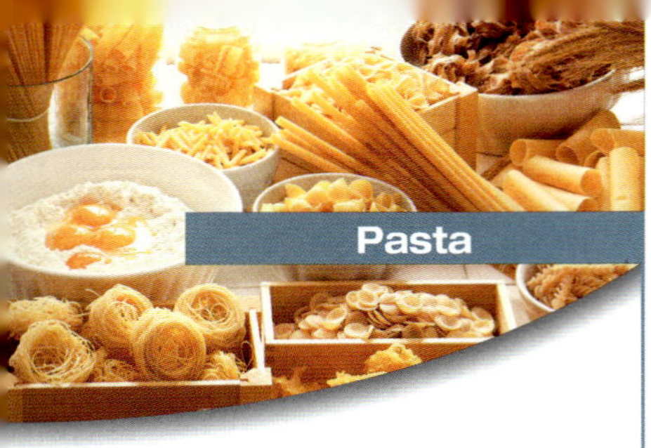

Bromatological evaluation per portion

Kcal	488
Protein (%)	13
Fats (%)	41.7
Carbohydrates (%)	45.3
Fiber (g)	2.1
Cholesterol (mg)	112.5

Valuable contents for the eye: ★

Caviar contains a large quantity of sodium and cholesterol, but also a large quantity of protein, iron, and particularly selenium.

Butter is made from milk and contains high quantities of saturated fatty acids.

Cream has a high fat content but is also extremely delicious.

Lemon contains high quantities of vitamin C, β-carotene, and also flavonoids (particularly in the pith or albedo, underneath the peel).

Spaghetti with caviar

Ingredients and amounts for 4 people

✓ 10½ oz (1⅓ cups) spaghetti

✓ 7 tablespoons black caviar, hard, small grain

✓ 3½ tablespoons heavy cream

✓ 3½ tablespoons butter

✓ cracked black pepper to taste

✓ juice of ½ lemon

Preparation

Cook the spaghetti al dente; drain and pour into a bowl.
Add the cream and butter, and mix well.
Add the caviar and the pepper, and mix well.
Drizzle with the lemon juice, and serve.

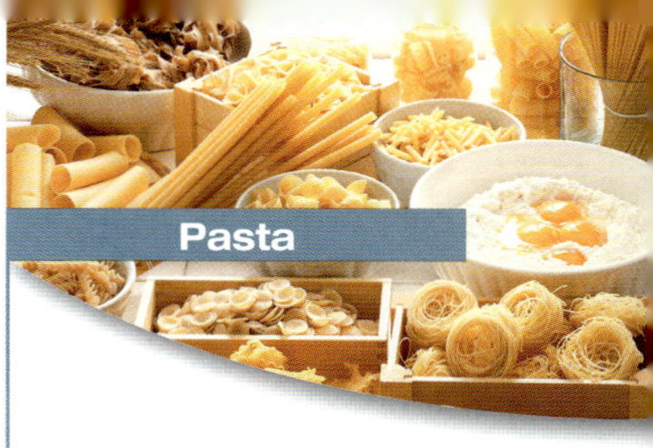

Spaghetti with tuna

Ingredients and amounts for 4 people

- ✓ 10½ oz (1⅓ cups) spaghetti
- ✓ 7 oz canned tuna, with oil drained
- ✓ 6 ripe cherry tomatoes
- ✓ 8 tablespoons extra virgin olive oil
- ✓ 16 stoned olives
- ✓ 2 tablespoons desalted capers
- ✓ 1 clove of garlic
- ✓ 2 sprigs of parsley
- ✓ salt and pepper to taste

Preparation

Heat the oil with the chopped garlic. Before the garlic changes color, add the tomato, capers, and parsley. Allow to cook for 4 to 5 minutes. Add the mashed tuna and the olives cut into disks, and cook for 5 to 6 minutes.

In the meantime, cook the spaghetti al dente, drain, and add to a bowl containing the sauce and mix well.

Bromatological evaluation per portion

Kcal	591
Protein (%)	14.9
Fats (%)	47.5
Carbohydrates (%)	37.6
Fiber (g)	4.4
Cholesterol (mg)	32.5

Valuable contents for the eye: ★★

Tuna is a fish rich in protein; it contains a good quantity of omega-3.

Tomatoes are rich in vitamins and oligominerals, but particularly they contain carotenoids and are the most important source of lycopene.

Olives are rich in monounsaturated fats, vitamin E, and potassium.

Capers contain vitamins A, C, and E and also a considerable quantity of sodium.

Garlic contains selenium, zinc, and alline, which is responsible for the taste and the penetrating, persistent odor of garlic. When alline is transformed into allicine, it has an antibacterial action and it lowers cholesterol and blood pressure levels.

Parsley contains flavonoids and is also an apiol, an anti-spastic, and an anti-pyretic. It also stimulates uterine contractions.

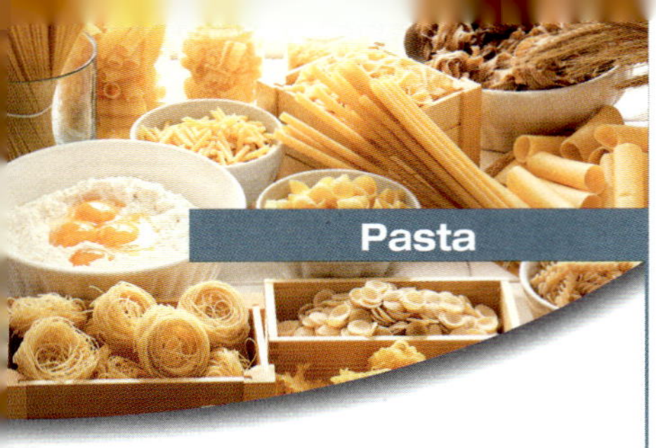

Tagliatelle pasta with radicchio

Ingredients and amounts for 4 people

- ✓ 10½ oz (1⅓ cups) egg tagliatelle or spaghetti
- ✓ 2 heads of red radicchio (or other tart radicchio)
- ✓ 1 medium-small onion
- ✓ 3½ tablespoons butter
- ✓ 1 tablespoon of extra virgin olive oil
- ✓ 3 tablespoons heavy cream
- ✓ 3½ oz pancetta, cut into fine strips
- ✓ ½ glass red wine
- ✓ 1 to 2 ripe tomatoes or 3 to 4 tablespoons fresh tomato pulp
- ✓ juice of ½ lemon
- ✓ salt and pepper to taste

Preparation

Finely slice the onion, and cook it in oil for a few minutes without browning.

Add the sliced pancetta and the sliced radicchio (only the lower part of the heads). Cook for 5 to 8 minutes.

Add the red wine, and allow it to evaporate.

Add the tomato, and cook for a further 7 to 8 minutes; add salt and pepper to taste.

Cook the pasta al dente; place into a dish, and add the remaining ingredients (cream, butter, lemon juice) and finally the sauce with the radicchio.

Mix and serve.

Bromatological evaluation per portion

Kcal	500
Protein (%)	13.9
Fats (%)	40.4
Carbohydrates (%)	45.7
Fiber (g)	4.6
Cholesterol (mg)	60

Valuable contents for the eye: ★

Egg pasta contains a greater number of nutrients than the common durum wheat pasta: eggs are rich in saturated fatty acids but also contain a good quantity of mono- and polyunsaturated fats. Unfortunately, they contain cholesterol but they are also an important source of lutein.

Radicchio contains flavonoids and vitamins A, B, and C.

Onion contains vitamin C and a good quantity of flavonoids (quercetin).

Red wine contains resveratrol and flavonoids.

Cream has a high fat content but is also extremely delicious.

Lemon contains high quantities of vitamin C, β-carotene, and flavonoids (particularly in the pith or albedo underneath the peel).

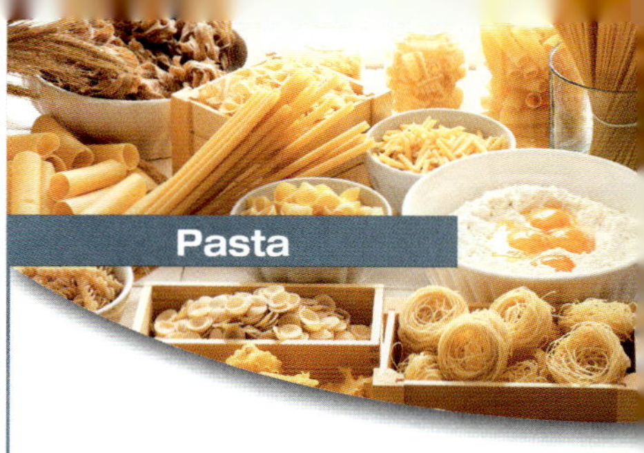

Tagliolini pasta with artichokes

Ingredients and amounts for 4 people

- ✓ 10½ oz (1⅓ cups) tagliolini pasta
- ✓ 4 to 6 artichokes, depending on the size
- ✓ 2 egg yolks
- ✓ 2 oz pecorino cheese, grated
- ✓ ½ onion
- ✓ ½ glass white wine
- ✓ 2 tablespoons butter
- ✓ 1 teaspoon oil
- ✓ salt and pepper to taste

Preparation

Prepare the artichokes by removing the external leaves, the tough parts, and any tufts in the heart; slice and place in water with a few drops of lemon juice.

Gently cook the onion in olive oil. Then, add the artichokes, salt, and pepper, and cook for a couple of minutes.

Next, add the white wine and a ladleful of hot water; cook for 15 to 20 minutes.

Beat the egg yolks with the peccorino cheese and butter in a preheated bowl.

Pour the hot pasta into the bowl and mix well.

Add the artichokes and the remainder of the cheese.

Serve immediately.

Bromatological evaluation per portion

Kcal	502
Protein (%)	14.8
Fats (%)	37.8
Carbohydrates (%)	47.4
Fiber (g)	4.8
Cholesterol (mg)	381

Valuable contents for the eye: ★

Artichokes are rich in fiber, mineral salts, and folic acid.

Eggs are rich in saturated fatty acids but also contain a good quantity of mono- and polyunsaturated fats. Unfortunately, they contain cholesterol, but they are also an important source of lutein.

Sheep's milk cheese has a strong taste and is rich in calcium.

Onion contains vitamin C and a good quantity of flavonoids (quercetin).

Wine contains small amounts of flavonoids.

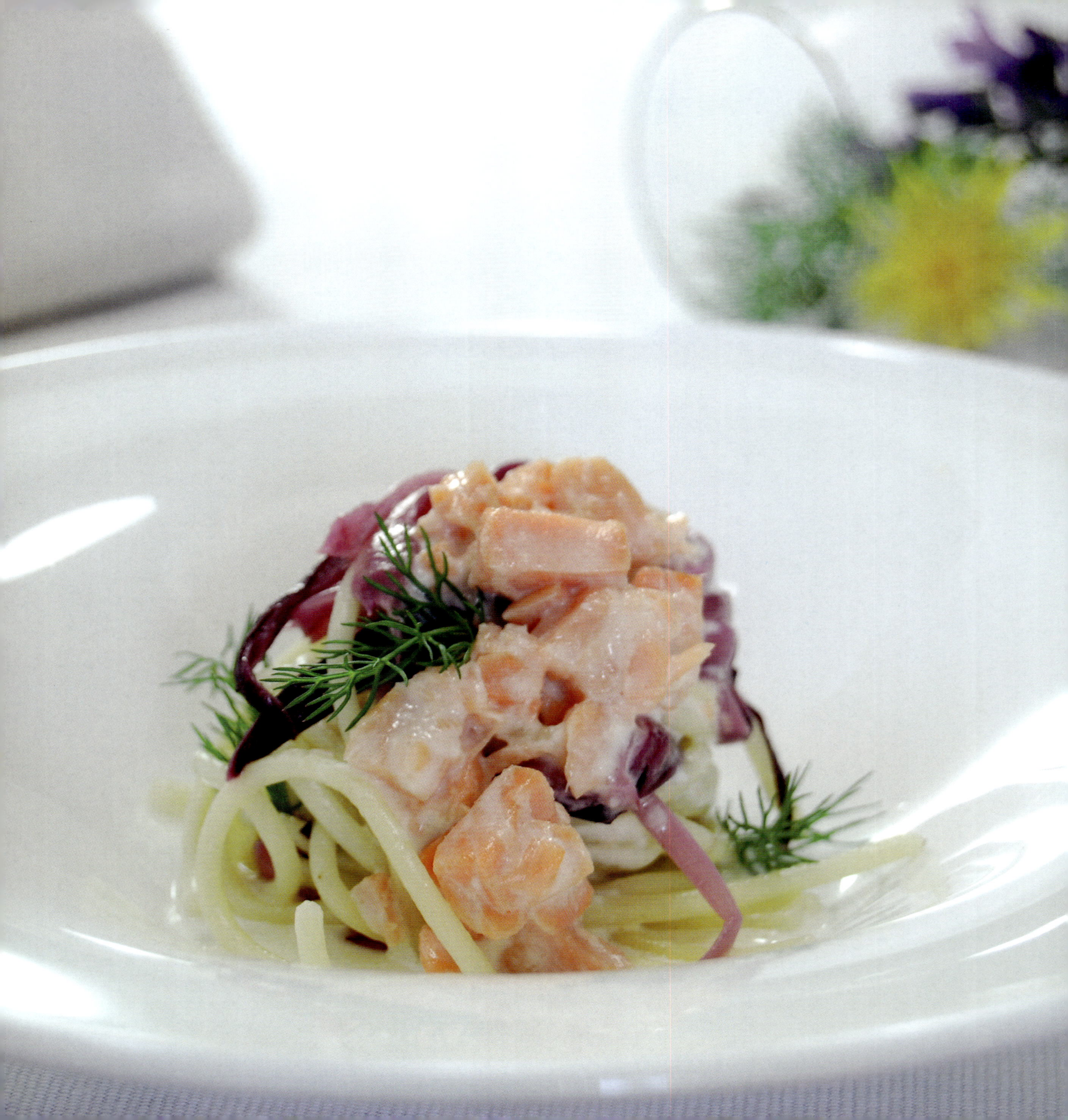

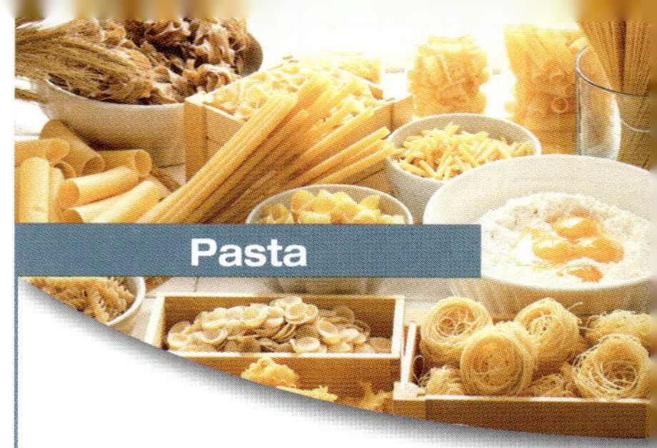

Tagliatelle pasta with radicchio and smoked salmon

Ingredients and amounts for 4 people

- ✓ 10½ oz (1⅓ cups) egg tagliatelle or spaghetti
- ✓ 3 heads of radicchio
- ✓ ⅔ cups smoked salmon
- ✓ 3½ tablespoons butter
- ✓ 4 tablespoons extra virgin olive oil
- ✓ 2 tablespoons cream
- ✓ 1 sprig of parsley
- ✓ 1½ oz (2¾ tablespoons) Parmesan cheese
- ✓ cracked black pepper
- ✓ salt to taste

Preparation

Cut the radicchio into sections 1 inch long; cook in a pan with the butter and the oil for 3 to 4 minutes.
Add the salmon cut into strips, and cook over high heat.
Add the chopped parsley and cream.
Cook the tagliatelle in abundant salted water, drain, and pour into the pan with the radicchio; cook over high heat for 2 minutes.
When ready for serving, sprinkle with Parmesan and cracked black pepper.

Bromatological evaluation per portion

Kcal	624
Protein (%)	16.9
Fats (%)	46.5
Carbohydrates (%)	36.6
Fiber (g)	4.6
Cholesterol (mg)	71.6

Valuable contents for the eye: ★★

Radicchio contains flavonoids and vitamins A, B, and C.
Salmon is a fish rich in omega-3 and oligominerals, particularly astaxanthin, which it obtains from the crustaceans it eats.
Parmesan cheese is rich in easily digestible protein, is low in fat, and contains vitamin A and some vitamins of the B group.
Cream has a high fat content but is also extremely delicious.
Egg pasta contains a greater number of nutrients than the common durum wheat pasta: eggs are rich in saturated fatty acids but also contain a good quantity of mono- and polyunsaturated fats. Unfortunately, they contain cholesterol but they are also an important source of lutein.

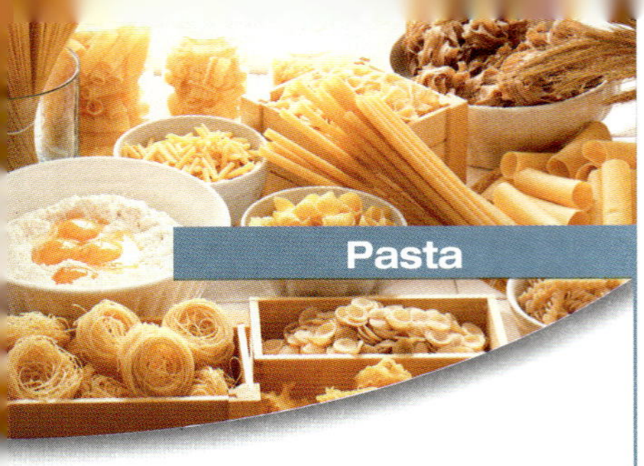

Tagliolini pasta with asparagus

Bromatological evaluation per portion

Kcal	487
Protein (%)	12.9
Fats (%)	38
Carbohydrates (%)	49.1
Fiber (g)	3.5
Cholesterol (mg)	84.3

Valuable contents for the eye: ★★

Asparagus is rich in fiber and contains vitamins B6 and C, folic acid, carotenoids, and flavonoids.

Pine nuts are very small but rich in flavonoids and omega-6.

Parmesan cheese is rich in easily digestible protein, is low in fat, and contains vitamin A and some vitamins of the B group.

Olive oil is an excellent source of unsaturated fatty acids.

Marjoram is rich in essential oils.

Ingredients and amounts for 4 people

✓ 10½ oz (1⅓ cups) tagliolini or linguine pasta
✓ 12 asparagus shoots
✓ 1½ oz (2¾ tablespoons) grated Parmesan cheese
✓ ¾ oz (1½ tablespoons) pine nuts
✓ 1 sprig of marjoram
✓ 6 tablespoons extra virgin olive oil

Preparation

Wash and peel the asparagus; remove the woody part of the stalk.
Cook the tagliolini pasta al dente in abundant boiling salted water along with half the asparagus tips (in the same water). The tips must remain firm and crunchy.
While the pasta is cooking, prepare the sauce by cooking the remainder of the asparagus in water; then, in a bowl, blend together with the Parmesan cheese, pine nuts, marjoram, and oil.
Add 2 tablespoons of the boiling water used to cook the pasta to make the sauce more liquidy.
Mix the pasta and the sauce.
Serve immediately.

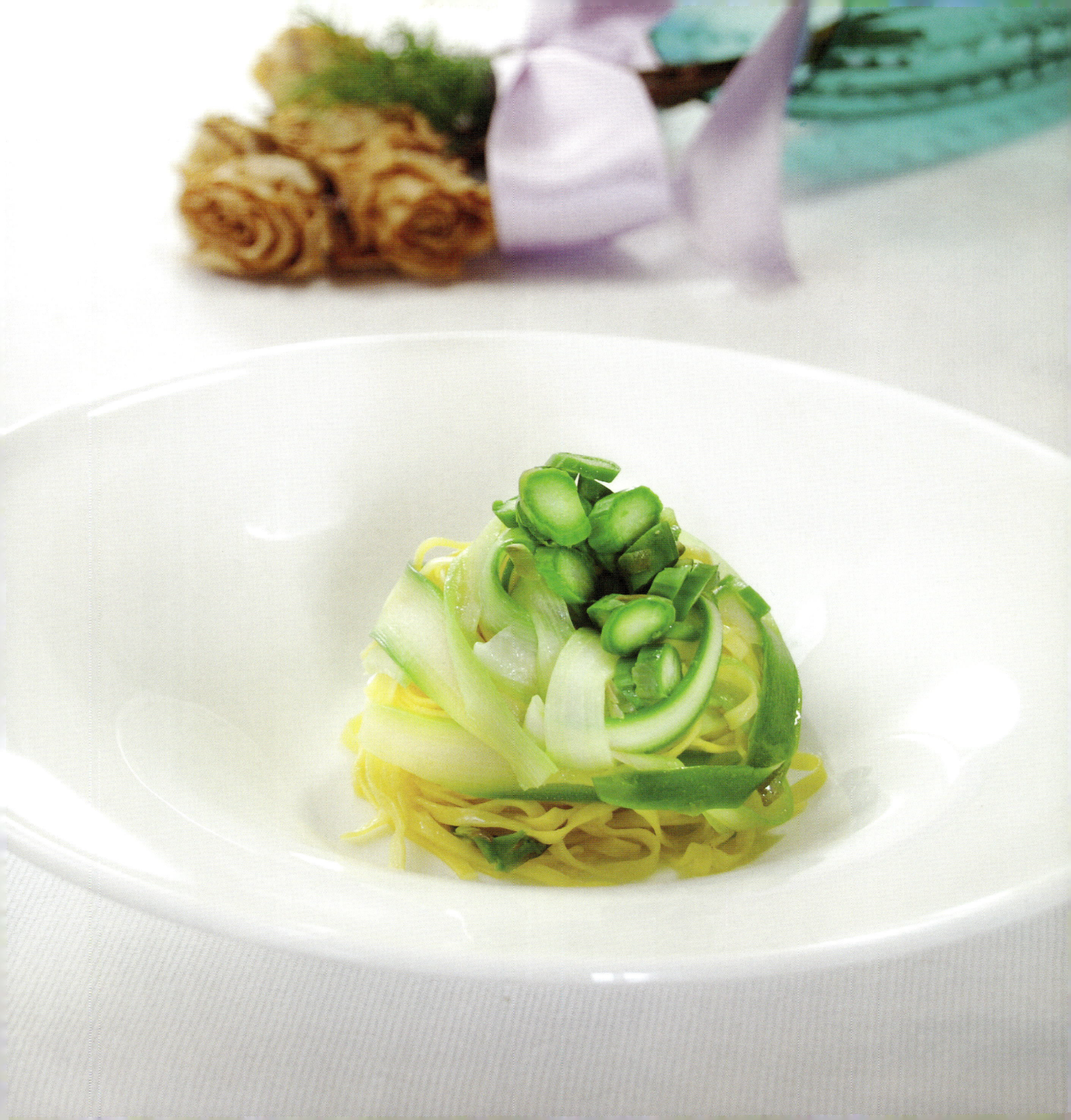

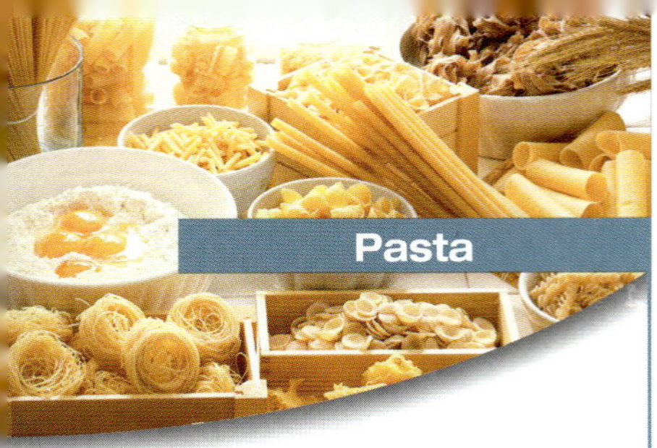

Gnocchi di patate (tiny potato dumplings)

Ingredients and amounts for 4 people

- ✓ 28 oz (3½ cups) yellow potatoes
- ✓ a pinch of salt
- ✓ 1 egg
- ✓ ¾ cup flour
- ✓ salt to taste

Preparation

Boil the potatoes, and peel them when they are still hot. Mash them thoroughly, and then add salt.

Add the flour and the egg; knead on a floured cutting board until a soft compact mixture is obtained.

The ratio of potato to flour depends largely on the consistency of the potatoes.

Split into portions and hand-roll into long "sausages" as thick as a finger.

Cut the "sausages" into ¾ to 1¼ inch pieces; rub each piece over the back of a dinner fork to create ridges.

Place the flour-covered dumplings onto a tray or, better still, onto a damp tea towel, taking care not to overlap them.

Fill a large saucepan with water, and bring to the boil; add 8 to 10 dumplings at a time, and when they rise to the surface, skim them from the surface and place them on a plate.

They can be served with meat sauce, gorgonzola cream, melted butter and grated cheese, or fresh tomato sauce.

Bromatological evaluation per portion

Kcal	504
Protein (%)	8.3
Fats (%)	43
Carbohydrates (%)	48.7
Fiber (g)	3.5
Cholesterol (mg)	67.9

Valuable contents for the eye: ★

Made from flour, eggs, and potatoes, these dumplings are very nutritious.

Potatoes are rich in starch and contain considerable quantities of potassium and vitamins C and B5.

The important protein in **flour** is gluten; flour also contains a varying amount of fiber depending on the quality of the flour, and a large quantity of carbohydrate.

Eggs are rich in saturated fatty acids but also contain a good quantity of mono- and polyunsaturated fats Unfortunately, they contain cholesterol but they are also an important source of lutein.

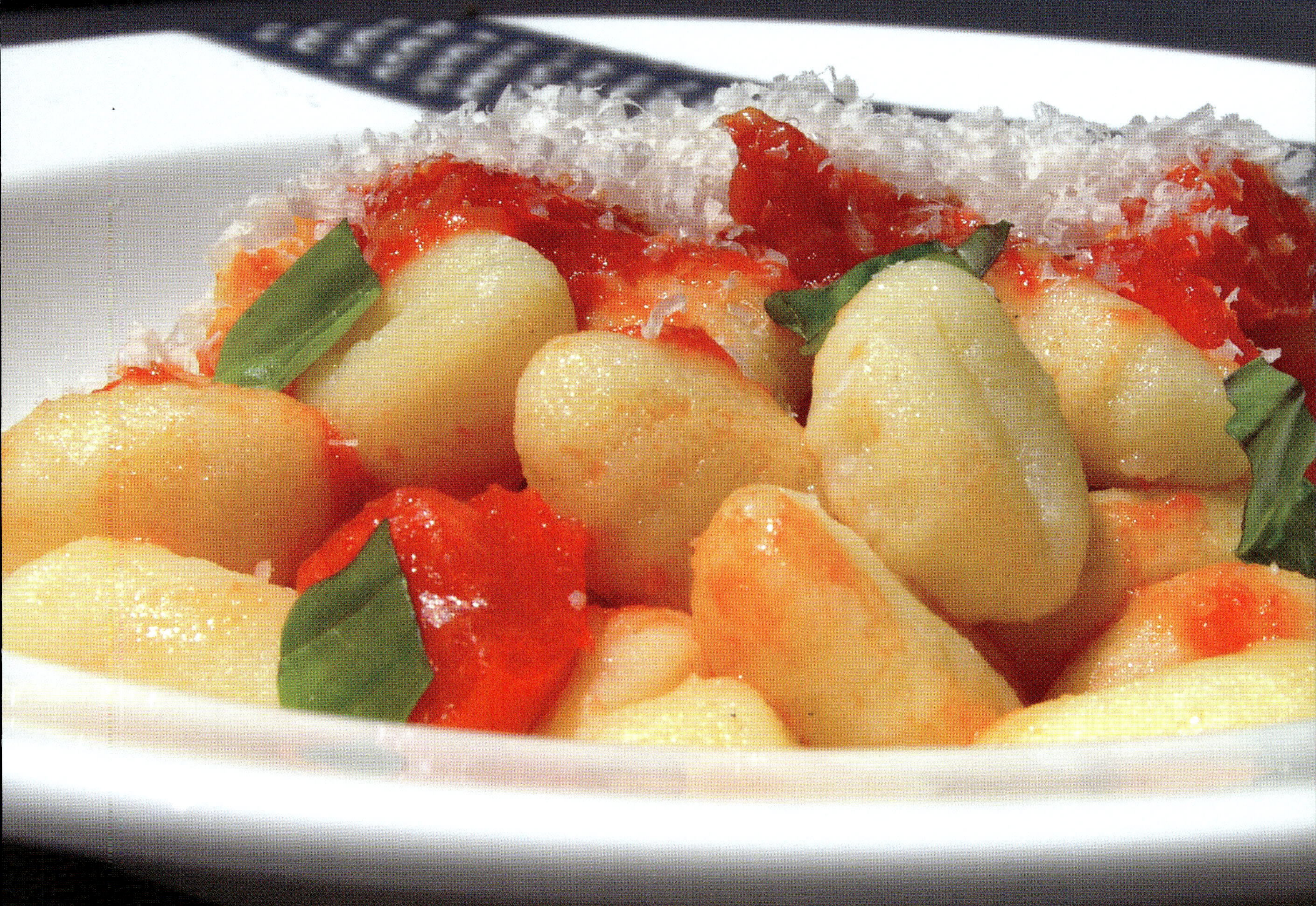

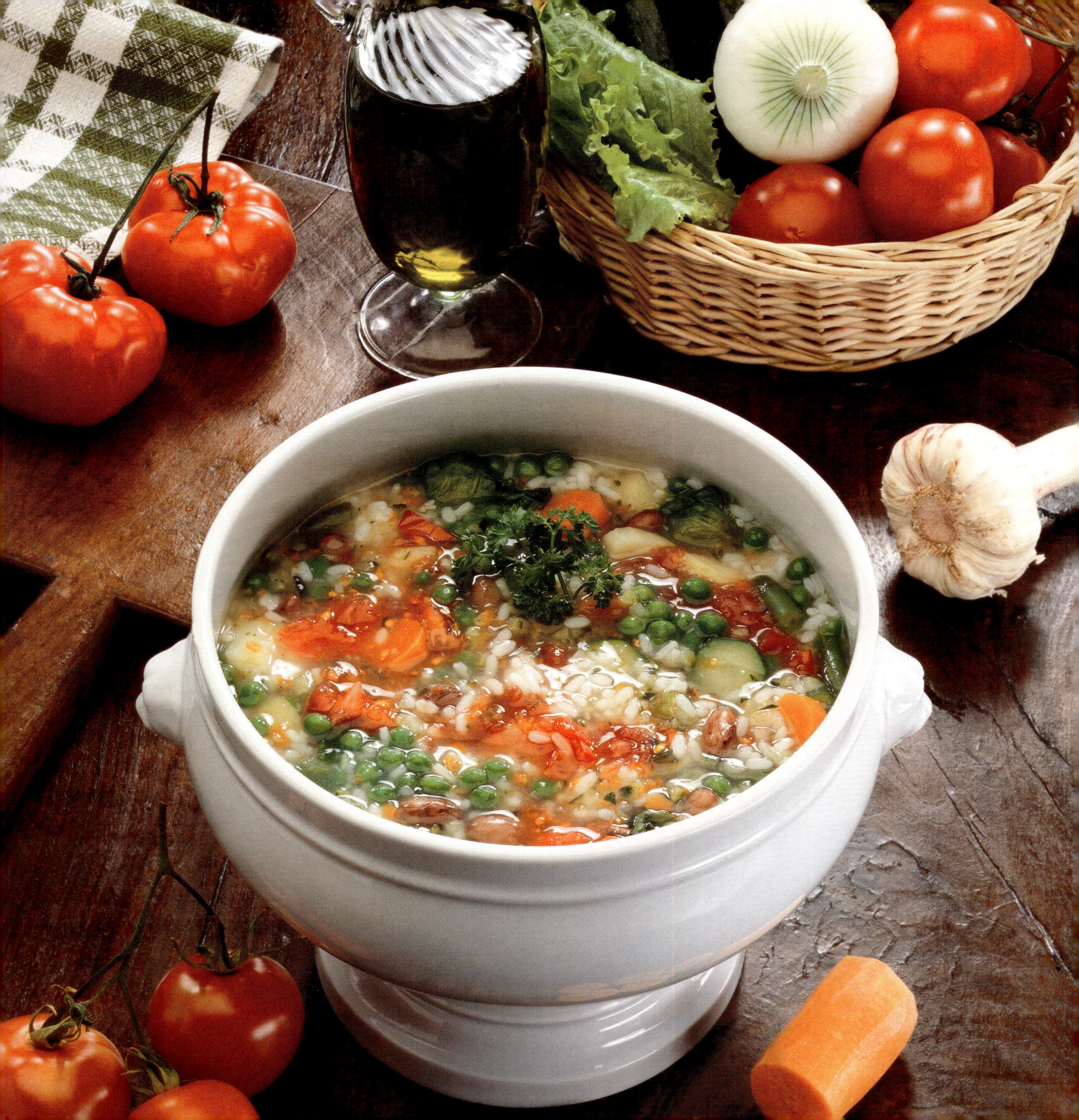

Soups

Soup is made by boiling meat, fish, or vegetables in water with spices, herbs, and salt. It can be described as something halfway between a meal and a condiment. In actual fact, it can be eaten on its own or used to season some types of fresh pastas or risotto and pasta dishes.

Vegetable soup is almost free from calories and fat; however, a meat- or fish-based soup can be very low in calories (particularly when the top layer that contains the dissolved fats has been skimmed off). A bowl of hot soup has proved to have relaxing properties on the nervous system; it is recommended to combat episodes of tiredness, listlessness, and fever and is advised generally when a liquid or low-calorie diet is prescribed.

Stock cubes or granules should not be used in the preparation of soup because these contain large quantities of flavor enhancers such as monosodium glutamate, inosinate, disodium guanylate, and fat; they also contain a high level of salt (sodium chloride).

Soup is used as a base to produce dishes that contain a number of other fairly high-calorie ingredients such as meat, bacon, mushrooms, and cheese, alongside vegetables and legumes, which are almost always present.

Minestrone consists of a mixture of vegetables and fats (oil and butter) simply cooked in boiling water. In any case, minestrones will also contain a variety of vegetables, both the simple ones and other and little-known ingredients (such as the potato, chicory, pumpkin, or cucumber).

Frequently, many minestrones have pasta or rice added just before the mealtime; preferably, this ingredient is cooked separately and mixed in at the last minute.

Soups are more ancient preparations: characteristically, they are served with slices of dry bread, which can also be toasted; the bread is dipped into the liquid or semi-liquid preparation, which frequently contains legumes; these soups are based on a base of meat, poultry, fish, giblets, and eggs.

Soups, pasta dishes, and minestrones have excellent nutritional characteristics for a number of reasons: they are generally very filling and low in calories (naturally if we exclude the richer and more elaborate recipes); they can be extremely varied and are available in a wide range of flavors; and they add a considerable quantity of vegetables to the diet, with the intrinsic vitamin, mineral salt, and fiber content.

The number of calories associated with these dishes can be increased by adding legumes, potatoes, cereals, and oil; when pasta or rice are added, the dish can be considered to be more or less complete in nutritional terms.

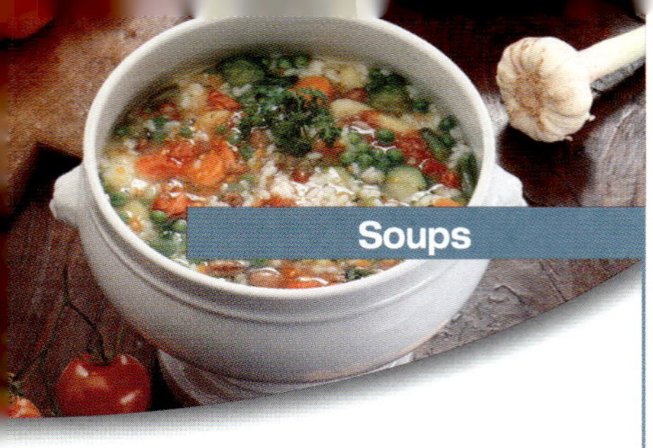

Bromatological evaluation per portion (250 ml)

Kcal	17
Protein (%)	62.8
Fats (%)	25.7
Carbohydrates (%)	11.5
Fiber (g)	0
Cholesterol (mg)	0

Valuable contents for the eye: ★

Beef broth contains mineral salts and simple proteins such as albumin, and is low in fat.

Beef broth

Ingredients and amounts for 4 people

✓ 2¼ lbs mixed cuts of beef
✓ 2¼ lbs beef bones
✓ 1 carrot
✓ 1 onion
✓ 1 stalk of celery
✓ 2 to 3 bay leaves
✓ 2 cloves of garlic
✓ 1 leek
✓ 1 ripe tomato
✓ 1 sprig of parsley
✓ 2 to 3 cloves
✓ 3 to 4 liters (¾ to 1 gallon) of water
✓ salt and black pepper to taste

Preparation

Pour the water and all the ingredients into a large stock pot and boil gently for approximately 2 hours, skimming the surface foam every 10 minutes.

Strain through a sieve, and let cool.

Place in the refrigerator overnight; remove the layer of fat that solidifies on the surface.

Note: Beef broth can be used for the preparation of risotto, soups, and other dishes. It can be stored in the freezer.

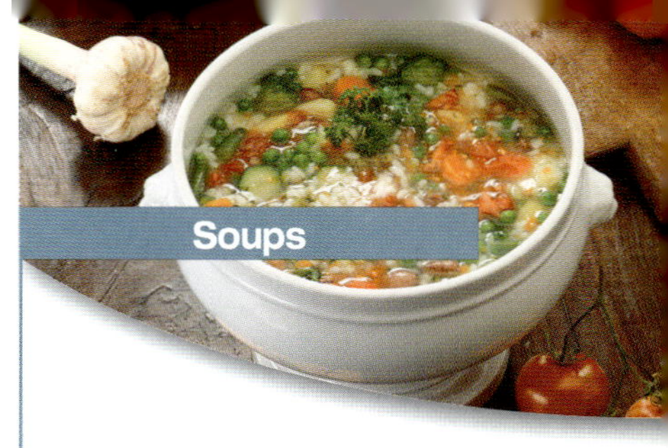

Fish broth

Ingredients and amounts for 4 people

- ✓ 1⅓-1½ lbs mixed fresh fish, cleaned and cut into pieces (sea bass, bass, hake, plaice)
- ✓ 1 carrot
- ✓ 1 onion
- ✓ 2 stalks of celery
- ✓ 2 ripe tomatoes
- ✓ 2 cloves of garlic
- ✓ 1 bunch of parsley
- ✓ 1 liter (33.8 oz) water
- ✓ salt and pepper to taste

Preparation

Fill a large saucepan with water. Add the fish and boil for a couple of minutes to clean the fish.

Fill a clean saucepan with new, clean water and add all the ingredients, including the fish that was scalded earlier.

Cook slowly for 1 hour.

Strain the broth through a sieve.

Note: Fish broth can be used for fish-based risotto.

Bromatological evaluation per portion (250 ml)

Kcal	16
Protein (%)	60
Fats (%)	24
Carbohydrates (%)	16
Fiber (g)	0
Cholesterol (mg)	0

Valuable contents for the eye: ★ ★

Fish broth contains mineral salts, simple proteins such as albumin, and a few fats, including omega-3.

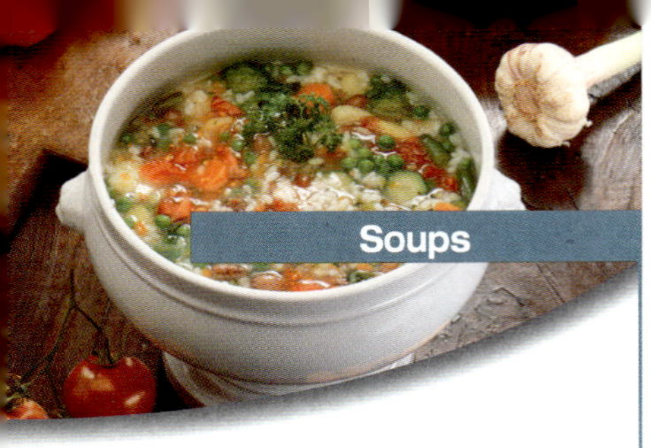

Bromatological evaluation per portion (250 ml)

Kcal	12
Protein (%)	24
Fats (%)	72
Carbohydrates (%)	4
Fiber (g)	0
Cholesterol (mg)	0

Valuable contents for the eye: ★

Vegetable broth contains mineral salts and water-soluble vitamins; it preserves some but not of all the beneficial substances contained in vegetables. The temperature can denature some of the vitamins.

Vegetable broth

Ingredients and amounts for 4 people

- ✓ 2 to 3 leeks
- ✓ 4 carrots
- ✓ 2 scallions or 1 onion
- ✓ 3 to 4 stalks of celery
- ✓ ½ bay leaf
- ✓ 2 liters (67.6 oz) water
- ✓ salt and pepper to taste

Preparation

Place all the ingredients in a saucepan, and boil for approximately 1 hour.

Strain through a sieve to filter.

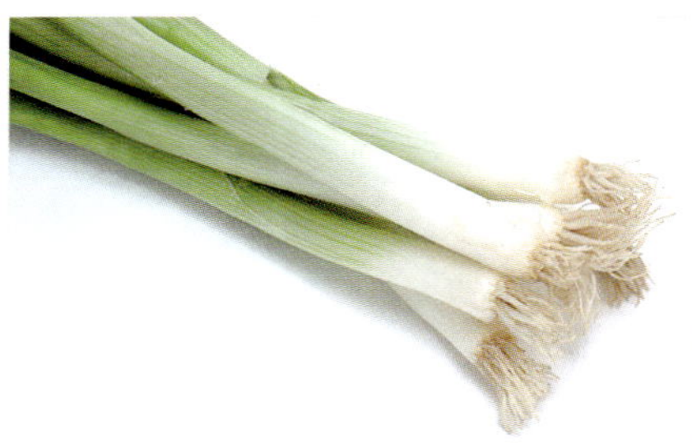

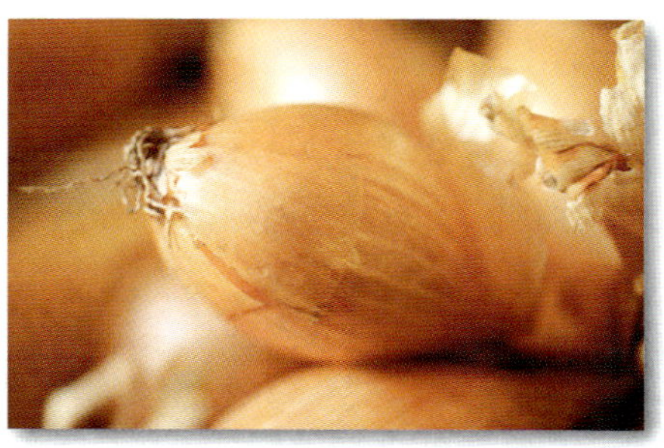
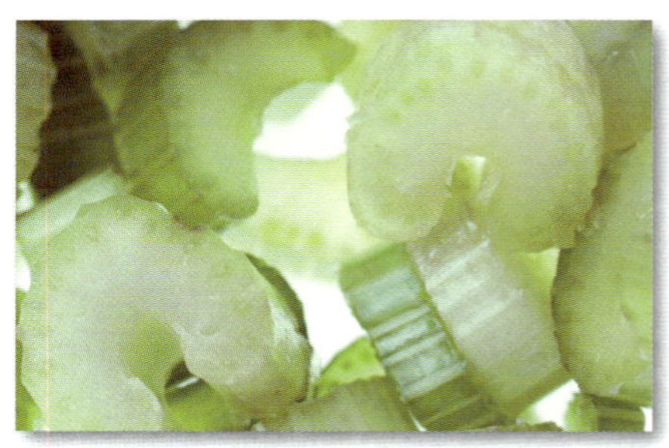

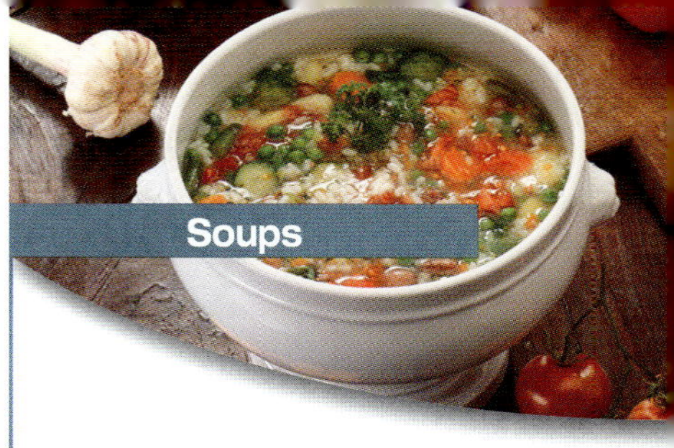

Cream of Belgian endive lettuce soup

Ingredients and amounts for 4 people

- ✓ 10½ oz (1⅓ cups) Belgian endive lettuce
- ✓ 1 potato
- ✓ 4 spring onions
- ✓ 7 oz milk
- ✓ 7 oz water
- ✓ grated nutmeg
- ✓ 2 tablespoons oil

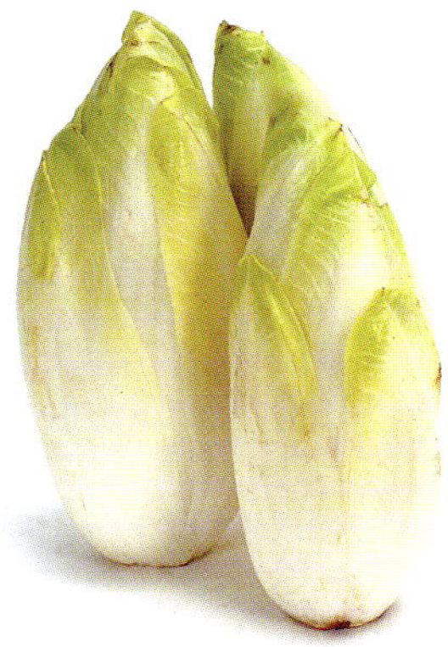

Preparation

Chop the lettuce, onions, and potato.
Cook in a pot with some oil.
Add salt, and cook until the potato is cooked.
Add the water, milk, and some grated nutmeg.
Cook for another 5 minutes; blend well to produce a smooth cream.
Serve hot.

Bromatological evaluation per portion

Kcal	125
Protein (%)	11.5
Fats (%)	45.9
Carbohydrates (%)	42.6
Fiber (g)	2
Cholesterol (mg)	3.5

Valuable contents for the eye: ★ ★ ★

Endive lettuce is an excellent source of fiber and carotenoids (lutein).
Potatoes are rich in starch and contain potassium and vitamins C and B5.
Milk (particularly whole milk) has a good balance of sugars, fats, and proteins; it contains high quantities of calcium and phosphorous, but particularly fat-soluble anti-oxidant vitamins and water-soluble vitamins.
Spring onions contain vitamin C and a good quantity of flavonoids (quercetin).
Nutmeg contains essential oil and has digestive properties.

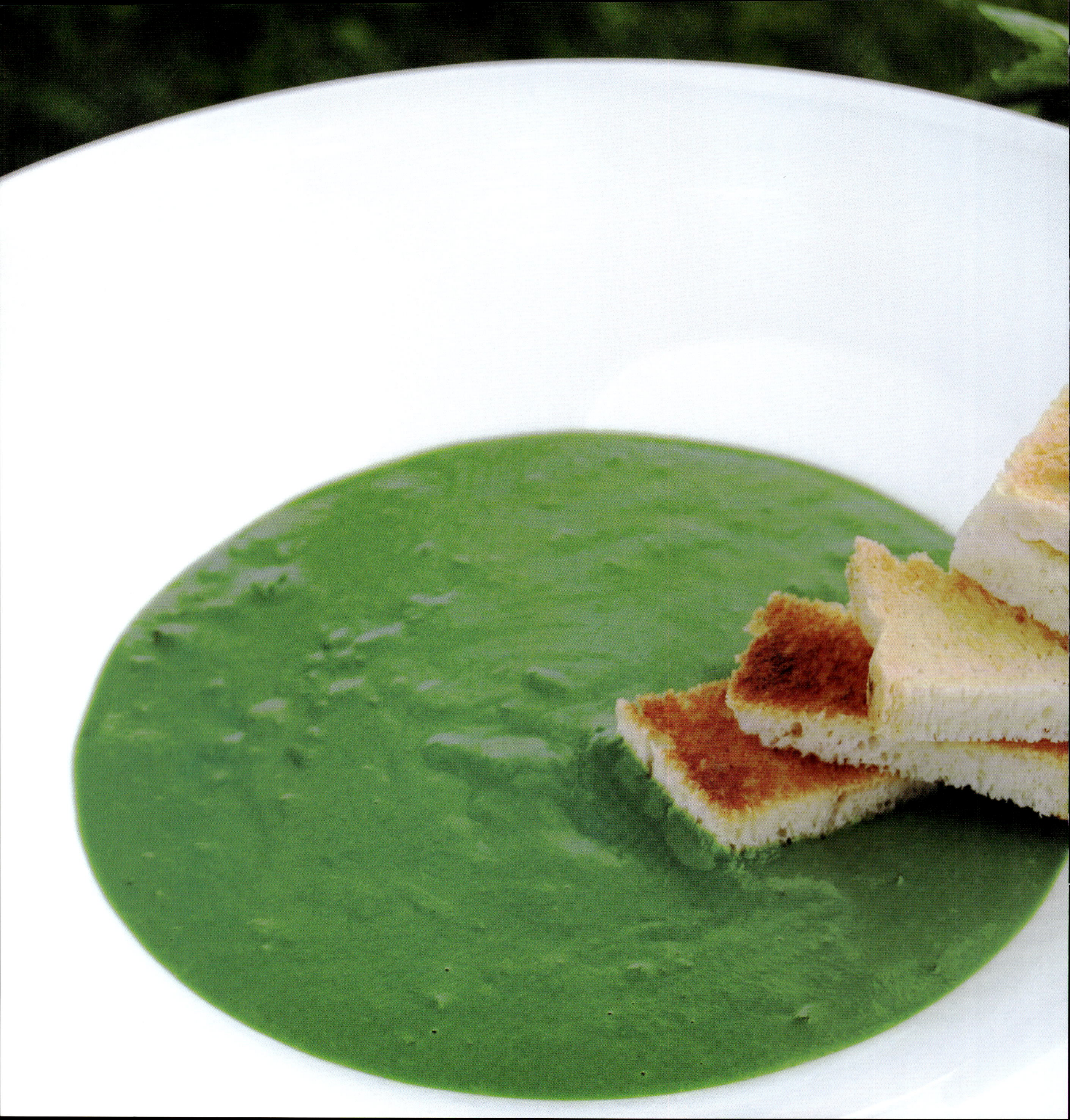

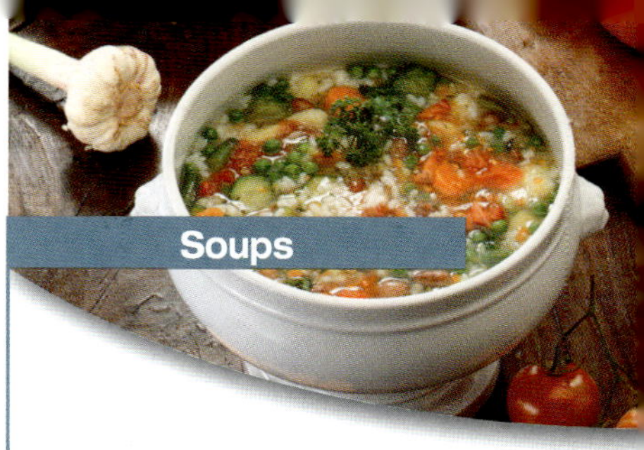

Cream of pea soup with lettuce and spinach

Ingredients and amounts for 4 people

- ✓ 1 cup peas
- ✓ 5 oz (2/3 cup) lettuce
- ✓ 5 oz (2/3 cup) spinach
- ✓ ½ liter (16.9 oz) vegetable broth
- ✓ ½ an onion
- ✓ 2 to 3 mint leaves
- ✓ 5 oz (2/3 cup) grated Parmesan cheese
- ✓ 2¾ tablespoons butter
- ✓ salt and pepper to taste

Preparation

Chop the onion, and soften in a saucepan with some melted butter. Add the peas and salt, and let everything blend for a few minutes. Pour in the boiling vegetable broth, and cook until the peas are soft. Finely slice the lettuce and the spinach and add to the peas.
Blend, add salt to taste, add a pat of butter, and cook for a few minutes.
Just before serving, add the grated Parmesan cheese, some mint leaves,and ground black pepper to taste.
Serve with toasted bread; rub the bread with mint leaves to give the bread a pleasant flavor.

Bromatological evaluation per portion

Kcal	248
Protein (%)	24.8
Fats (%)	69.5
Carbohydrates (%)	5.7
Fiber (g)	2.7
Cholesterol (mg)	56.8

Valuable contents for the eye: ★★★

Peas are rich in vitamin C and carotenoids; they also contain phytosterols (which lower the cholesterol level).
Lettuce is an excellent source of fiber and carotenoids (lutein).
Spinach is rich in vitamin C and lutein; it is rich in iron but also contains a considerable quantity of oxalate that reduces iron absorption.
Parmesan cheese is rich in easily digestible protein, is low in fat, and contains vitamin A and some vitamins of the B group.
Mint contains flavonoids and its essential oil has an antispastic effect.
Onions contain vitamin C and a good quantity of flavonoids (quercetin).

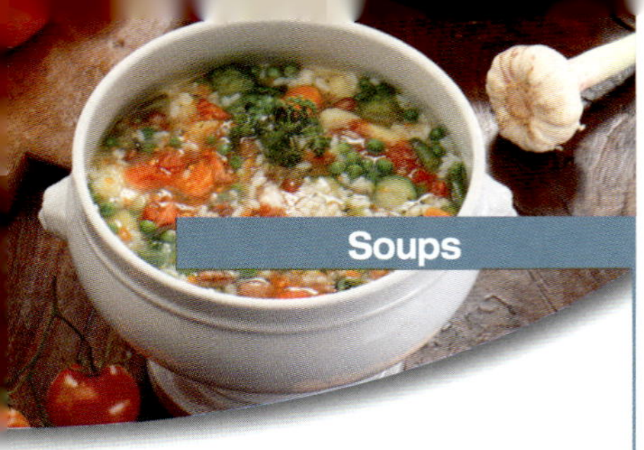

Lentil soup

Bromatological evaluation per portion

Kcal	187
Protein (%)	30.7
Fats (%)	7.7
Carbohydrates (%)	61.6
Fiber (g)	8.2
Cholesterol (mg)	0

Valuable contents for the eye: ★ ★ ★

Lentils are a good source of zinc. They contain thiamine and iron. Moreover, they are a good source of carotenoids and cathechines.

Tomatoes are rich in vitamins and oligominerals, but particularly they contain carotenoids and are the most important source of lycopene.

Carrots are an excellent source of β-carotene; they stimulate diuresis and intestinal motility.

Onion contains vitamin C and a good quantity of flavonoids (quercetin).

Garlic contains selenium, zinc, and alline, which is responsible for the taste and the penetrating, persistent odor of garlic. When alline is transformed into allicine, it has an antibacterial action, and it lowers cholesterol levels and blood pressure.

Ingredients and amounts for 4 people

✓ 1 cup lentils
✓ 1 clove of garlic
✓ 1 stalk of celery
✓ 4 to 5 cherry tomatoes, chopped
✓ 1 carrot, diced
✓ 1 medium onion, chopped
✓ 1 liter (33.8 oz) of water
✓ salt to taste

Preparation

Soak the lentils in water for approximately 6 hours.

Fill a saucepan with salted water, add the lentils and the vegetables (onion, carrot, peeled tomatos, garlic, and celery), and bring to a boil.

Cook for approximately 1 hour.

When done, remove the garlic, celery, carrot, and onion, and serve.

These vegetables can be eaten along with the lentils. If that is the case, they should all be diced.

Season with a small amount of olive oil poured directly into the serving dish.

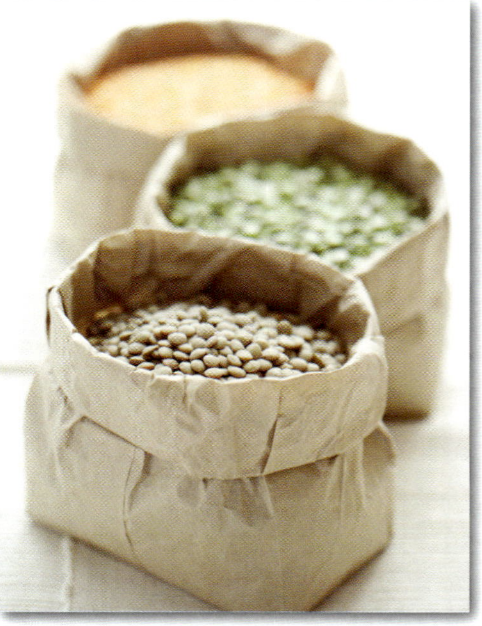

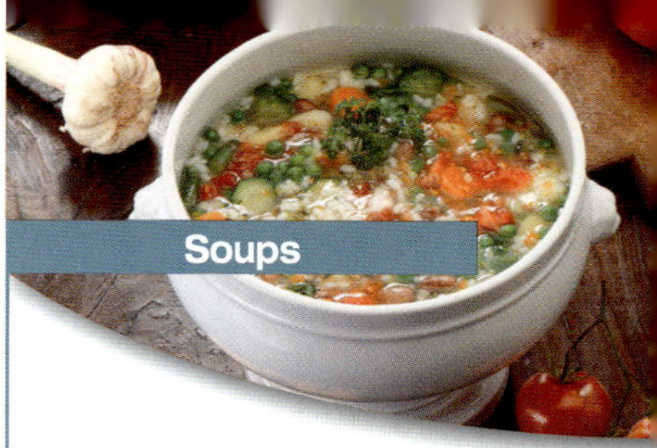

Heavenly soup

Ingredients and amounts for 4 people

- ✓ 1 liter (33.8 oz) beef broth
- ✓ 1 whole egg, separated
- ✓ 1 tablespoon Parmesan cheese
- ✓ 1 tablespoon breadcrumbs
- ✓ small amount of grated nutmeg
- ✓ table salt to taste

Preparation

Whip the egg white until stiff, and gently add the yolk, Parmesan cheese, breadcrumbs, and nutmeg. Mix all the ingredients together. Heat the broth, and when boiling, pour in the egg mixture, whisking with a fork to dissolve the ingredients.

Cook for 2 minutes. Turn off the heat, and stop the cooking procedure by adding some cold water.

Bromatological evaluation per portion (250 ml)

Kcal	61
Protein (%)	39.5
Fats (%)	40.7
Carbohydrates (%)	19.8
Fiber (g)	0
Cholesterol (mg)	52

Valuable contents for the eye: ★

Beef broth contains mineral salts and simple proteins, such as albumin, and is low in fat.

Eggs are rich in saturated fatty acids but also contain a good quantity of mono- and polyunsaturated fats. Unfortunately, they contain cholesterol but they are also an important source of lutein.

Parmesan cheese is rich in easily digestible protein, is low in fat, and contains vitamin A and some vitamins of the B group.

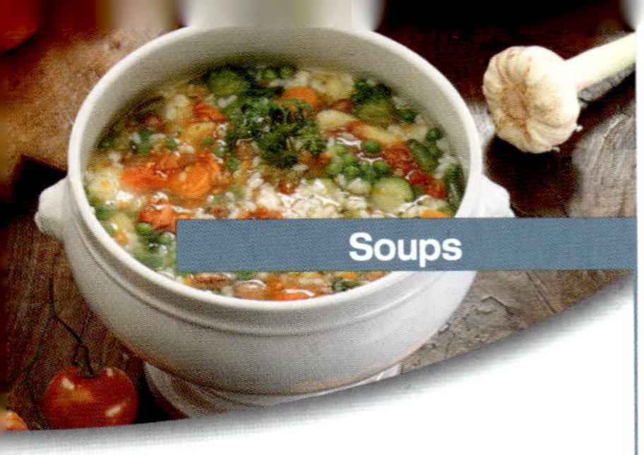

Soups

Bromatological evaluation per portion

Kcal	210
Protein (%)	30.1
Fats (%)	38.2
Carbohydrates (%)	31.7
Fiber (g)	4.7
Cholesterol (mg)	23.9

Valuable contents for the eye: ★ ★

Beans contain protein and fiber and are a good source of carotenoids and flavonoids.
Carrots are an excellent source of β-carotene; they stimulate diuresis and intestinal motility.
Potatoes are rich in starch and contain potassium and vitamins C and B5.
Onion contains vitamin C and a good quantity of flavonoids (quercetin).
Tomatoes are rich in vitamins and oligominerals, but particularly they contain carotenoids and are the most important source of lycopene.
Parmesan cheese is rich in easily digestible protein, is low in fat, and contains vitamin A and some vitamins of the B group.

Mamma's recipe for bean soup

Ingredients and amounts for 4 people

- ✓ 21 oz (2⅔ cups) fresh borlotti beans
- ✓ 1¾ oz piece of salami
- ✓ 1¾ oz Parmesan cheese rind in a single piece
- ✓ 2 stalks of celery, diced
- ✓ 2 carrots, diced
- ✓ 2 potatoes, diced
- ✓ 1 onion
- ✓ 4 to 5 tablespoons concentrated tomato paste (optional)
- ✓ 4 to 5 sage leaves
- ✓ 2 sprigs of rosemary
- ✓ 1½ liters (50½ oz) water
- ✓ salt and pepper to taste

Preparation

Fry the onion until soft. Add the carrots, celery, and potatoes.
Add the water, beans, sage, and rosemary.
Add salt and pepper to taste, and cook for 2 hours.
Add the salami and the Parmesan, and cook for a further 5 to 10 minutes.
Before serving, blend the soup with a handheld blender to increase the density.

Note: If dried beans are used, 10½ oz (1⅓ cups) are sufficient. These should be soaked in cold water for at least 6 hours; eliminate those that float to the surface.

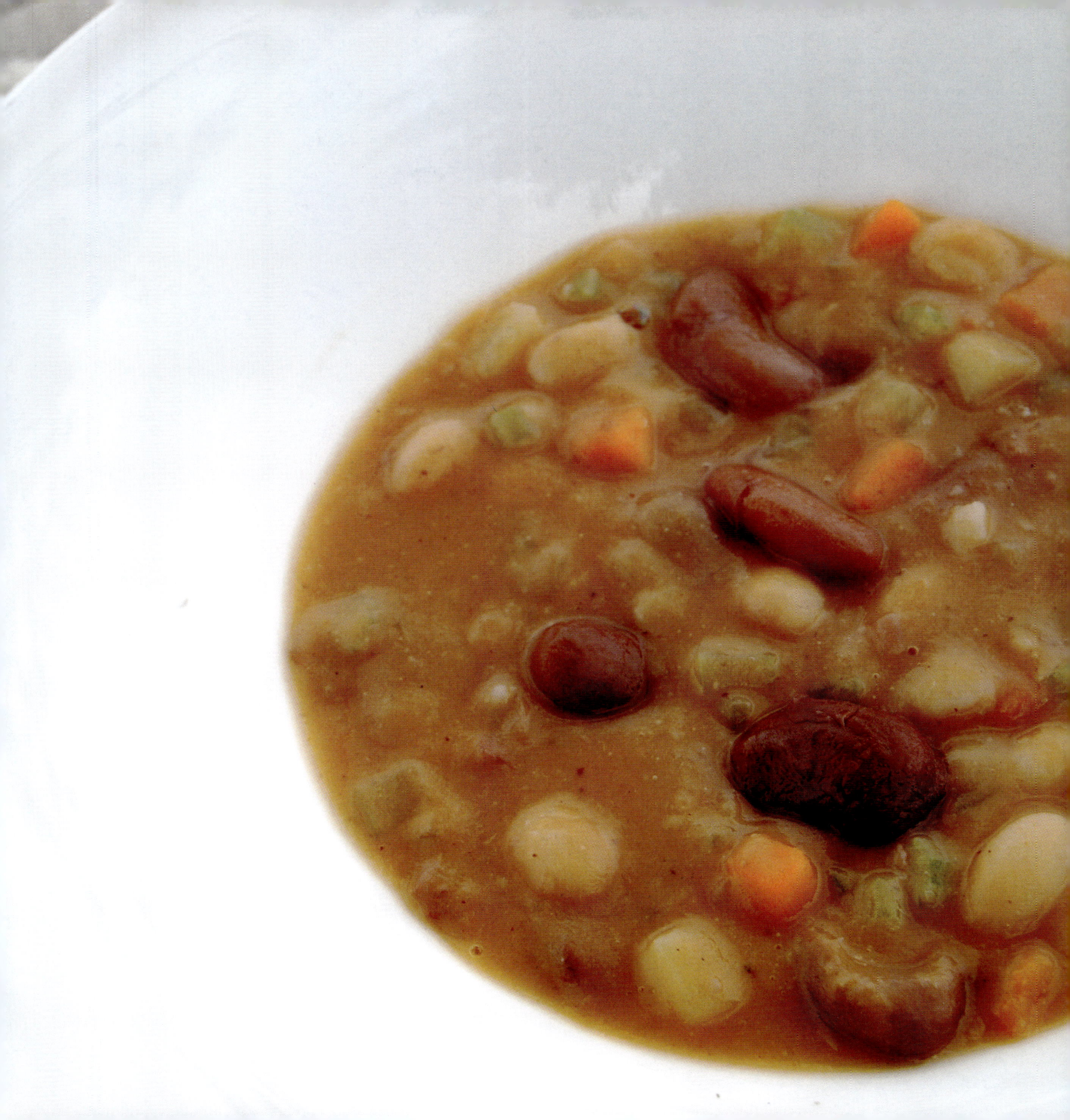

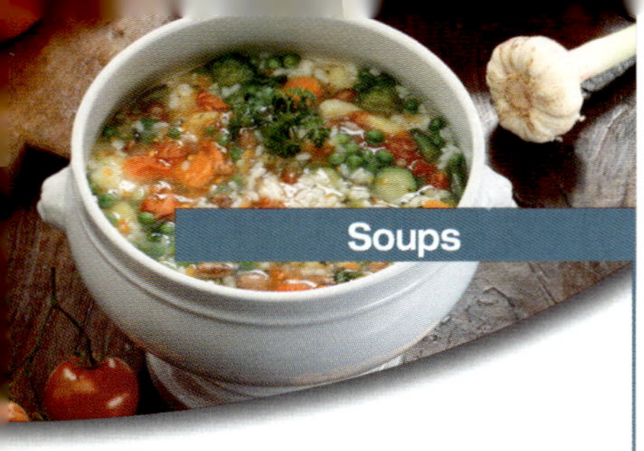

Potato and parsley soup

Bromatological evaluation per portion

Kcal	236
Protein (%)	6.4
Fats (%)	45.9
Carbohydrates (%)	47.7
Fiber (g)	2.6
Cholesterol (mg)	0

Valuable contents for the eye: ★★

Potatoes are rich in starch and contain potassium and vitamins C and B5.
Onion contains vitamin C and a good quantity of flavonoids (quercetin).
Parsley contains flavonoids and is also an apiol, an antispastic, and an antipyretic. It also stimulates uterine contractions.

Ingredients and amounts for 4 people

✓ 4 potatoes, finely sliced
✓ 1 onion
✓ 2 sprigs of fresh parsley
✓ 2 tablespoons extra virgin olive oil
✓ 1 liter (33.8 oz) boiling water
✓ salt and pepper to taste

Preparation

Heat the oil, and soften the onion.
Add the potatoes and cook until the potatoes stick to the bottom of the casserole dish. Add boiling water, salt, and pepper and cook for 20 to 30 minutes until the potatoes start crumbling.
Blend gently with the handheld blender to increase the density.
Add the chopped parsley, and mix well.
Serve hot, which enhances the aroma of the fresh parsley.

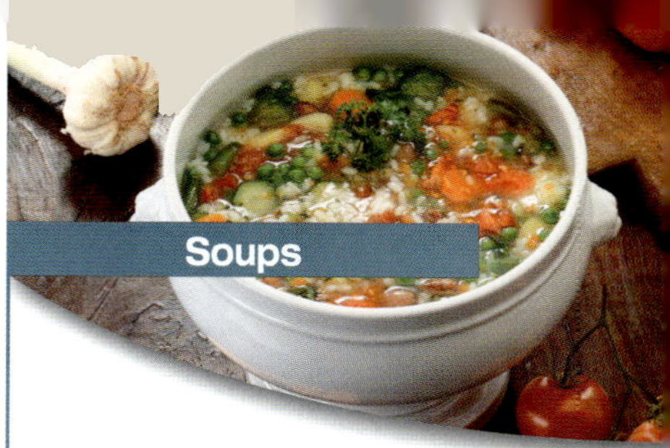

Potato and leek soup

Ingredients and amounts for 4 people

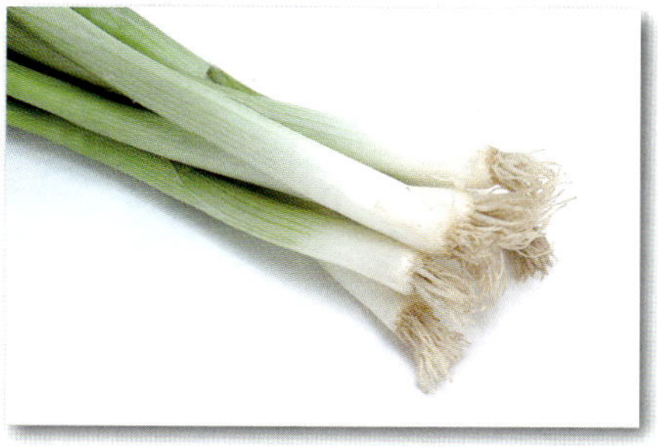

- ✓ 3 potatoes
- ✓ 3 leeks
- ✓ 2 tablespoons extra virgin olive oil
- ✓ 1 tablespoon butter
- ✓ 3½ tablespoons grated Parmesan cheese
- ✓ 2 cups boiling water
- ✓ salt and pepper to taste

Preparation

Finely slice the leeks and potatoes; fry gently in butter and oil.
When the potatoes stick to the bottom of the casserole dish, add the boiling water. Cook over high heat for 15 minutes.
Add salt to taste, and blend with a handheld blender.
This soup can be sprinkled with grated Parmesan cheese before serving.

Bromatological evaluation per portion

Kcal	339
Protein (%)	10.7
Fats (%)	50.7
Carbohydrates (%)	38.6
Fiber (g)	5.3
Cholesterol (mg)	21.6

Valuable contents for the eye: ★ ★

Potatoes are rich in starch and contain potassium and vitamins C and B5.
Leeks are low in calories and vitamins but contain carotenoids.
Olive oil is an excellent source of unsaturated fatty acids.
Parmesan cheese is rich in easily digestible protein, is low in fat, and contains vitamin A and some vitamins of the B group.

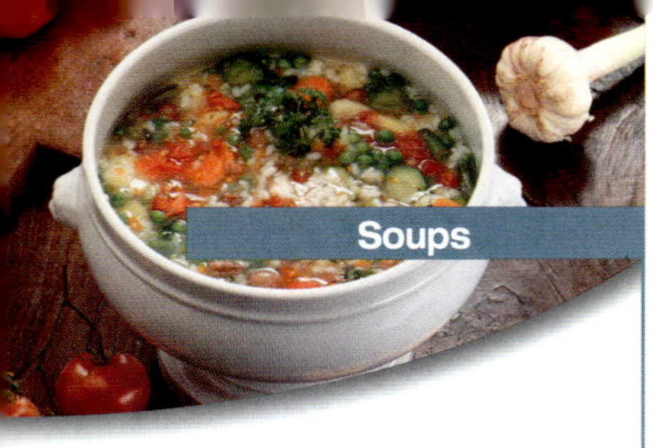

Bromatological evaluation per portion

Kcal	324
Protein (%)	13.4
Fats (%)	42.7
Carbohydrates (%)	43.9
Fiber (g)	5.4
Cholesterol (mg)	13.5

Valuable contents for the eye: ★ ★ ★

Potatoes are rich in starch and contain potassium and vitamins C and B5.

Pumpkin is an excellent source of carotenoids, vitamin C, and vitamins of the B group.

Leeks are low in calories and vitamins but contain carotenoids.

Olive oil is an excellent source of unsaturated fatty acids.

Vegetable broth contains mineral salts and water-soluble vitamins; it preserves some but not all the beneficial substances contained in vegetables. The temperature can denature some of the vitamins.

Potato, leek, and pumpkin soup

Ingredients and amounts for 4 people

- ✓ 10½ oz (1⅓ cups) diced potatoes
- ✓ ¾ cup chopped leeks
- ✓ 1¾ cups diced pumpkin pulp
- ✓ 2 oz bacon, cut into pieces
- ✓ 1 liter (33.8 oz) vegetable broth
- ✓ 1 sprig of parsley
- ✓ 4 tablespoons extra virgin olive oil
- ✓ 1 clove of garlic
- ✓ salt and pepper to taste

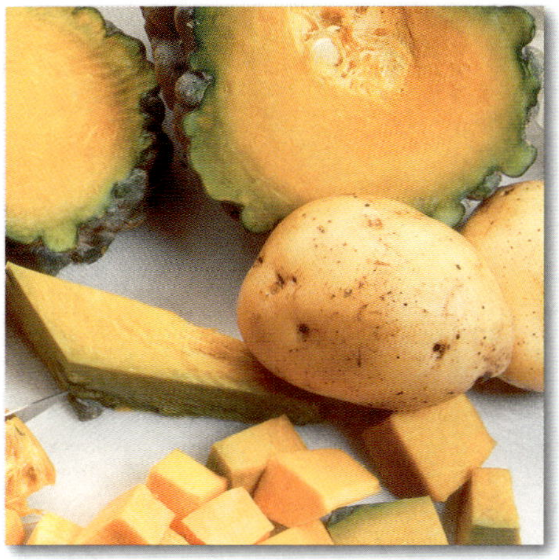

Preparation

Brown the garlic in oil; remove the garlic and brown the vegetables (potatoes, leeks, pumpkin) in the oil.
Add the hot broth, and cook for 30 minutes.
Add the bacon; add salt and black pepper to taste.
Two minutes before serving, add 2 tablespoons of chopped parsley.
Serve with toasted bread.

Cabbage soup

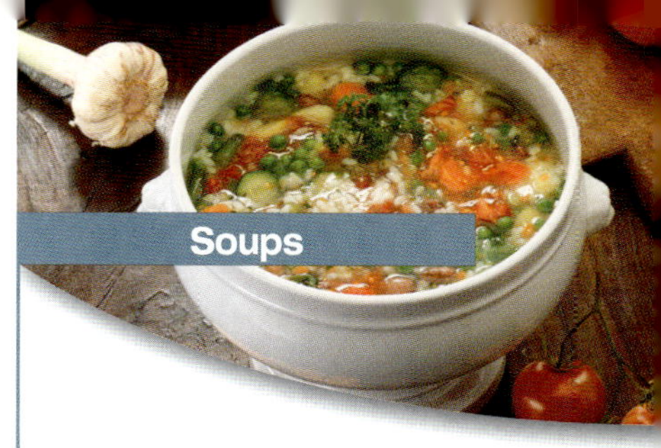

Ingredients and amounts for 4 people

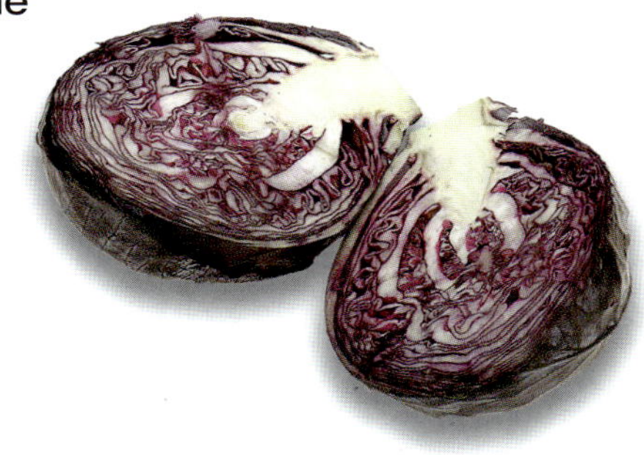

- ✓ 1¾ cups finely chopped cabbage
- ✓ 2 carrots, sliced
- ✓ 2 potatoes, chopped
- ✓ 1 onion
- ✓ 2 tablespoons extra virgin olive oil
- ✓ 1 liter (33.8 oz) water
- ✓ 1¾ oz very thinly-sliced pancetta (cured meat)
- ✓ 1¾ oz Parmesan cheese rind in a single piece
- ✓ salt and pepper to taste

Preparation

Gently fry the onion in the oil.
Add the cabbage, potatoes, carrots, and water.
Add salt and pepper to taste.
Cook for approximately 30 minutes; add the pancetta and the cheese.
Cook for another 5 minutes, and serve hot.

Bromatological evaluation per portion

Kcal	181
Protein (%)	18.5
Fats (%)	76.2
Carbohydrates (%)	5.3
Fiber (g)	2.4
Cholesterol (mg)	18.1

Valuable contents for the eye: ★★★

Cabbage is rich in vitamin C and has a particularly high quantity of carotenoids, such as luteine.
Carrots are an excellent source of β-carotene; they stimulate diuresis and intestinal motility.
Onion contains vitamin C and a good quantity of flavonoids (quercetin).
Olive oil is an excellent source of unsaturated fatty acids.
Parmesan cheese is rich in easily digestible protein, is low in fat, and contains vitamin A and some vitamins of the B group.

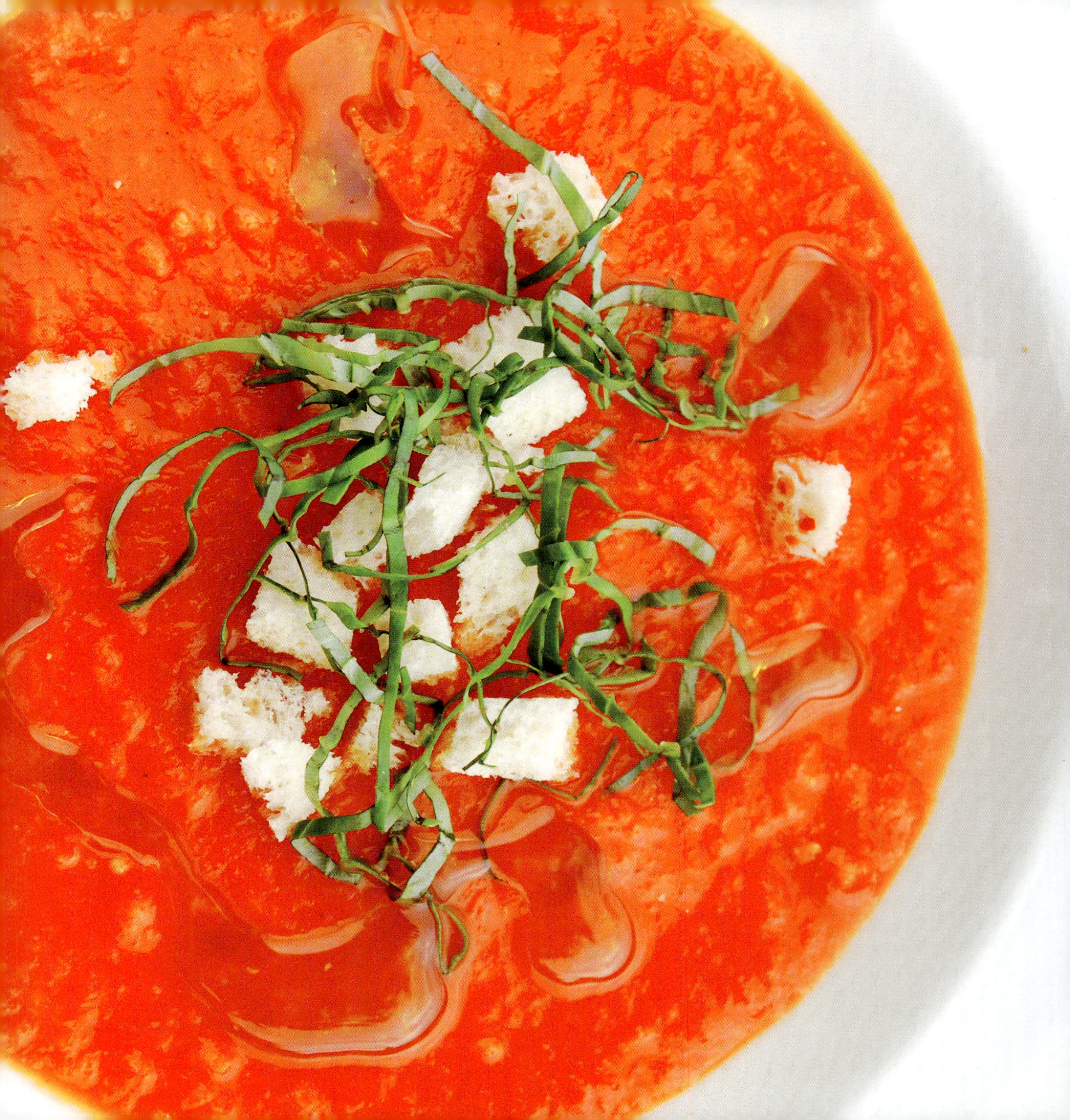

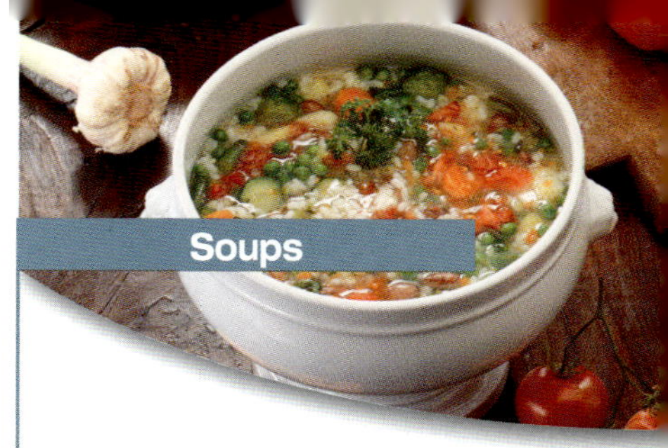

Tomato soup

Ingredients and amounts for 4 people

- ✓ 10½ oz (1⅓ cups) sweet ripe tomatoes
- ✓ 1 clove of garlic
- ✓ 12 fresh basil leaves
- ✓ 1 stalk of celery
- ✓ 1 liter (33.8 oz) water
- ✓ 6 tablespoons grated Parmesan cheese
- ✓ 2 tablespoons extra virgin olive oil
- ✓ 4 slices dry homemade bread
- ✓ salt and pepper to taste

Preparation

Peel the tomatoes, cut into pieces, and remove the seeds.

Heat the oil, and gently brown the garlic and the finely sliced celery. Add the tomatoes and then the water, salt, and pepper. Cook for at least 30 minutes until the tomatoes are liquid; cool.

Before serving, cut the bread into cubes. Add to the tomato soup, and cook again for another 15 to 20 minutes.

Pour into the soup bowls, and garnish with a basil leaf.

Serve with a large quantity of grated Parmesan cheese.

Bromatological evaluation per portion

Kcal	288
Protein (%)	16.3
Fats (%)	31.8
Carbohydrates (%)	51.9
Fiber (g)	2
Cholesterol (mg)	13.6

Valuable contents for the eye: ★ ★ ★

Tomatoes are rich in vitamins and oligominerals, but particularly they contain carotenoids and are the most important source of lycopene.

Parmesan cheese is rich in easily digestible protein, is low in fat, and contains vitamin A and some vitamins of the B group.

The greater the whole-grain content of the **bread**, the greater the vitamin and fiber content.

Garlic contains selenium, zinc, and alline, which is responsible for the taste and the penetrating, persistent odor of garlic. When alline is transformed into allicine, it has an antibacterial action and it lowers the cholesterol levels and the blood pressure.

Celery has diuretic and aphrodisiac properties; it contains minerals, water-soluble vitamins, and favonoids.

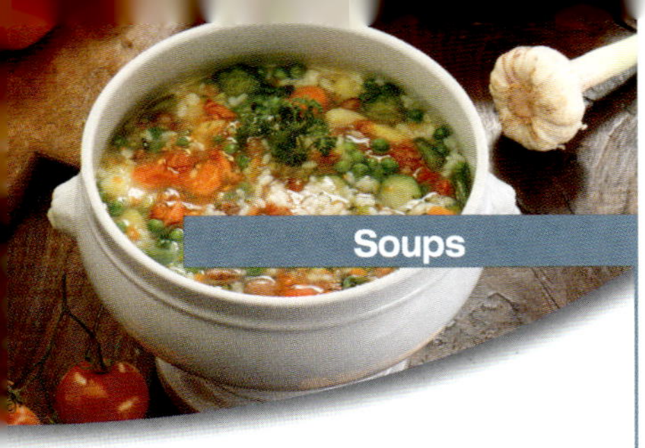

Chickpea soup

Bromatological evaluation per portion

Kcal	267
Protein (%)	21.9
Fats (%)	31.7
Carbohydrates (%)	46.4
Fiber (g)	9.3
Cholesterol (mg)	0

Valuable contents for the eye: ★ ★ ★

Chickpeas are rich in carbohydrates and protein, vitamins A and C, and linoleic acid (omega-6); they also contain carotenoids and flavonoids.

Parsley contains flavonoids and is also an apiol, an antispastic, and an antipyretic. It also stimulates uterine contractions.

Ingredients and amounts for 4 people

- ✓ 10½ oz (1⅓ cups) dried chickpeas
- ✓ 1 clove of garlic
- ✓ 2 tablespoons extra virgin olive oil
- ✓ 1 sprig of rosemary
- ✓ 1 sprig of parsley
- ✓ salt and pepper to taste

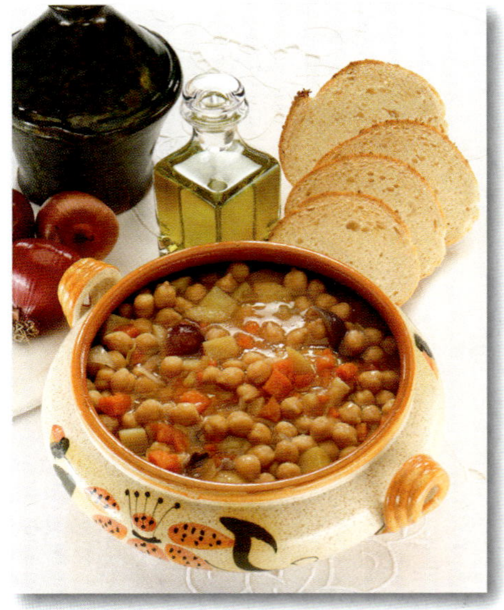

Preparation

Soak the chickpeas in cold water for approximately 6 hours.
Warm the oil, garlic, and rosemary in a pan, and then remove the garlic.
Add the chickpeas; add salt and pepper to taste.
Cover with a good quantity of water; cook for 2½ hours.
When completely cooked, blend partially using the handheld blender.
Serve in soup bowls garnished with fresh parsley, 1 tablespoon of oil, and ground black pepper to taste.

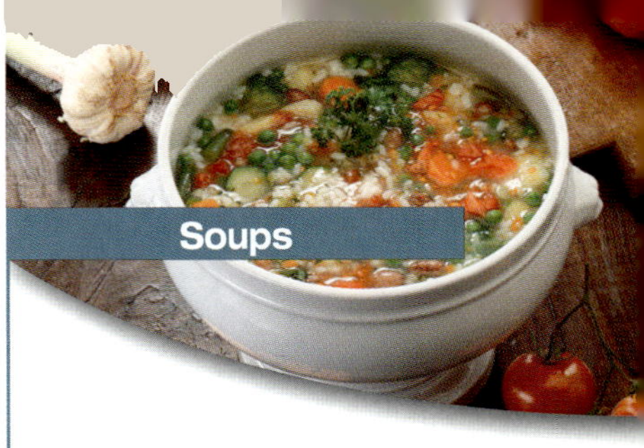

Onion soup

Ingredients and amounts for 4 people

- ✓ 2¼ lbs chopped red onions
- ✓ 4 slices dry bread
- ✓ 4 tablespoons of pecorino (sheep's milk) cheese
- ✓ 1 liter (33.8 oz) beef broth
- ✓ 1 tablespoon flour
- ✓ 2 tablespoons butter
- ✓ salt and pepper to taste

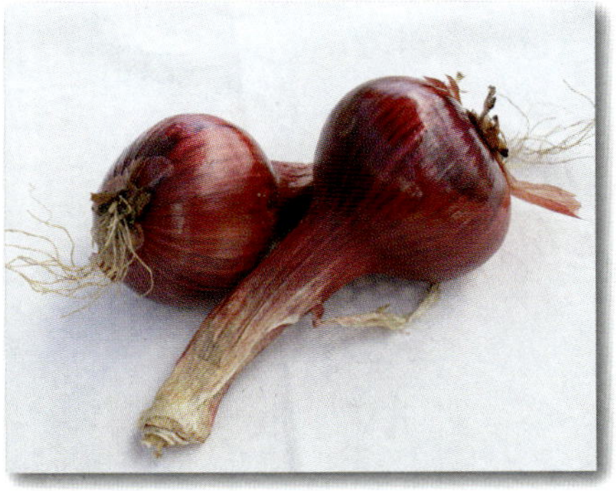

Preparation

In a terracotta casserole, heat the flour with the butter until the mixture becomes golden brown.
Add the finely chopped onion, and continue stirring and cooking for approximately 20 minutes.
Add the hot broth. Place bread and grated pecorino on the top; add salt and pepper to taste.
Place in the oven, and cook for approximately 1 hour, until the soup browns and thickens.

Bromatological evaluation per portion

Kcal	344
Protein (%)	14.2
Fats (%)	31.2
Carbohydrates (%)	54.6
Fiber (g)	2.1
Cholesterol (mg)	34.1

Valuable contents for the eye: ★★

Onion contains vitamin C and a good quantity of flavonoids (quercetin).
Pecorino (sheep's milk cheese) has a strong flavor and is rich in calcium.
The greater the whole-grain content of the **bread**, the greater the vitamin and fiber content.
Beef broth contains mineral salts and simple proteins, such as albumin, and is low in fat.

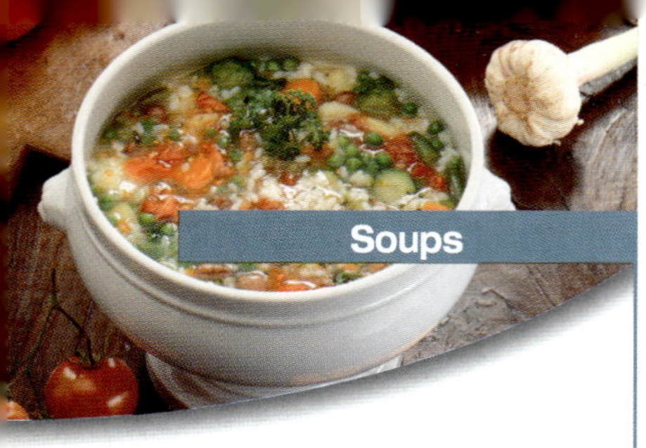

Cream of pumpkin soup

Bromatological evaluation per portion

Kcal	54
Protein (%)	19.3
Fats (%)	13
Carbohydrates (%)	67.7
Fiber (g)	1
Cholesterol (mg)	0

Valuable contents for the eye: ★★★

Pumpkin is an excellent source of carotenoids, vitamin C, and vitamins of the B group.
Potatoes are rich in starch and contain potassium and vitamins C and B5.
Leeks are low in calories and vitamins, but they contain carotenoids.
Cream has a high fat content, but is also extremely delicious.
Vegetable broth contains mineral salts and water-soluble vitamins; it preserves some but not all the beneficial substances contained in vegetables. The temperature can denature some of the vitamins.

Ingredients and amounts for 4 people

✓ 1¾ cups cleaned pumpkin
✓ 1 small leek, chopped
✓ 1¾ cups cleaned pumpkin
✓ 2 tablespoons olive oil
✓ 1 potato, chopped
✓ 3 cups vegetable broth
✓ ½ glass fresh cream (optional)
✓ salt and pepper to taste

Preparation

In a casserole, stew the leek in the oil, add the finely chopped pumpkin and potato, and continue to cook until the potato tends to stick to the bottom of the casserole.
Add the hot vegetable broth, and cook for 20 minutes.
Remove from the heat, and blend all the ingredients together.
Add the fresh cream (optional).
Add salt and pepper to taste.
Serve with a tablespoon of extra virgin olive oil and Parmesan cheese shavings.

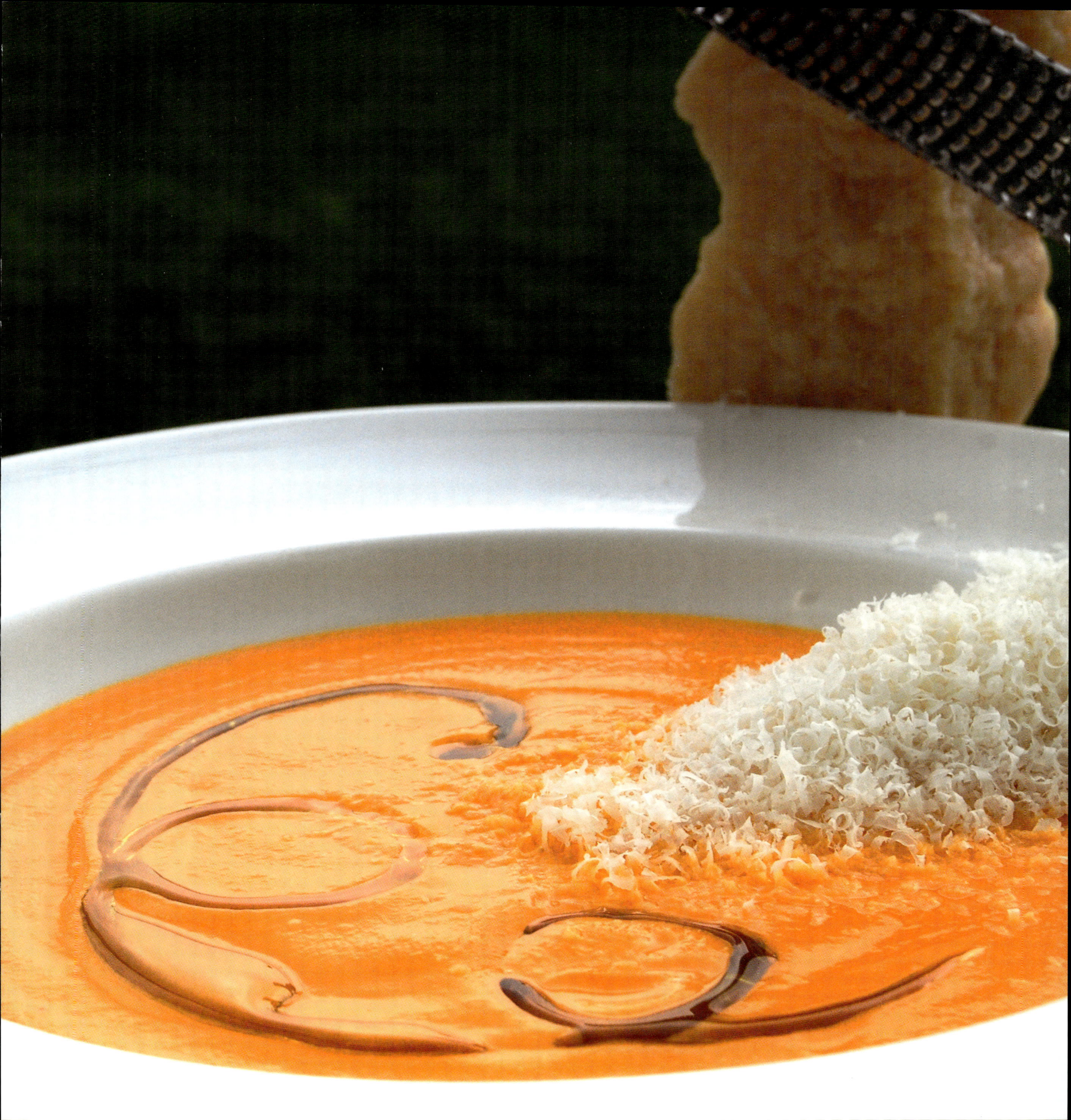

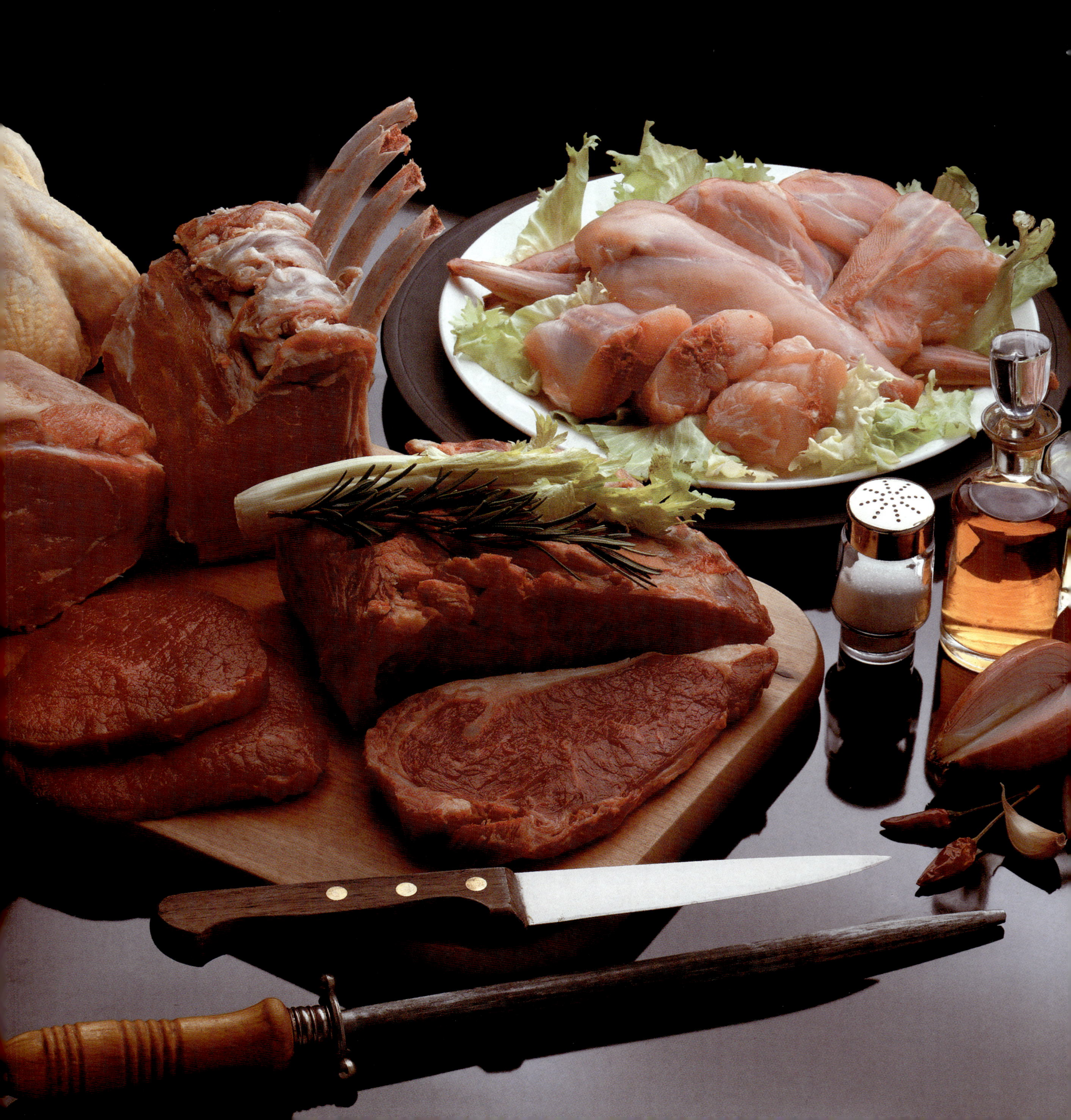

Meat

Everyone is aware that protein is essential for life. It is very likely that teachers start talking about protein in elementary schools, and it would be absolutely impossible to reach adulthood without realizing that in order to grow and live healthily, the daily diet must be rich in protein.

The muscles, organs, cells, hormones, and enzymes are nothing more than a complex combination of proteins, where 20 or so amino acids combine like pieces of a jigsaw puzzle to form the pattern and give each protein an unmistakable specificity.

When proteins are mentioned, thoughts run immediately to muscles and meat that symbolize the prototype of foods rich in protein. It is no coincidence that meat was something of a legend for the athletes in Olympia, but even in the bourgeois society, meat was a mark of social wellness, with no scientific logic. Things changed in the 1960s and 1970s when scientific societies warned about the dangers associated with animal fats and therefore the negative aspects of excessive consumption of fatty meat.

Due to the incessant repair work, the body requires 1 g of protein per kg of body weight every day. So a person weighing 70 kg requires 70 g of protein per day.

In times of famine, man can survive just as well with 0.75 g of protein per kg body weight per day (56 g of protein for a person weighing 70 kg) because according to physiology, this quantity should be sufficient, as long as part of the protein is of animal origin, which will supply proteins that are "complete" with all essential amino acids.

The dietary benefits of meat go beyond the completeness of the proteins because no other food is in a position to supply a suitably high quantity of bioavailable iron, zinc, carnitine, and the B complex. There is less dietary interest in the old commercial distinction between red and white meats because the amount of fat, which at one time was much higher in red meats, has been greatly reduced by genetic selection and suitable feeds, to attenuate the "fat-phobias" of modern consumers. The advantages of easier mastication and greater ease of digestion of the white meats still applies as this type of meat generally has a lower quantity of connective tissue. Good chefs will choose the cut of meat that is most suitable for roasting, braising, grilling, or boiling.

Meat is undoubtedly a precious food; however, it is not indispensable, as vegetarians are well aware. However, eating a few portions of meat each week is still a guarantee for nutritional completeness and should not be considered as a health or diet risk.

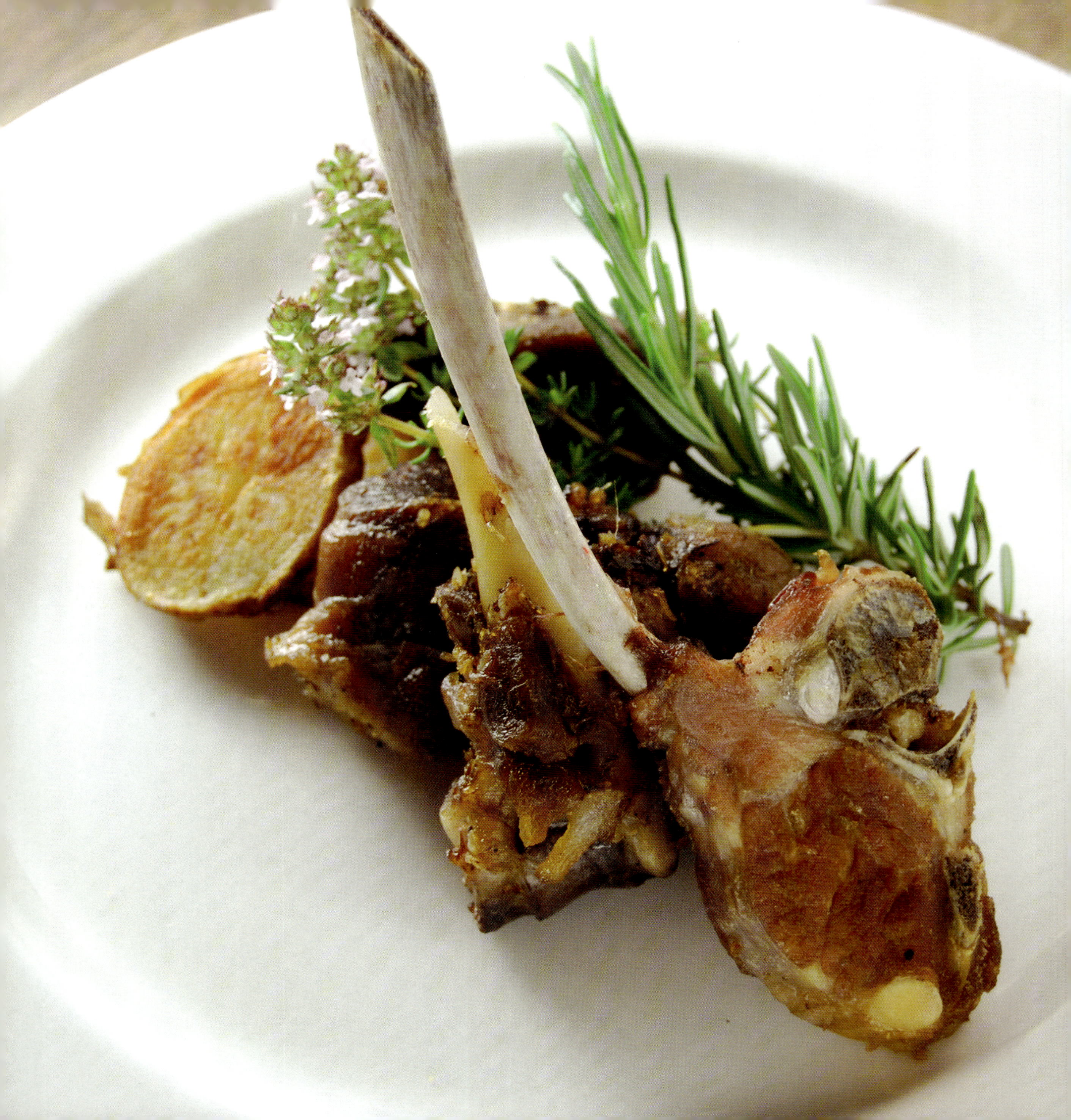

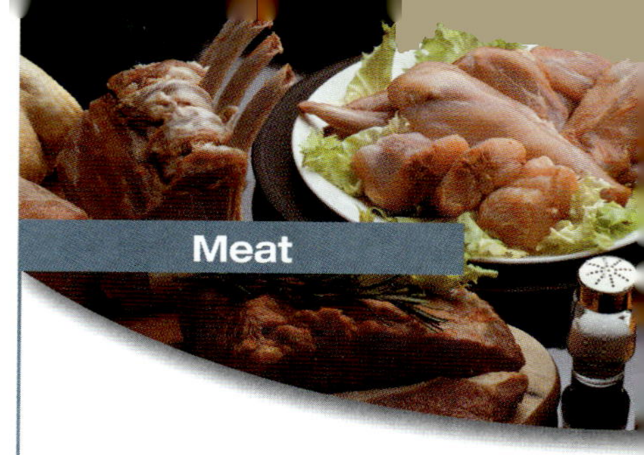

Meat

Roast lamb

Ingredients and amounts for 4 people

✓ 12 to 16 lamb cutlets

✓ 2 tablespoons extra virgin olive oil

✓ 1 tablespoon mixed herbs from Provence

✓ 1 sprig of rosemary

✓ 1 clove of garlic

✓ 2 teaspoons butter

✓ salt and pepper to taste

Preparation

Brush the cutlets with some oil, salt, and pepper, and brown well on both sides in an oven dish.

Place the oven dish in a preheated oven and cook at 425°F for 10 minutes. When the dish is still hot, add the herbs, garlic, and butter. Mix well and serve.

Garnish with a sprig of rosemary.

Bromatological evaluation per portion

Kcal	244
Protein (%)	34
Fats (%)	66
Carbohydrates (%)	0
Fiber (g)	0
Cholesterol (mg)	82.5

Valuable contents for the eye: ★

Lamb is a meat that is extremely rich in zinc.

Olive oil is an excellent source of unsaturated fatty acids.

Mixed herbs from Provence are thyme, rosemary, summer savory, marjoram, and oregano.

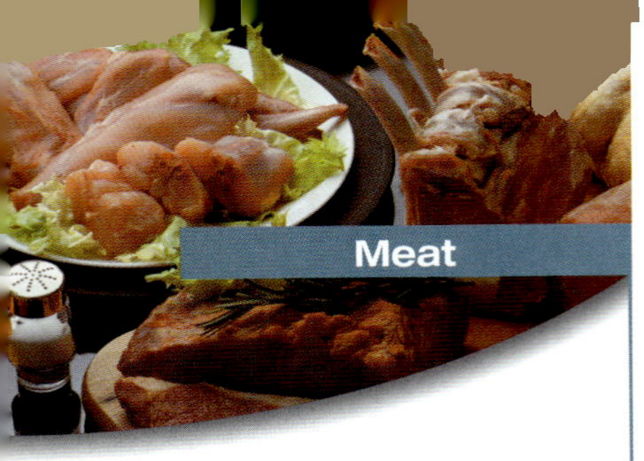

Lamb stew with beans

Bromatological evaluation per portion

Kcal	560
Protein (%)	34.9
Fats (%)	50.6
Carbohydrates (%)	14.5
Fiber (g)	4.9
Cholesterol (mg)	165

Valuable contents for the eye: ★

Lamb is a meat that is extremely rich in zinc.
Beans contain protein and fiber and are a good source of carotenoids and flavonoids.
Onion contains vitamin C and a good quantity of flavonoids (quercetin).
Garlic contains selenium, zinc, and alline, which is responsible for the taste and the penetrating, persistent odor of garlic. When alline is transformed into allicine, it has an antibacterial action and it lowers cholesterol and blood pressure levels.
Parsley contains flavonoids and is also an apiol, an antispastic, and an antipyretic.. It also stimulates uterine contractions.
Butter is made from milk and contains high quantities of saturated fatty acids.

Ingredients and amounts for 4 people

- ✓ 1¾ lbs shoulder or breast of lamb, deboned, cut into pieces
- ✓ 3 onions
- ✓ 3½ tablespoons butter
- ✓ 3½ tablespoons flour
- ✓ 1 liter (33.8 oz) water
- ✓ 1 teaspoon aromatic herbs (sage, rosemary, marjoram, thyme)
- ✓ 1 clove of garlic, finely chopped
- ✓ 1¾ cups precooked beans
- ✓ 1 sprig of parsley, finely chopped
- ✓ salt and pepper to taste

Preparation

Sprinkle the meat with flour.
Peel and slice the onions; soften in the butter and then add the meat and brown.
Add the water, the aromatic herbs, the garlic, salt, and pepper.
Put the lid on the casserole and cook in the oven for 1 hour at 300°F.
Add the beans and cook for a further 10 minutes.
Prior to serving, add the parsley.

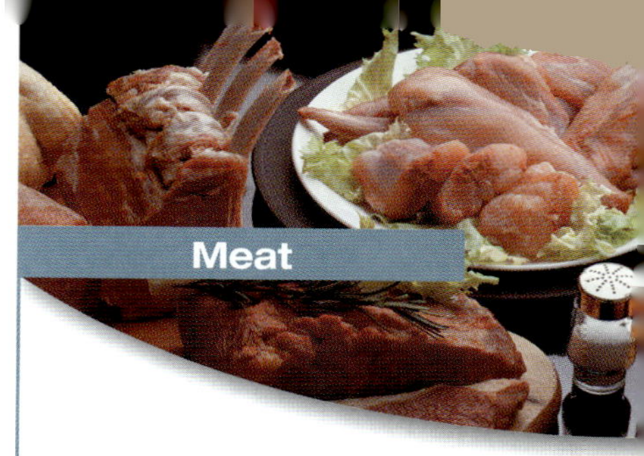

Lamb stew with red wine

Ingredients and amounts for 4 people

- ✓ 1¾ lbs lamb, cut into pieces
- ✓ 1½ glasses red wine
- ✓ 3 tablespoons seed oil
- ✓ 4 cloves of garlic, finely chopped
- ✓ 1 onion, sliced into large pieces
- ✓ 2 bay leaves
- ✓ ½ glass tomato concentrate
- ✓ 4 chili peppers
- ✓ 1 tablespoon flour
- ✓ salt to taste

Preparation

Marinate the lamb pieces in the wine for at least 3 hours; remove the meat and keep the wine to one side.
Heat the oil in a large casserole dish; add the lamb that has been dried and dusted with flour.
Cook until the meat has been browned well on all sides.
Add the garlic, onion, bay leaves, tomato concentrate, salt, wine and chili peppers.
Cook slowly until the lamb is tender.

Bromatological evaluation per portion

Kcal	455
Protein (%)	37.8
Fats (%)	54.8
Carbohydrates (%)	7.4
Fiber (g)	1.1
Cholesterol (mg)	140

Valuable contents for the eye: ★

Lamb is a meat that is extremely rich in zinc.
Red wine contains resveratrol and flavonoids.
Garlic contains selenium, zinc, and alline, which is responsible for the taste and the penetrating, persistent odor of garlic. When alline is transformed into allicine, it has an antibacterial action and it lowers cholesterol and blood pressure levels.
Tomatoes are rich in vitamins and oligominerals, but particularly they contain carotenoids and are the most important source of lycopene.
Chili pepper is a good source of carotenoids, particularly lutein.
Onion contains vitamin C and a good quantity of flavonoids (quercetin).

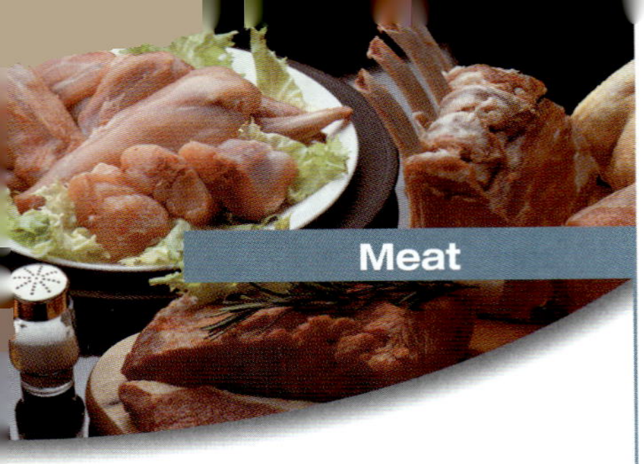

Roast leg of lamb

Bromatological evaluation per portion

Kcal	574
Protein (%)	30.4
Fats (%)	57.8
Carbohydrates (%)	11.8
Fiber (g)	1.5
Cholesterol (mg)	165

Valuable contents for the eye: ★

Lamb is a meat that is extremely rich in zinc.
The **potato** is rich is starch and contains potassium and vitamins C and B5.
Garlic contains selenium, zinc, and alline, which is responsible for the taste and the penetrating, persistent odor of garlic. When alline is transformed into allicine, it has an antibacterial action and it lowers cholesterol and blood pressure levels.
Sunflower seed oil contains omega-6 and vitamin E, even though a portion of this vitamin is lost during the industrial refining process.
Butter is made from milk and contains high quantities of saturated fatty acids.

Ingredients and amounts for 4 people

✓ 1 leg of lamb
✓ 2 tablespoons rosemary, finely cut
✓ 6 to 7 potatoes sliced
✓ 2 cloves of garlic
✓ 4 tablespoons sunflower seed oil
✓ 2¾ tablespoons butter
✓ salt to taste

Preparation

Salt the lamb meat well once the femoral bone has been removed.
Brown the meat well in hot oil.
Place the leg of lamb at the center of a roasting pan with the potatoes to the side.
Cook in the oven for 40 minutes at 390°F, turning the joint and the potatoes occasionally.
Add the seasoning and butter.
Turn off the heat and leave the pan in the oven for approximately 10 minutes.
It can be served on a carving dish with the potatoes.

Rabbit with olives

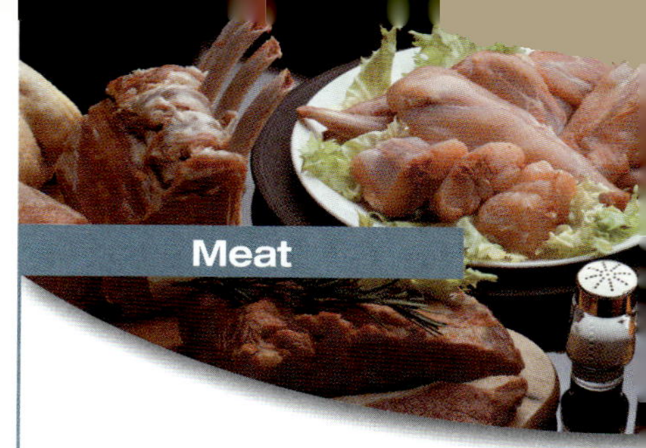

Ingredients and amounts for 4 people

- ✓ 1 cleaned and skinned rabbit, cut into pieces
- ✓ 6 tablespoons extra virgin olive oil
- ✓ 1 onion
- ✓ 2 cloves of garlic
- ✓ 1 tablespoon rosemary, finely chopped
- ✓ 2 cups red wine
- ✓ 1 can (14 oz) tomato pulp or 4 large ripe tomatoes, skinned and cut into pieces
- ✓ 3½ oz stoned Taggia olives (small, tasty black olives)
- ✓ salt and black pepper to taste

Preparation

Brown the rabbit meat for a few minutes in the oil; add the onion, garlic, and rosemary.

Add the wine, salt, and pepper and cook for approximately 30 minutes over low heat.

Add the tomatoes and Taggia olives.

Cook for at least 1 hour over low heat on the stove or in the oven at 285°F, adding some hot water if necessary.

Bromatological evaluation per portion

Kcal	475
Protein (%)	25.2
Fats (%)	51.5
Carbohydrates (%)	23.3
Fiber (g)	1.1
Cholesterol (mg)	73.8

Valuable contents for the eye: ★ ★

Rabbit is a very lean meat.
Red wine contains resveratrol and flavonoids.
Tomatoes are rich in vitamins and oligominerals, but particularly they contain carotenoids and are the most important source of lycopene.
Olives are rich in mono-unsaturated fats, vitamin E, and potassium.
Onion contains vitamin C and a good quantity of flavonoids (quercetin).
Olive oil is an excellent source of unsaturated fatty acids.

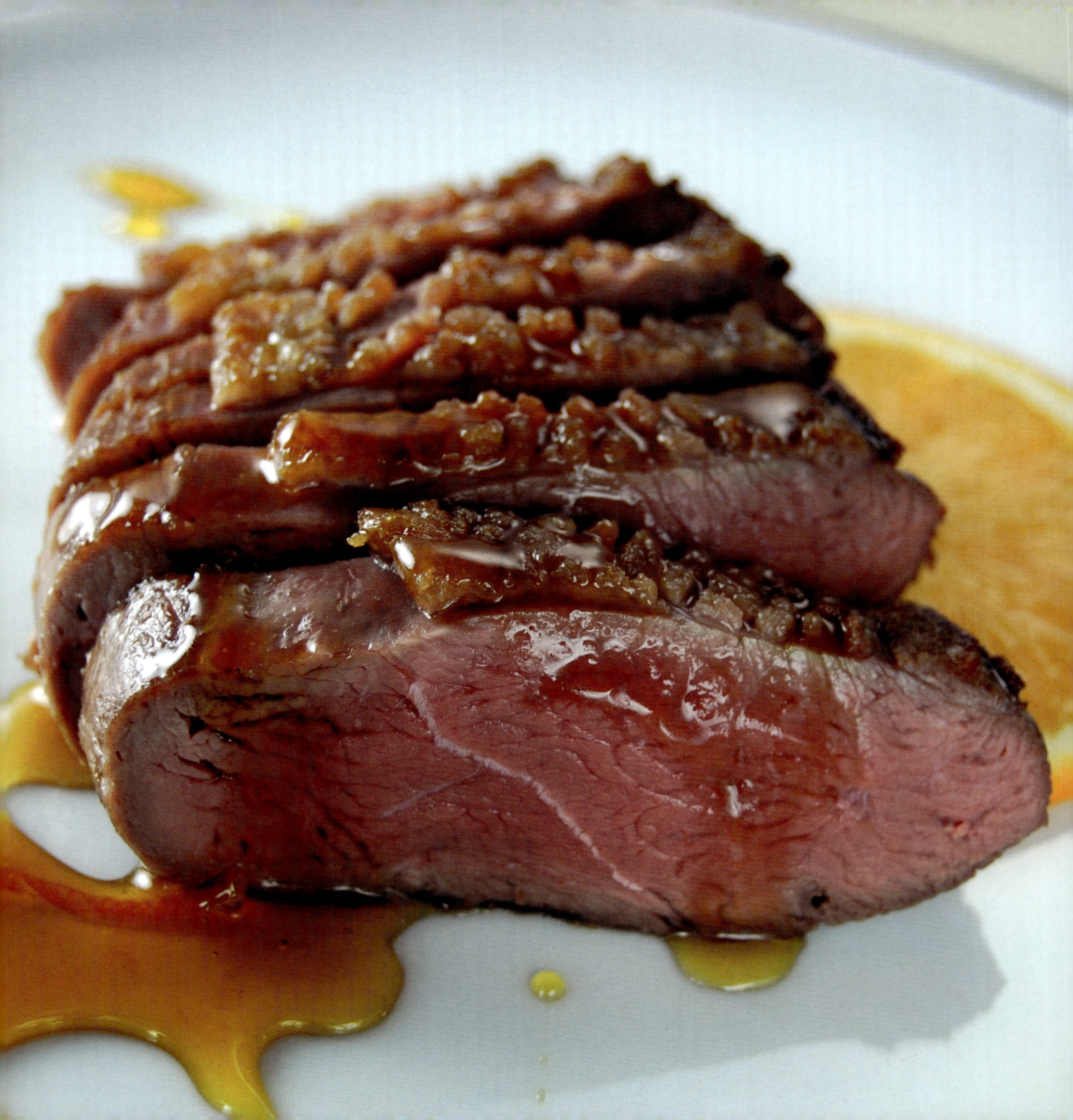

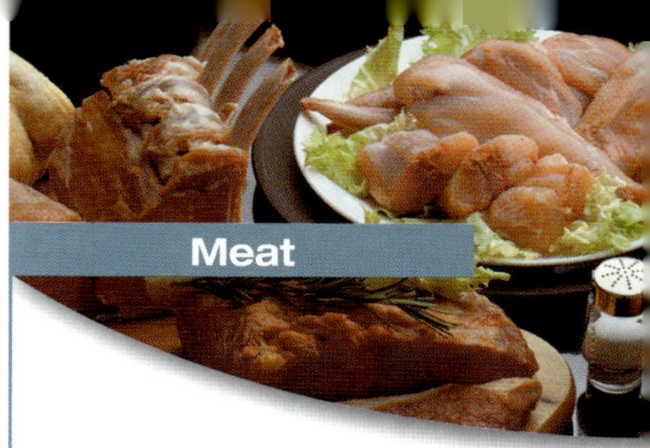

Duck à l'orange

Ingredients and amounts for 4 people

- ✓ 1 duck weighing approximately 3 lbs
- ✓ 3 oranges
- ✓ 2 tablespoons extra virgin olive oil
- ✓ 1 clove of garlic
- ✓ 1 sprig of rosemary
- ✓ ½ onion
- ✓ ½ carrot
- ✓ ½ rib of celery
- ✓ 5 oz lean bacon, sliced
- ✓ 1 glass white wine
- ✓ 7 tablespoons sugar
- ✓ salt and pepper to taste

Preparation of the duck

Remove the head, neck, and feet of the duck. Put salt, pepper, garlic, rosemary, and the chopped peel of an orange inside.
In an oven dish, add the oil, some pepper, onion, carrot, celery, and bacon; brown the duck evenly.
Drizzle the remainder of the oil over the bird.
Place in the oven for 1½ hours at 340°F.
Pour on some white wine every 10 minutes.
Add the juice of 2 oranges over a 30-minute period; when the duck is cooked, remove the garlic, rosemary, and orange peel from inside the duck.
Cut the bird into pieces and place on a preheated plate.
Pour on the orange sauce *(see below)*.

Orange sauce

Peel another 2 oranges and cut the external peel into strips.
Boil in a small amount of water twice to remove the bitter taste.
In a separate pot, add sugar, 1 to 2 tablespoons water, and caramelize (with no mixing).
Add the orange peel and mix for approximately 2 minutes.
Pour the orange sauce over the duck or serve on the side.

Bromatological evaluation per portion

Kcal	471
Protein (%)	37.5
Fats (%)	48
Carbohydrates (%)	14.5
Fiber (g)	1.8
Cholesterol (mg)	25

Valuable contents for the eye: ★★

Duck is a strong-flavored meat, particularly when wild; most of the fat is found in the skin.
The **orange** is rich in sucrose and contains high quantities of vitamin C and β-carotene. It also contains flavonoids (particularly in the pith or albedo underneath the peel).
Olive oil is an excellent source of unsaturated fatty acids.
White wine contains small quantities of flavonoids.

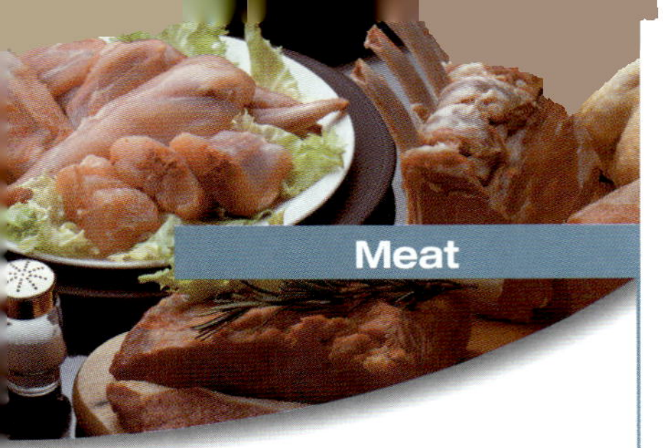

Chicken in red wine

Bromatological evaluation per portion

Kcal	356
Protein (%)	33.5
Fats (%)	47.4
Carbohydrates (%)	19.1
Fiber (g)	0.9
Cholesterol (mg)	93

Valuable contents for the eye: ★★

Chicken contains digestible proteins and has a good ratio of saturated and unsaturated fatty acids.

Red wine contains resveratrol and flavonoids.

Tomatoes are rich in vitamins and oligominerals, but particularly they contain carotenoids and are the most important source of lycopene.

Onion contains vitamin C and a good quantity of flavonoids (quercetin).

Garlic contains selenium, zinc, and alline, which is responsible for the taste and the penetrating, persistent odor of garlic. When alline is transformed into allicine, it has an antibacterial action and it lowers cholesterol and blood pressure levels.

Ingredients and amounts for 4 people

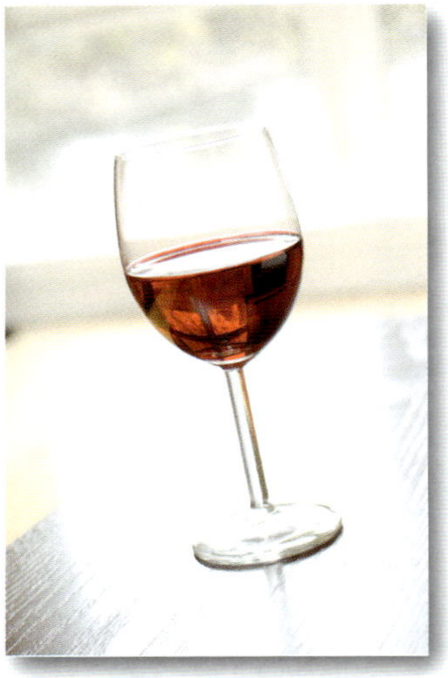

- ✓ 14 oz chicken, cut into small pieces
- ✓ 3 onions
- ✓ 1¾ oz Parma ham in a single slice
- ✓ 1¾ oz minced beef
- ✓ 2 tablespoons extra virgin olive oil
- ✓ 1 clove of garlic, chopped
- ✓ ½ teaspoon rosemary, chopped
- ✓ 2 glasses red wine
- ✓ 3½ oz tomato pulp
- ✓ salt to taste

Preparation

Heat the oil and cook the chicken until browned; reduce the heat and add the ham diced into small pieces, minced beef, the sliced onion, the garlic, and the rosemary.

Add salt, pepper, red wine, and tomato to cover all of the meat; cook slowly for at least 1 hour over low heat, adding water if necessary.

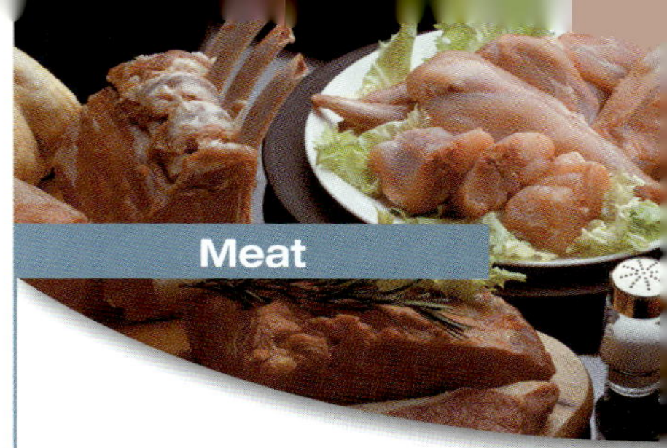

Chicken and tomato stew

Ingredients and amounts for 4 people

✓ 1 whole chicken, cut into pieces
✓ 28 oz tomato pulp
✓ 1¾ oz bacon, thinly sliced
✓ 2 carrots, diced
✓ 2 stalks of celery, cut into pieces
✓ 1 onion, cut into pieces
✓ 8 basil leaves
✓ 1 teaspoon marjoram
✓ 4 tablespoons extra virgin olive oil
✓ 2 tablespoons butter
✓ 2 cups hot water or egetable stock
✓ salt and pepper to taste

Optional: 4 to 5 potatoes cut into pieces, 1 ⅓ cups fresh peas, or 20 black olives.

Preparation

In hot butter and oil, cook the chicken until well browned.
Add the onion, celery, carrots, and bacon.
Add salt and pepper to taste.
Cook for 20 minutes.
Add the tomato, basil, and marjoram, and then add the stock (and potatoes, peas, or olives if desired).
Cook for at least another 30 minutes.

Bromatological evaluation per portion

Kcal	420
Protein (%)	29.2
Fats (%)	60.2
Carbohydrates (%)	10.6
Fiber (g)	3.7
Cholesterol (mg)	130

Valuable contents for the eye: ★ ★

Chicken contains digestible proteins and has a good ratio of saturated and unsaturated fatty acids.
Tomatoes are rich in vitamins and oligominerals, but particularly they contain carotenoids and are the most important source of lycopene.
Carrots are an excellent source of β-carotene; they also stimulate diuresis and intestinal motility.
Onion contains vitamin C and a good quantity of flavonoids (quercetin).
Olive oil is an excellent source of unsaturated fatty acids.
Celery has diuretic properties; is also an aphrodisiac; and contains minerals, water-soluble minerals, and flavonoids.
Marjoram is rich in essential oils.

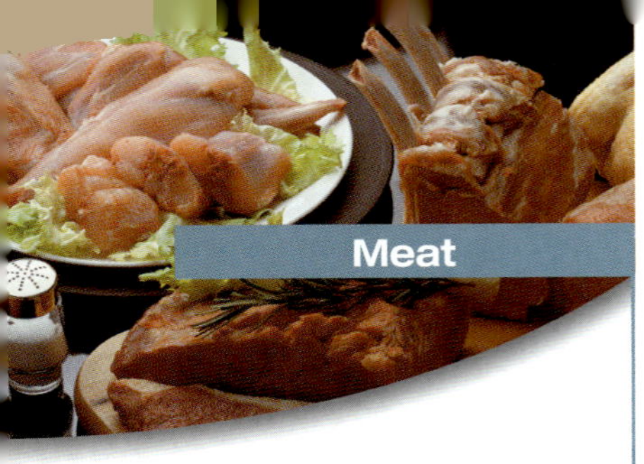

Roast pork with Golden Delicious apples

Bromatological evaluation per portion

Kcal	425
Protein (%)	31.8
Fats (%)	44.9
Carbohydrates (%)	23.3
Fiber (g)	2.7
Cholesterol (mg)	96.3

Valuable contents for the eye: ★

Lean **pork** is an excellent source of protein and is rich in the vitamins of the B group.
Apples are rich in fructose; they contain flavonoids (quercetin) and also oligo-elements such as zinc and selenium.
White wine contains small quantities of flavonoids.
Olive oil is an excellent source of unsaturated fatty acids.

Ingredients and amounts for 4 people

- ✓ 1¾ lbs pork filet, tied to form a roast
- ✓ 4 to 5 Golden Delicious apples
- ✓ ½ bottle dry white wine
- ✓ 4 tablespoons extra virgin olive oil
- ✓ salt and pepper to taste

Preparation

Wash the apples and cut in half.
Remove the cores but do not peel. Place into a container.
Pour the wine over the apples and marinate for 1 to 2 hours.
Pour the oil into a roasting pan, heat, add the pork roast, and brown the meat on all sides.
Add salt and pepper to taste.
Place the pan in the oven at 390°F to 425°F for approximately 30 minutes; pour some white wine used to marinate the apples over the meat every 10 minutes.
After cooking for 30 to 40 minutes, remove the pan with the meat from the oven and surround the roast pork with the apples; pour the remainder of the wine on the pork.
Return to the oven for a further 15 to 20 minutes.
Put the apples and the gravy into a blender, and blend to produce a tasty sauce.
Cut the meat into slices and pour the sauce over before serving.

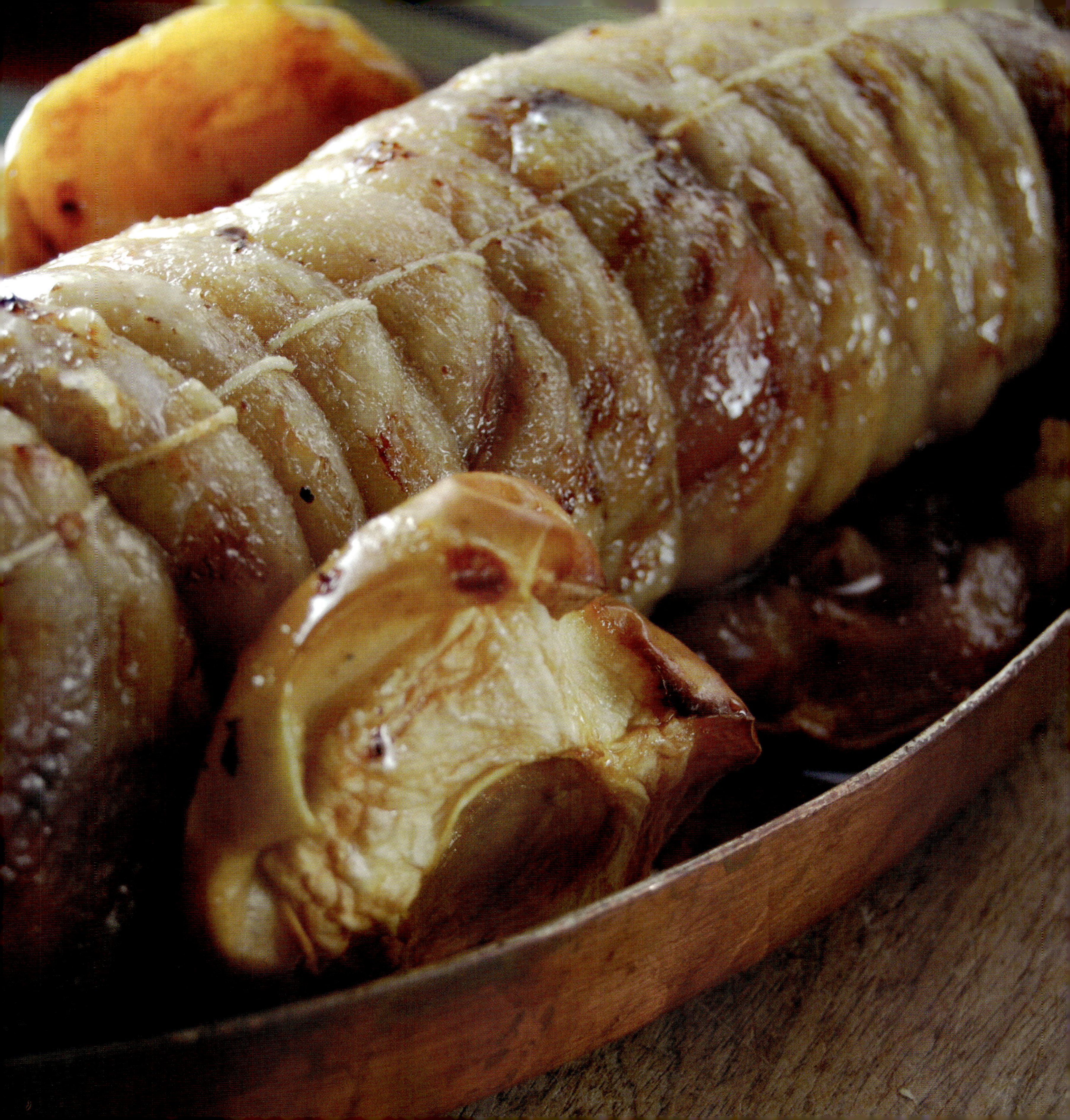

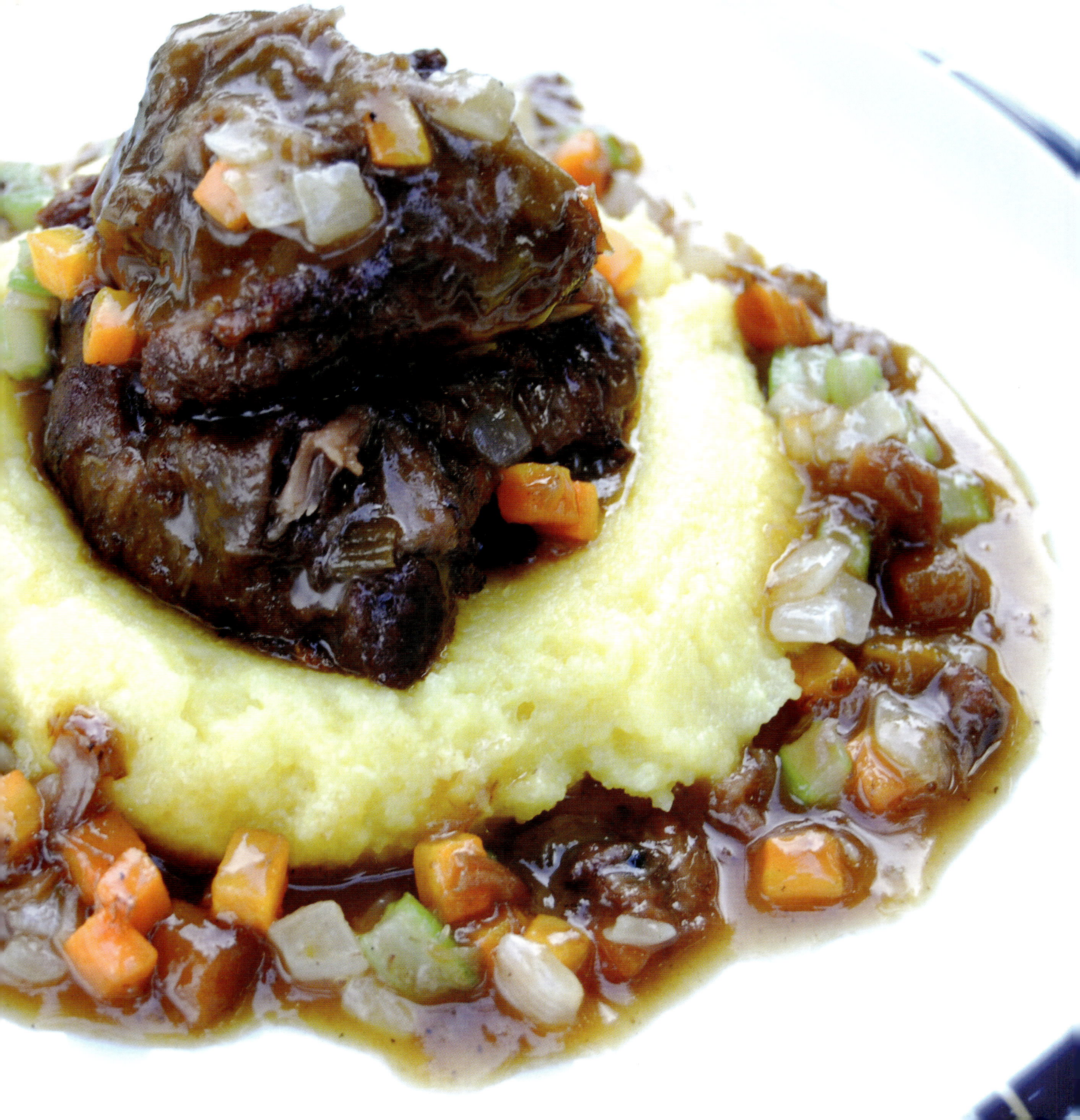

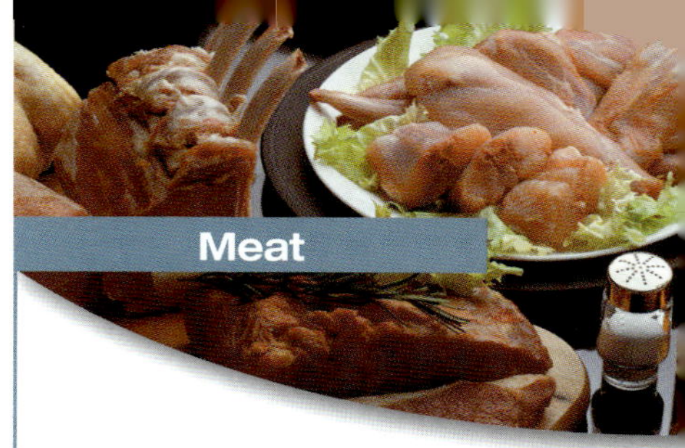

Braised beef in red wine

Ingredients and amounts for 4 people

- ✓ 1¾ lbs beef
- ✓ 2 cups Barbera red wine
- ✓ 2 cups water
- ✓ 2 tablespoons flour
- ✓ 2 onions, cut into pieces
- ✓ 2 carrots, diced
- ✓ 2 stalks of celery, cut into pieces
- ✓ 2 to 3 bay leaves, finely chopped
- ✓ 3 to 4 sage leaves, finely chopped
- ✓ 1 bunch of rosemary, marjoram, and sage
- ✓ 1 clove of garlic, chopped
- ✓ 4 tablespoons extra virgin olive oil
- ✓ 3½ tablespoons butter
- ✓ salt and pepper to taste

Preparation

Soak the beef in the wine for at least 4 hours at room temperature or for a couple of days in the refrigerator.
Roll the meat in the flour poured onto a cutting board; place in a roasting pan and brown for 2 to 3 minutes in oil and butter. Add the mixture of onion, celery, carrot, garlic, sage, rosemary, marjoram, bay leaves, salt, and pepper; cook 1 to 2 more minutes.
Then add the red wine used to soak the meat.
Cook for 3 to 4 hours over low heat or in the oven at 300°F, occasionally adding a ladleful of hot water.
Serve with steamed potatoes, polenta, or basmati rice.

Bromatological evaluation per portion

Kcal	543
Protein (%)	33.2
Fats (%)	44
Carbohydrates (%)	22.8
Fiber (g)	0.3
Cholesterol (mg)	157.5

Valuable contents for the eye: ★

Beef is a meat that is rich in iron with a moderate fat content.
Red wine contains resveratrol and flavonoids.
Onion contains vitamin C and a good quantity of flavonoids (quercetin).
Carrots are an excellent source of β-carotene; they also stimulate diuresis and intestinal motility.
Olive oil is an excellent source of unsaturated fatty acids.
Butter is made from milk and contains high quantities of saturated fatty acids.
Garlic contains selenium, zinc, and alline, which is responsible for the taste and the penetrating, persistent odor of garlic. When alline is transformed into allicine, it has an antibacterial action and it lowers cholesterol and blood pressure levels.

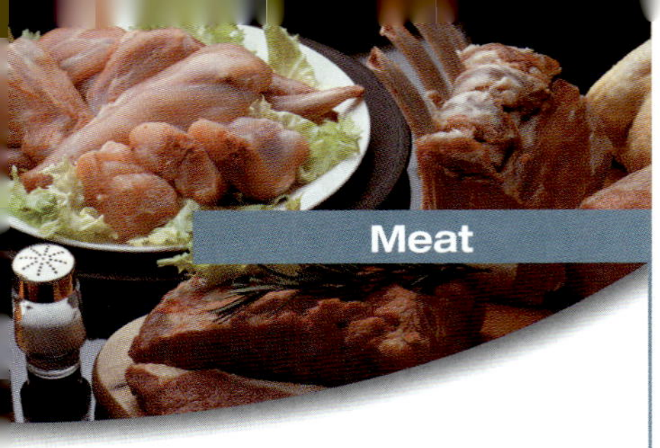

Bromatological evaluation per portion

Kcal	515
Protein (%)	41.3
Fats (%)	58.6
Carbohydrates (%)	0.1
Fiber (g)	0
Cholesterol (mg)	175

Valuable contents for the eye: ★

Beef is a meat that is rich in iron with a moderate fat content.

Olive oil is an excellent source of unsaturated fatty acids.

Butter is made from milk and contains high quantities of saturated fatty acids.

Oven-cooked T-bone steak

Ingredients and amounts for 4 people

✓ 1 1¾ to 2¼ lbs T-bone steak

✓ 2 tablespoons extra virgin olive oil

✓ 2 tablespoons butter

✓ salt and pepper to taste

Preparation

Let the meat sit out at room temperature for 1 hour.

Preheat the oven to 480°F.

Pour a small amount of oil over the meat and place it on the grill rack inside the oven.

Place a roasting pan beneath the meat.

Cook the meat for approximately 10 minutes; remove it from the oven, salt and pepper to taste and spread a small amount of butter on both sides. Return to the oven for another 7 to 8 minutes; serve on a very hot plate.

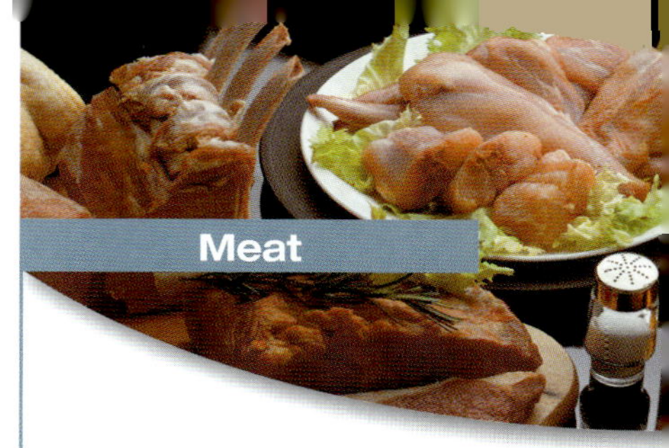

Filet of beef in balsamic vinegar

Ingredients and amounts for 4 people

- ✓ 4 slices of beef (each filet 5 oz)
- ✓ 2 small shallots
- ✓ 6 tablespoons balsamic vinegar
- ✓ 3½ tablespoons butter

Preparation

Brown the meat in butter for 4 minutes on each side.
Remove from the pan and keep warm.
Add the finely sliced shallots to the pan and cook over low heat for 5 minutes.
Add the balsamic vinegar and cook until the liquid has been reduced by half.
Pour the gravy over the hot filets (optional: the gravy can be filtered) and serve.

Bromatological evaluation per portion

Kcal	298
Protein (%)	39
Fats (%)	58.9
Carbohydrates (%)	2.1
Fiber (g)	0
Cholesterol (mg)	121

Valuable contents for the eye: ★

Beef is a meat that is rich in iron with a moderate fat content.
Balsamic vinegar is low in calories but has a very intense flavor.
Like the onion, **shallots** contain flavonoids.
Butter is made from milk and contains high quantities of saturated fatty acids.

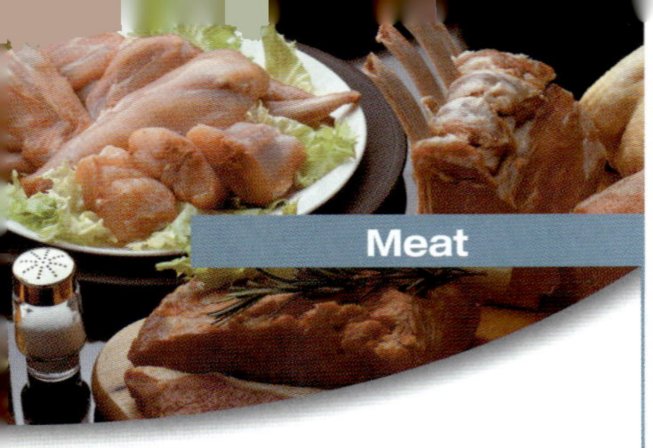

Filet of beef with radicchio

Bromatological evaluation per portion

Kcal	310
Protein (%)	37.7
Fats (%)	62.3
Carbohydrates (%)	0
Fiber (g)	0
Cholesterol (mg)	96.5

Valuable contents for the eye: ★

Beef is a meat that is rich in iron with a moderate fat content.
Radicchio is rich in flavonoids and vitamins A, B, and C.
Olive oil is an excellent source of unsaturated fatty acids.
Butter is made from milk and contains high quantities of saturated fatty acids.

Ingredients and amounts for 4 people

✓ 4 slices of beef (each filet 5 oz)
✓ 4 heads of radicchio, finely sliced
✓ 4 tablespoons flour
✓ 3 tablespoons extra virgin olive oil
✓ 1½ tablespoons butter
✓ ½ glass red wine
✓ salt and pepper to taste

Preparation

In a pan, cook the slices of beef for 4 minutes on each side in a small amount of oil and a slightly larger quantity of butter.
Remove the meat from the pan and keep warm.
Cook the radicchio over high heat in the oil/butter mixture until soft, then add flour, and mix; add the salt, pepper, and the red wine, and cook for an additional 2 to 3 minutes.
Season the meat with the radicchio gravy and serve on very hot plates.

Filet of beef in red wine gravy

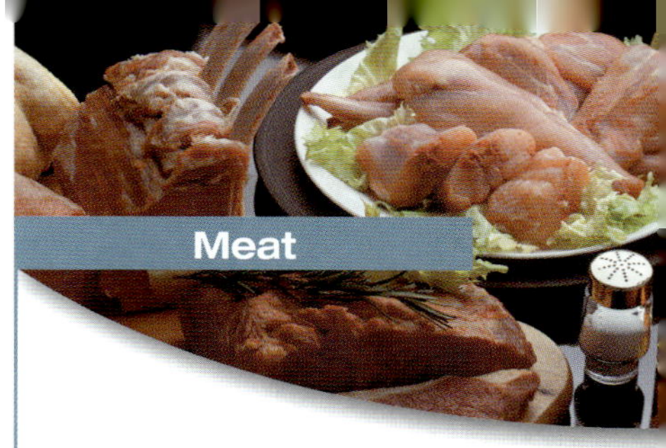

Ingredients and amounts for 4 people

- ✓ 4 slices of beef (each filet 5 oz)
- ✓ 2 tablespoons extra virgin olive oil
- ✓ 1½ tablespoons butter
- ✓ 2 ½ glasses red wine
- ✓ 1 carrot, diced
- ✓ 1 onion
- ✓ salt and pepper to taste

Preparation

Brown the meat in butter and oil for 4 minutes on each side.
Remove from the pan and keep warm.
Add salt, pepper, the onion and diced carrot to the pan and cook slowly for 5 minutes; then add the wine and reduce the liquid to a third.
Stir in ½ a spoon of butter.
Pour the gravy over the hot filet.

Bromatological evaluation per portion

Kcal	353
Protein (%)	32.9
Fats (%)	54
Carbohydrates (%)	13.1
Fiber (g)	0
Cholesterol (mg)	96.5

Valuable contents for the eye: ★

Beef is a meat that is rich in iron with a moderate fat content.
Red wine contains resveratrol and flavonoids.
Carrots are an excellent source of β-carotene; they also stimulate diuresis and intestinal motility.
Onion contains vitamin C and a good quantity of flavonoids (quercetin).
Olive oil is an excellent source of unsaturated fatty acids.
Butter is made from milk and contains high quantities of saturated fatty acids.

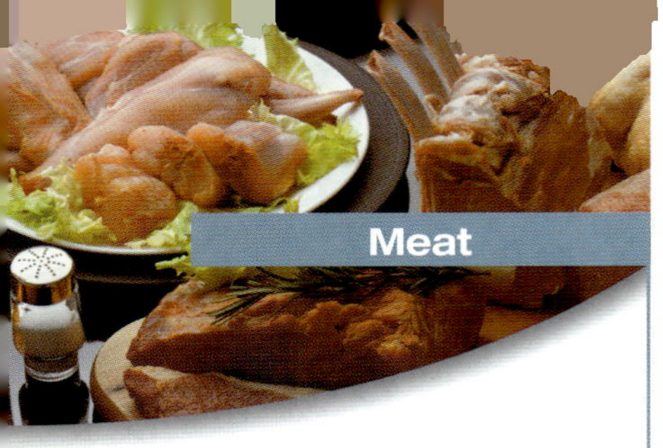

Mamma's beef-burger recipe

Bromatological evaluation per portion

Kcal	455
Protein (%)	17.7
Fats (%)	59.3
Carbohydrates (%)	23
Fiber (g)	1.7
Cholesterol (mg)	26.1

Valuable contents for the eye: ★

Beef is a meat that is rich in iron with a moderate fat content.

Parmesan cheese is rich in easily digestible protein, is low in fat, and contains vitamin A and some vitamins of the B group.

Lemon contains high quantities of vitamin C and β-carotene. It also contains flavonoids (particularly in the pith or albedo underneath the peel).

Parsley contains flavonoids and is also an apiol, an antispastic, and an antipyretic. It also stimulates uterine contractions.

Olive oil is an excellent source of unsaturated fatty acids.

Butter is made from milk and contains high quantities of saturated fatty acids.

Ingredients and amounts for 4 people

✓ 14 oz top-quality ground beef

✓ 2 sprigs of fresh parsley, finely chopped

✓ 4¼ tablespoons freshly grated Parmesan cheese

✓ juice of 1 lemon

✓ 3 tablespoons extra virgin olive oil

✓ 2 tablespoons butter

✓ salt to taste

Preparation

Mix the ground beef with the parsley, Parmesan, salt, and lemon juice.
Shape into 4 individual burgers.
Heat the oil and butter in a pan and cook the meat on both sides.

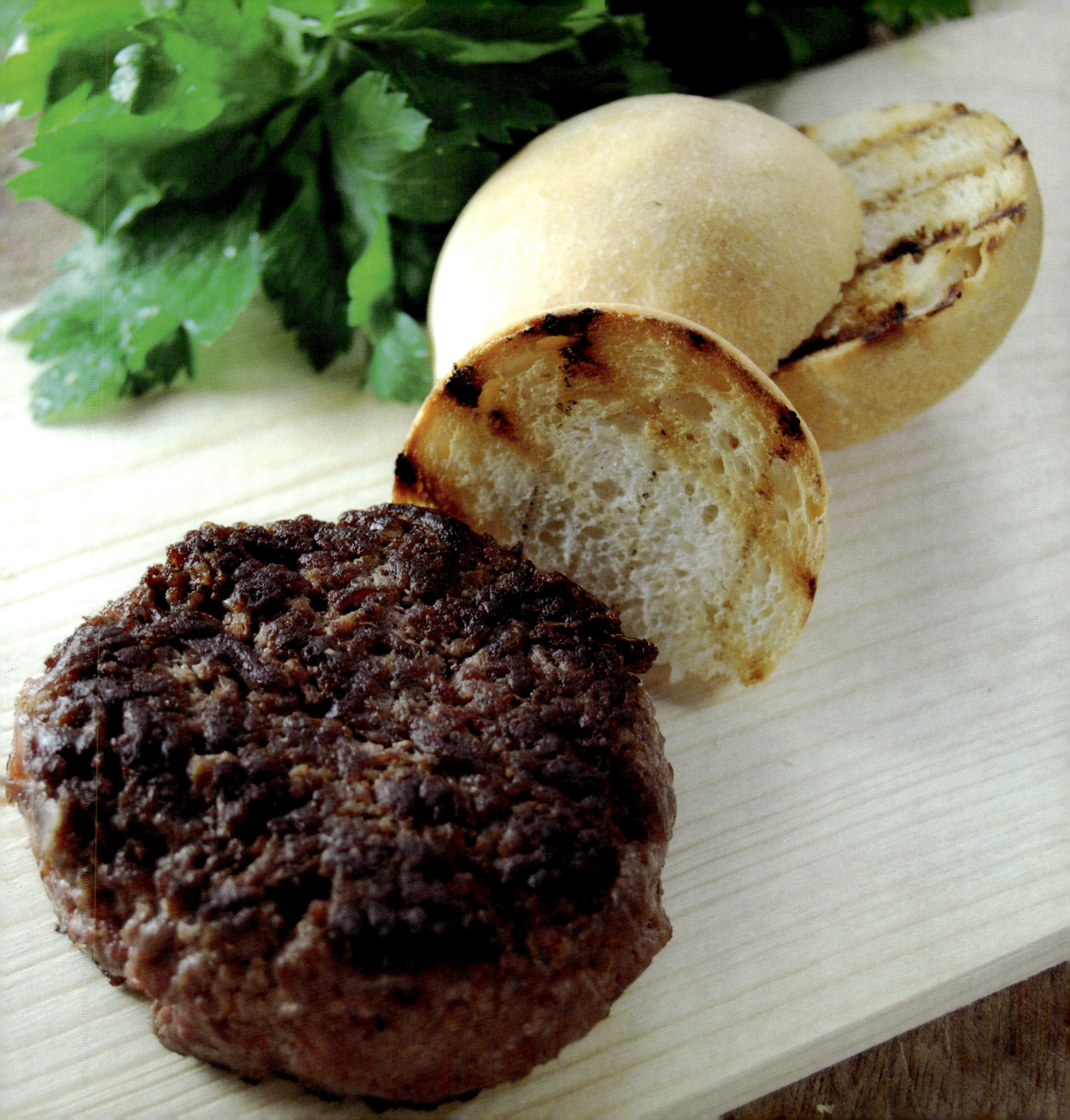

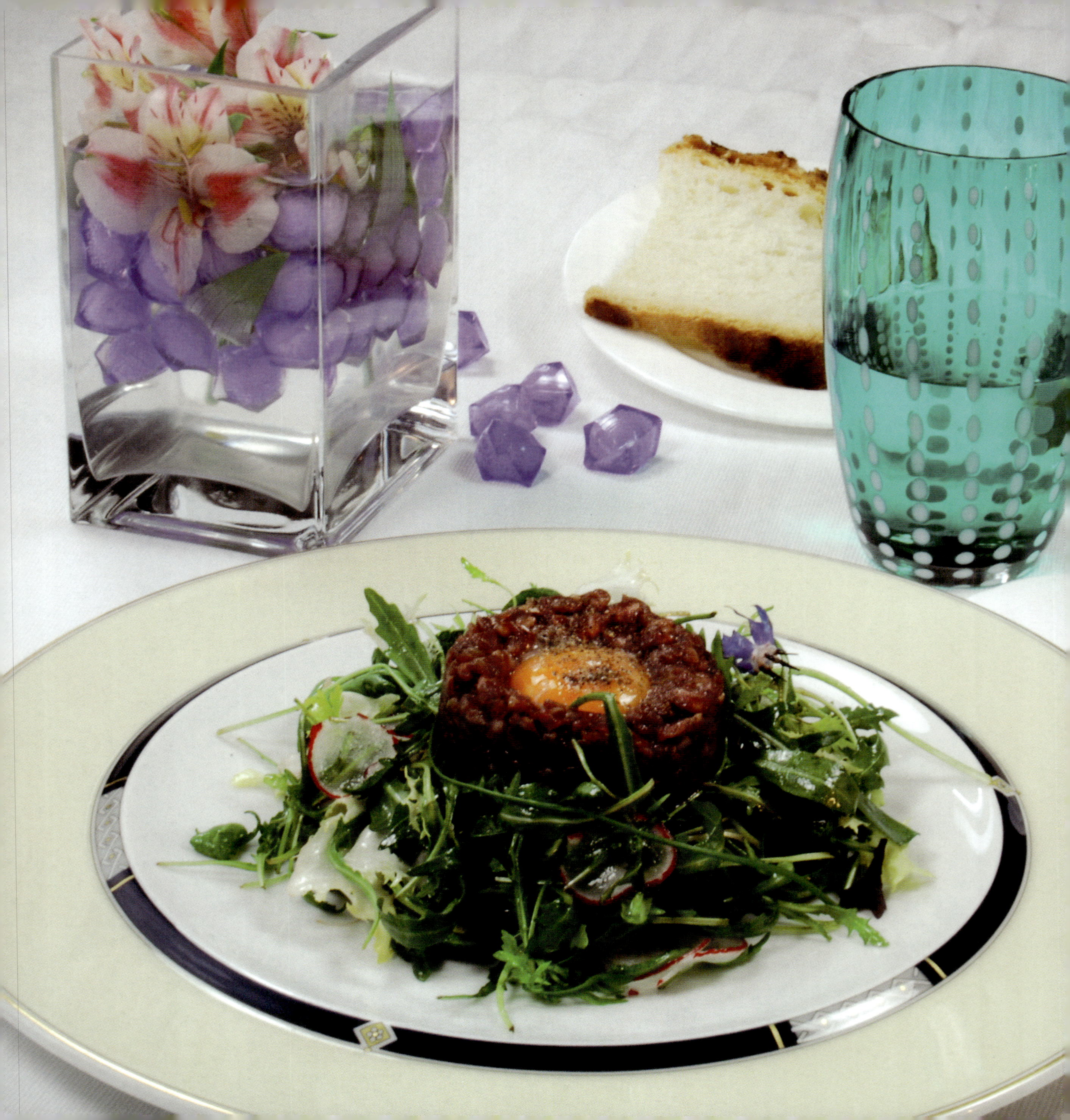

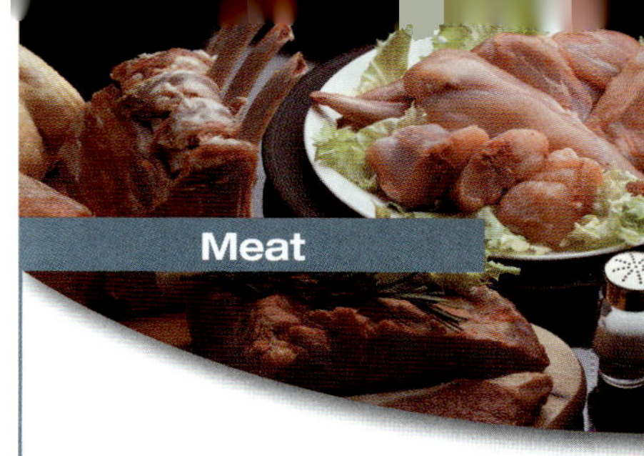

Filet of beef tartare

Ingredients and amounts for 4 people

- ✓ 21 oz ($1\frac{1}{3}$ lbs) filet of beef
- ✓ 1 very small scallion
- ✓ 1 teaspoon capers
- ✓ 1 sprig of parsley
- ✓ 4 teaspoons extra virgin olive oil
- ✓ juice of 1 lemon (approximately 4 tablespoons)
- ✓ 4 egg yolks
- ✓ 1 teaspoon very mature balsamic vinegar
- ✓ salt and black pepper to taste

Preparation

Cut the filet into slices, then into strips, and then slice into very small pieces.

Place the chopped meat into a container and season with oil and lemon juice; add the scallion, capers, and parsley, which have all been finely chopped, and the balsamic vinegar.

Mix well and let sit for a few minutes.

Place the intact egg yolks on top of the meat.

Before eating, the egg should be mixed with the meat.

This mixture can be served as a side with a small amount of mixed salad (or, for example, the "puntarelle alla romana," which belongs to the chicory family).

Bromatological evaluation per portion

Kcal	417
Protein (%)	36.2
Fats (%)	63.8
Carbohydrates (%)	0
Fiber (g)	0.6
Cholesterol (mg)	624

Valuable contents for the eye: ★

Beef is a meat that is rich in iron with a moderate fat content.

Eggs are rich in saturated fatty acids but also contain a good quantity of mono- and polyunsaturated fats. Unfortunately, they contain cholesterol, but they are also an important source of lutein.

Olive oil is an excellent source of unsaturated fatty acids.

Capers contain vitamins A, C, and E, and also a large quantity of sodium.

Lemon contains high quantities of vitamin C and β-carotene. It also contains flavonoids (particularly in the pith or albedo underneath the peel).

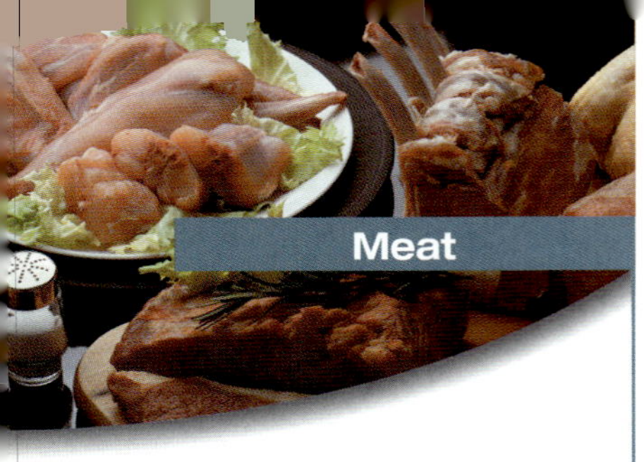

Roast curried veal

Bromatological evaluation per portion

Kcal	184
Protein (%)	90
Fats (%)	9.7
Carbohydrates (%)	0.3
Fiber (g)	0
Cholesterol (mg)	142

Valuable contents for the eye: ★

Veal is the most easily digested red meat.
Curry contains bi-demethoxycurcumrin, an efficacious neuroprotector.

Ingredients and amounts for 4 people

✓ 1¾ lbs very fresh veal filets
✓ 4½ lbs sea salt crystals
✓ 2 tablespoons curry

Preparation

Sprinkle the curry over all sides of the meat.
Place 1 lb sea salt crystals in a roasting pan.
Place the meat on the bed of salt and cover evenly with the rest of the salt.
Place the pan in the oven at 390°F and cook for 30 minutes.
Remove from the oven and let sit for 10 minutes.
Carefully remove all the salt. Cut the meat into slices and serve with steamed potatoes or basmati rice.

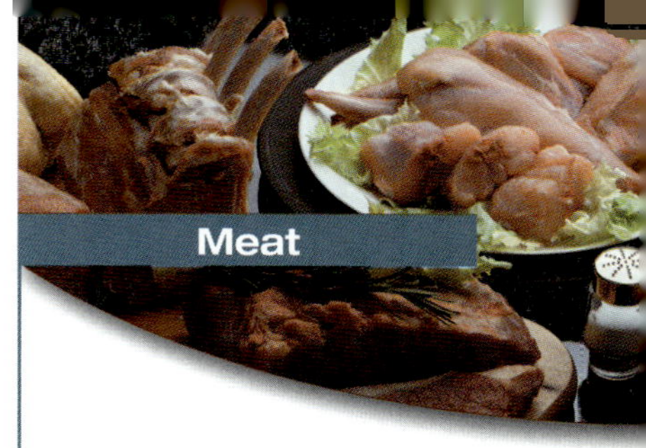

Veal stew with **red wine**

Ingredients and amounts for 4 people

- ✓ $1\frac{1}{3}$ lbs veal, cut into pieces
- ✓ 1 onion
- ✓ 1 tablespoon flour
- ✓ 4 tablespoons seed oil
- ✓ 2 glasses red wine (Barolo, Barbera, or Nebbiolo preferred)
- ✓ 1 liter (33.8 oz) meat stock
- ✓ 2 bay leaves
- ✓ 1 bunch of aromatic herbs (thyme, sage, and rosemary)
- ✓ salt and pepper to taste

Preparation

Dust the meat with flour.
Heat the oil well, brown the meat, and gradually add the onion.
Continue cooking for 10 minutes over low heat.
Add the wine and continue cooking until the wine has evaporated.
Add the bay leaves, aromatic herbs, salt, pepper, and the meat stock.
Cook slowly over low heat for at least 1 hour.

Bromatological evaluation per portion

Kcal	278
Protein (%)	38.7
Fats (%)	36.9
Carbohydrates (%)	24.4
Fiber (g)	0
Cholesterol (mg)	85.2

Valuable contents for the eye: ★

Veal is the most easily digested red meat.
Red wine contains resveratrol and flavonoids.
Onion contains vitamin C and a good quantity of flavonoids (quercetin).
Olive oil is an excellent source of unsaturated fatty acids.

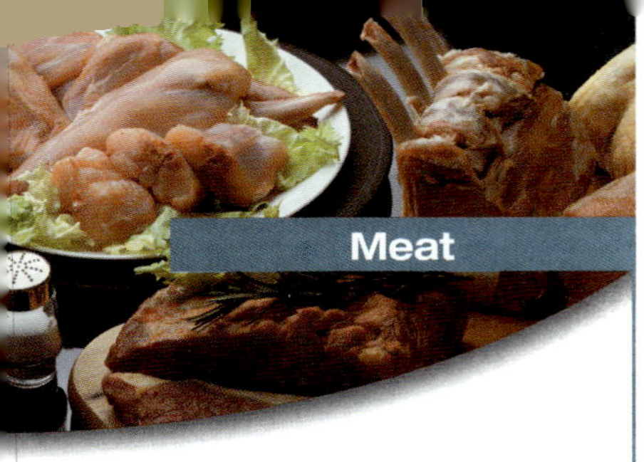

Veal alla Genovese

Bromatological evaluation per portion

Kcal	403
Protein (%)	40.7
Fats (%)	48.4
Carbohydrates (%)	10.9
Fiber (g)	1
Cholesterol (mg)	132.6

Valuable contents for the eye: ★

Veal is the most easily digested red meat.
Onion contains vitamin C and a good quantity of flavonoids (quercetin).
Garlic contains selenium, zinc, and alline, which is responsible for the taste and the penetrating, persistent odor of garlic. When alline is transformed into allicine, it has an antibacterial action and it lowers cholesterol and blood pressure levels.
Anchovies are low in fat and contain omega-3 fatty acids.
Parmesan cheese is rich in easily digestible protein, is low in fat, and contains vitamin A and some vitamins of the B group.
Olive oil is an excellent source of unsaturated fatty acids.

Ingredients and amounts for 4 people

- ✓ 1⅓ lbs veal rump
- ✓ 3 to 4 medium-sized onions
- ✓ 2 cloves of garlic
- ✓ 1 bunch of parsley
- ✓ 4 tablespoons extra virgin olive oil
- ✓ 1½ tablespoons butter
- ✓ 2 anchovies
- ✓ 3½ tablespoons Parmesan cheese shavings
- ✓ 1 glass white wine
- ✓ salt to taste

Preparation

Prepare the meat by making 5 to 6 deep cuts (small pouches).
In each cut, place a piece of garlic, some chopped parsley, and a piece of Parmesan cheese.
Put the extra virgin olive oil and the butter in a pan; heat slowly.
Add 3 to 4 finely sliced onions, the mashed or chopped anchovies, and the salt.
Add the meat.
Cook over low heat for 30 to 35 minutes.
When the meat is cooked and the gravy is reduced well, add the glass of white wine and allow it to evaporate.

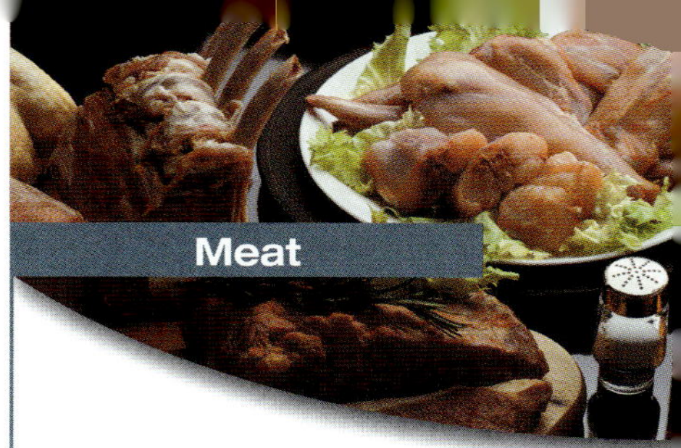

Mamma's recipe for Valdotaine-style veal

Ingredients and amounts for 4 people

✓ 4 thin slices of veal, trimmed of fat

✓ 4 thin slices Parma ham

✓ 4 sage leaves

✓ 4 thin slices Fontina cheese

✓ 2 tablespoons butter

✓ 1 teaspoon white flour

Preparation

Dust the slices of veal in the flour and brown in a pan with butter. When one side of the meat is cooked, turn over. To the cooked side add a slice of ham, placing a sage leaf between the pieces of meat; a toothpick can help you hold the meats together.

Return to the heat and place a slice of melting cheese (Fontina or cheese slice); grill well and serve.

No salt is needed for this dish.

Bromatological evaluation per portion

Kcal	391
Protein (%)	43.4
Fats (%)	56.6
Carbohydrates (%)	0
Fiber (g)	0
Cholesterol (mg)	105

Valuable contents for the eye: ★

Veal is the most easily digested red meat.

Fontina is a type of cheese made from whole milk and as a result is fairly high in fat. Its yellow color is due to a considerable quantity of carotenoids.

Sage is an aromatic plant, rich in essential oils. It also contains quantities of tannins and choline.

Butter is made from milk and contains high quantities of saturated fatty acids.

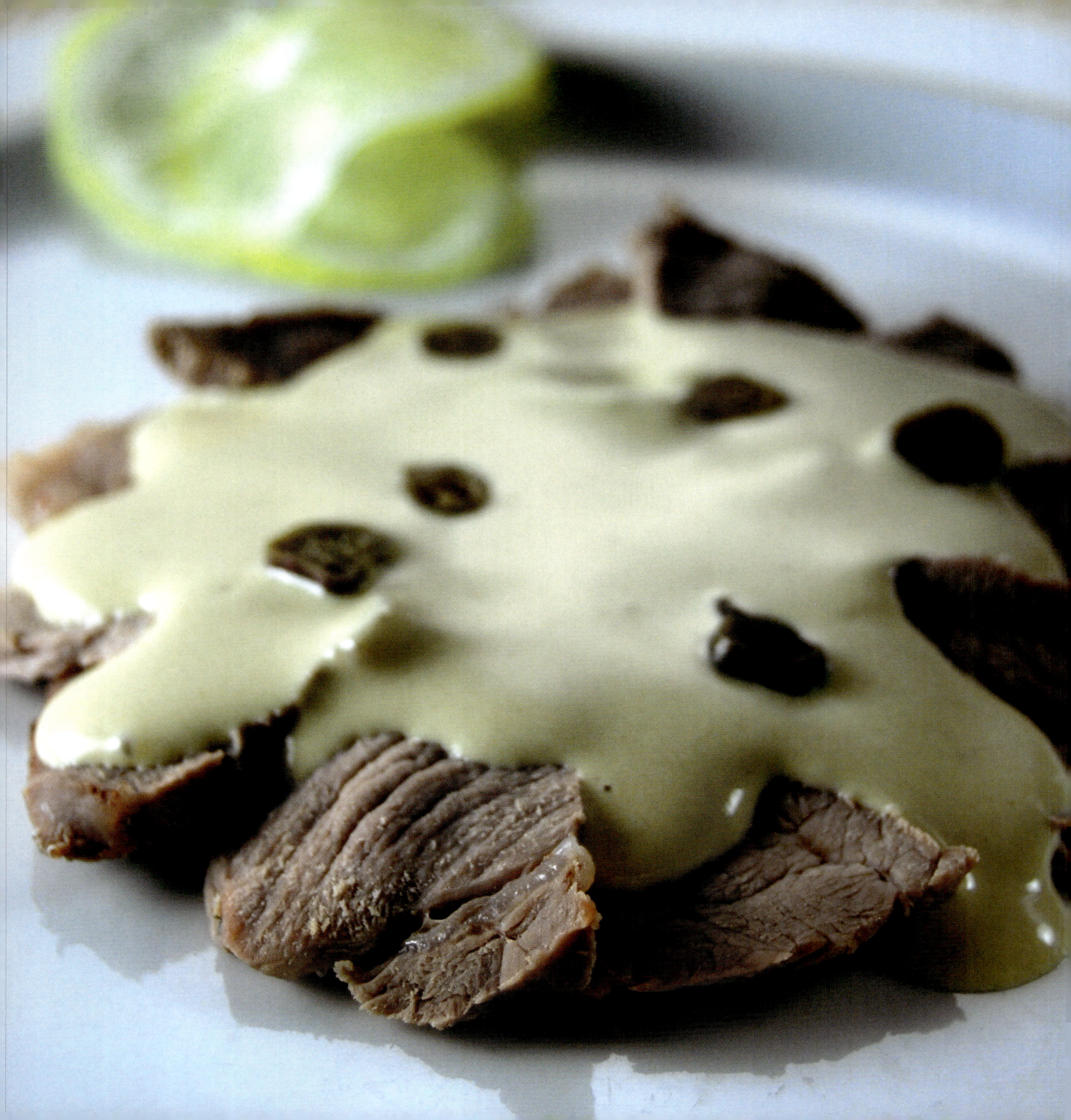

Vitel tonné

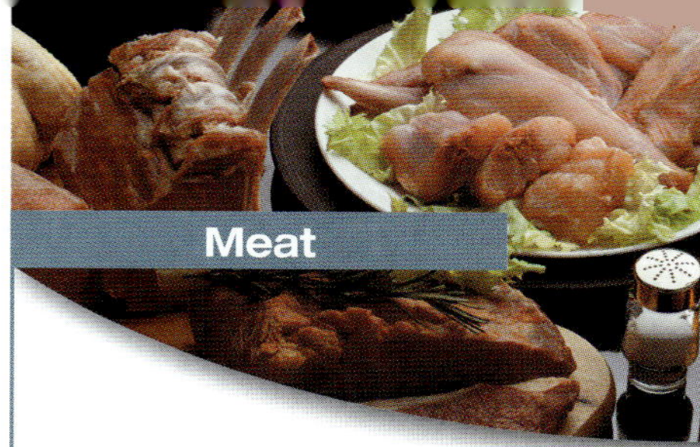

Meat

Ingredients and amounts for 4 people

- ✓ 1⅓ lbs filet of veal at room temperature
- ✓ 1½ liters (50.7 oz) water
- ✓ 1 carrot
- ✓ ½ onion, finely chopped
- ✓ 2 stalks of celery
- ✓ 2 bay leaves
- ✓ salt and pepper to taste
- ✓ 10½ oz good quality canned tuna, with no oil
- ✓ 3½ tablespoons capers
- ✓ juice of 1 lemon
- ✓ 6 tablespoons mayonnaise (recipe below)

Preparation of the veal

Make the stock with water, carrot, onion, celery, bay leaves, salt, and pepper. Once this mixture has been boiling for approximately 30 minutes, add the veal.

Turn the heat off after 10 minutes and allow to cool.

Cut the meat into thin slices and cover with the tuna sauce.

Serve garnished with capers and slices of lemon.

Preparation of mayonnaise

Note: The eggs should be at room temperature for at least 2 hours.

Place 2 whole eggs, the lemon juice, 1 teaspoon of vinegar, and a pinch of salt in the blender. Blend at the maximum speed and gradually add 10½ oz cold sunflower seed oil.

Tuna sauce

Put the mayonnaise in the blender, add the canned tuna (with no oil), capers, and pepper and blend at a very low speed to produce a smooth but consistent sauce.

Bromatological evaluation per portion

Kcal	449
Protein (%)	37
Fats (%)	60.8
Carbohydrates (%)	2.2
Fiber (g)	0.8
Cholesterol (mg)	130.8

Valuable contents for the eye: ★★

Veal is the most easily digested red meat.

Tuna is rich in protein and contains a good quantity of omega-3.

Capers contain vitamins A, C, and E, but also a large quantity of sodium.

Mayonnaise contains eggs that supply saturated fatty acids and also a good quantity of the mono- and polyunsaturated fats. Unfortunately, it contains cholesterol but is also a source of lutein.

Lemon contains high quantities of vitamin C and β-carotene and it also contains flavonoids (particularly in the pith or albedo underneath the peel).

Sunflower seed oil contains omega-6 and vitamin E, even though a portion of this vitamin is lost during the industrial refining process.

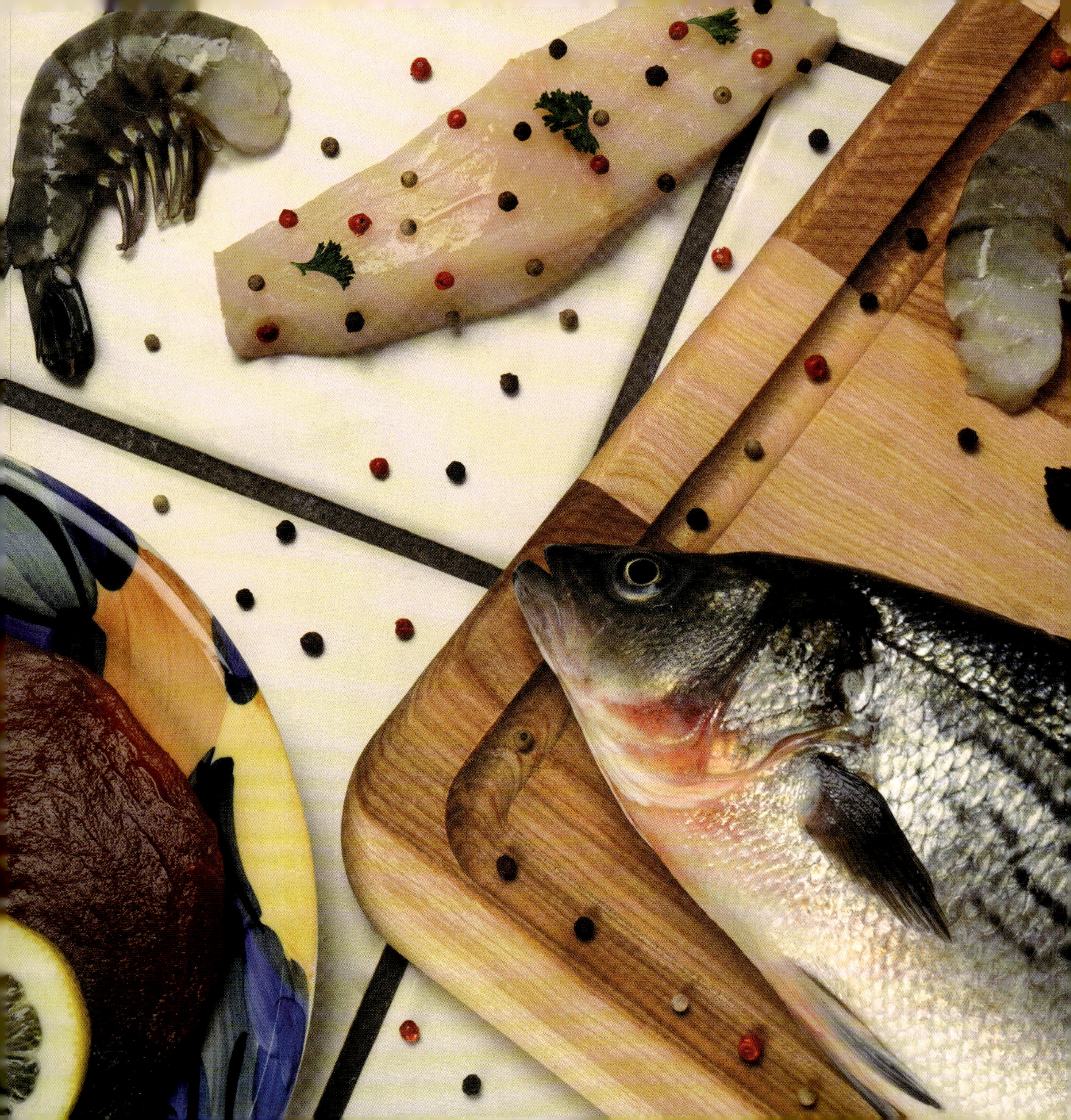

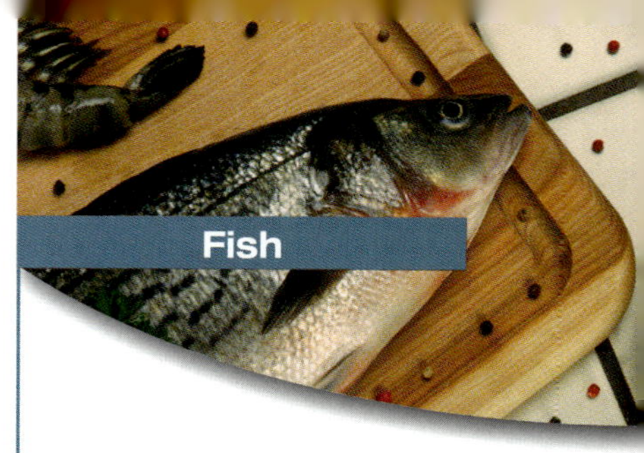

Marinated anchovies

Ingredients and amounts for 4 people

- ✓ 1 lb fresh anchovies
- ✓ 1 clove of garlic
- ✓ juice of 3 lemons
- ✓ 4 tablespoons white wine vinegar
- ✓ 2 teaspoons balsamic vinegar
- ✓ 1 bunch of fresh parsley
- ✓ 4 tablespoons extra virgin olive oil
- ✓ salt and black pepper to taste

Preparation

Remove the heads, the interiors, and the scales from the anchovies.
In a container, mix the lemon juice, white wine vinegar, the balsamic vinegar, garlic, salt, pepper, and the finely chopped parsley.
Add the anchovies.
Cover with clear plastic wrap and place in the refrigerator for 2 hours.
Drain the marinade liquid, add 4 tablespoons of good quality extra virgin olive oil and serve with pickled sweet peppers and basmati rice (optional).

Bromatological evaluation per portion

Kcal	189
Protein (%)	49.7
Fats (%)	46.5
Carbohydrates (%)	3.8
Fiber (g)	0.4
Cholesterol (mg)	47.6

Valuable contents for the eye: ★ ★

Anchovies are low in fat and contain omega-3 fatty acids.
Lemon contains high quantities of vitamin C and β-carotene and it also contains flavonoids (particularly in the pith or albedo underneath the peel).
Garlic contains selenium, zinc and alline, which is responsible for the taste and the penetrating, persistent odor of garlic. When alline is transformed into allicine, it has an antibacterial action and it lowers cholesterol and blood pressure levels.
Parsley contains flavonoids and is also an apiol and an antispastic. It also an antipyretic and stimulates uterine contractions.

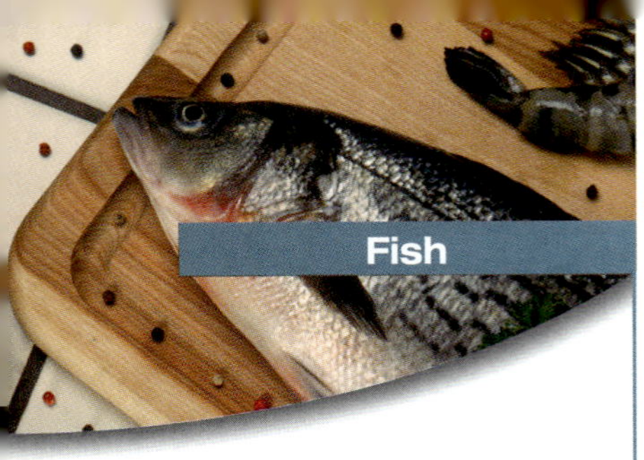

Fish

Anchovies or sardines (Genovese style)

Bromatological evaluation per portion

Kcal	300
Protein (%)	32.8
Fats (%)	65.4
Carbohydrates (%)	1.8
Fiber (g)	0.4
Cholesterol (mg)	31.8

Valuable contents for the eye: ★★

Anchovies and **sardines** are low in fat and contain omega-3 fatty acids.

Olive oil is an excellent source of unsaturated fatty acids.

Parmesan cheese is rich in easily digestible protein, is low in fat, and contains vitamin A and some vitamins of the B group.

Parsley contains flavonoids and is also an apiol, an antispastic, and an antipyretic. It also stimulates uterine contractions.

Garlic contains selenium, zinc and alline, which is responsible for the taste and the penetrating, persistent odor of garlic. When alline is transformed into allicine, it has an antibacterial action and it lowers cholesterol and blood pressure levels.

Ingredients and amounts for 4 people

✓ 14 oz anchovies or sardines

✓ 3 tablespoons extra virgin olive oil

✓ 7 tablespoons freshly grated Parmesan cheese

✓ 1 sprig of parsley

✓ 1 clove of garlic

Preparation

Carefully clean the very fresh anchovies (or sardines) (ie, remove the heads, the interiors ,and the scales and split them open).

Drizzle a small quantity of oil over the fish and coat them in cheese mixed with parsley and finely chopped garlic.

Fry in a pan with fresh boiling oil.

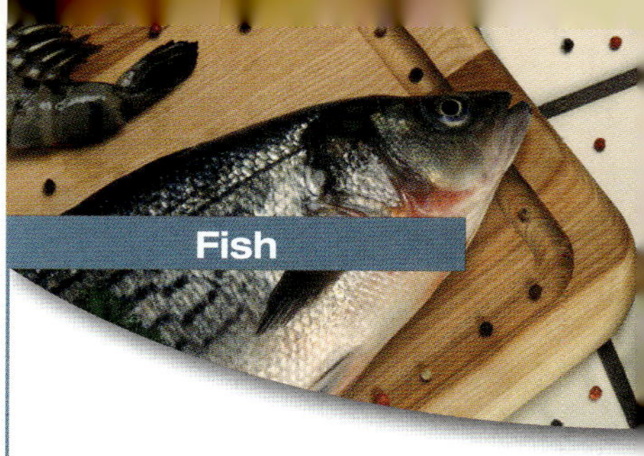

Dried salted cod in milk

Ingredients and amounts for 4 people

✓ 1⅓ lbs dried salted cod

✓ 8 tablespoons extra virgin olive oil

✓ 3½ tablespoons butter

✓ 1 cup milk

✓ 2 onions

Preparation

Wash the fish well to remove any excess salt. Break into pieces.
Soak for at least 24 hours in abundant cold water (if possible, change the water after 12 to 18 hours).
Thinly slice 2 onions and allow them to cook very slowly over a low heat in oil and butter.
Add the salted cod and cook for 3 to 4 minutes.
Gradually add the hot milk and then complete the cooking for 15 to 20 minutes.
Optional and only if the salt has been largely removed from the cod: Add a chopped anchovy and some capers.

Bromatological evaluation per portion

Kcal	477
Protein (%)	28.5
Fats (%)	65.6
Carbohydrates (%)	5.9
Fiber (g)	0.5
Cholesterol (mg)	37.5

Valuable contents for the eye: ★★★

The **cod** has been stored under salt. It is low in fat and rich in omega-3 and selenium; its liver oil contains large quantities of vitamins A and D.
Milk (particularly whole milk) has a good balance of sugars, fats, and proteins; it contains high quantities of calcium and phosphorous, but particularly fat-soluble anti-oxidant vitamins and water-soluble vitamins.
Butter is made from milk and contains high quantities of saturated fatty acids.
Onion contains vitamin C and a good quantity of flavonoids (quercetin).
Olive oil is an excellent source of unsaturated fatty acids.

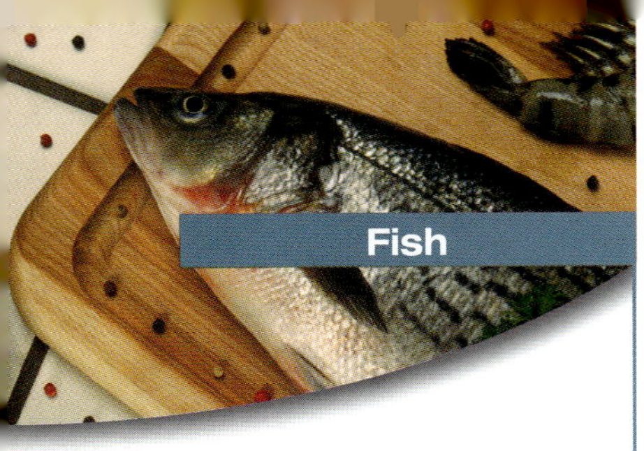

Bromatological evaluation per portion

Kcal	625
Protein (%)	21.6
Fats (%)	74.8
Carbohydrates (%)	3.6
Fiber (g)	1.8
Cholesterol (mg)	0

Valuable contents for the eye: ★★★

The **cod** has been stored under salt. It is low in fat and rich in omega-3 and selenium; its liver oil contains large quantities of vitamins A and D.
Tomatoes are rich in vitamins and oligominerals, but particularly they contain carotenoids and are the most important source of lycopene.
Onion contains vitamin C and a good quantity of flavonoids (quercetin).
Olive oil is an excellent source of unsaturated fatty acids.

Mother's recipe for dried salted cod stew

Ingredients and amounts for 4 people

✓ 1⅓ lbs dried salted cod
✓ 3 medium-sized onions
✓ 1¾ cups fresh tomato pulp
✓ 1 sprig of parsley
✓ 13½ tablespoons extra virgin olive oil
✓ salt and pepper to taste

Preparation

Cut the cod into bite-sized pieces and soak for 36 to 48 hours, changing the water several times; when it is well reconstituted in water, remove the skin.
Heat the olive oil and then fry the pieces of cod.
Add finely chopped onion and allow to brown.
Add the tomato, some pepper, chopped parsley and salt to taste.
Cook for at least 1 hour on low heat, stirring so that it does not stick to the pot.
As it cooks, remove any bones; do not worry if the cod disintegrates.
Polenta makes an excellent side dish to accompany the fish.

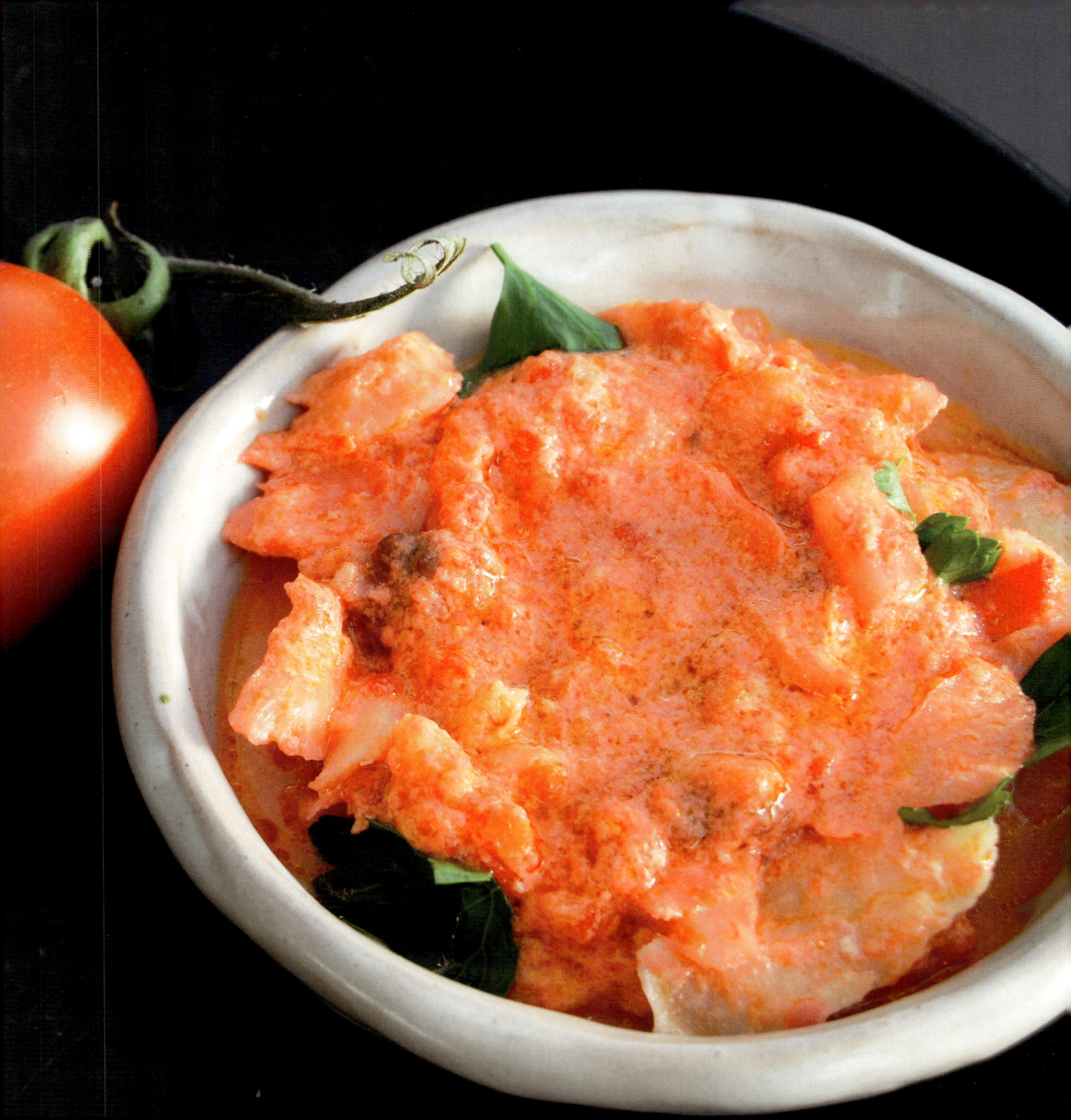

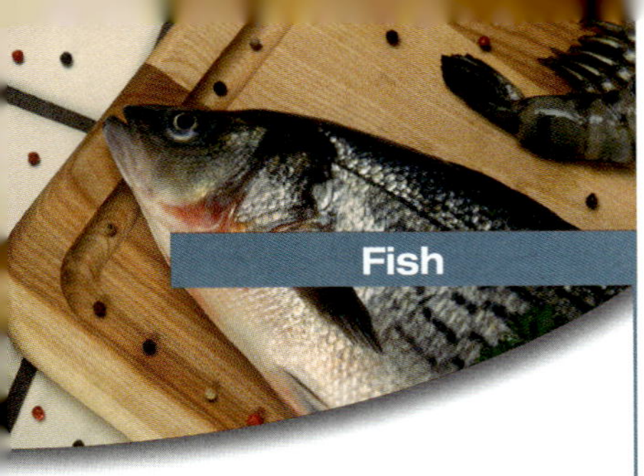

Bromatological evaluation per portion

Kcal	643
Protein (%)	34.6
Fats (%)	39.3
Carbohydrates (%)	26.1
Fiber (g)	6.2
Cholesterol (mg)	165

Valuable contents for the eye: ★ ★

Sea bass is low in fat, easily digested, high in protein and rich in omega-3 fatty acids..
Potatoes are rich in starch and contain potassium and vitamins C and B5.
Mushrooms are low in calories and rich in cellulose.

Sea bass with **potatoes, porcini mushrooms,** and **thyme**

Ingredients and amounts for 4 people

- ✓ 2 sea bass (1¾ lbs each)
- ✓ 8 potatoes
- ✓ 4 to 6 porcini mushrooms, cleaned and sliced
- ✓ 1 glass white wine
- ✓ 3 to 4 tablespoons extra virgin olive oil
- ✓ 1 sprig of parsley
- ✓ 1 teaspoon thyme
- ✓ salt and pepper to taste

Preparation

Prepare the fish for baking in the oven (ie, clean the inside, remove the scales, and wash in salty water).
Place the fish in a lightly oiled casserole dish.
Pour a tablespoon of oil and a handful of salt over the fish.
To the side, place the parboiled potatoes, cut into slices 6 to 7 mm thick, then add the mushrooms and the salt. After cooking for a few minutes, stir the potatoes and pour the wine onto the fish.
Cook in the oven at least for 15 minutes at 350°F.
Once cooked, sprinkle with finely sliced parsley and thyme.

Note: In this recipe, the porcini mushrooms can be replaced with cleaned artichokes cut into 8 segments.

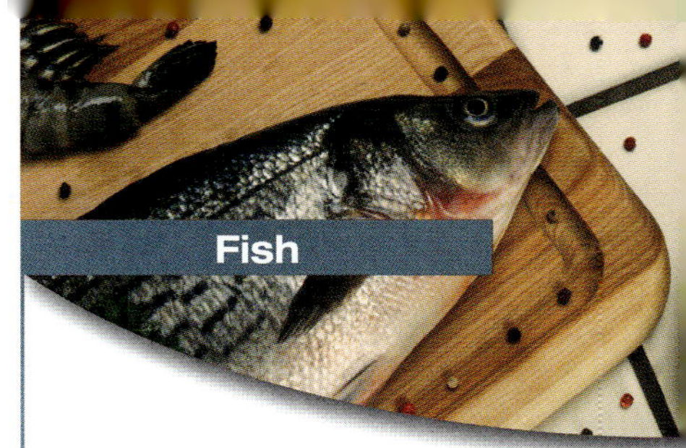

Sea bass under salt

Ingredients and amounts for 4 people

- ✓ $3\frac{1}{3}$ lbs sea bass, scaled and cleaned
- ✓ $6\frac{2}{3}$ lbs salt crystals
- ✓ 2 cloves of garlic
- ✓ 2 bay leaves
- ✓ 2 sprays of rosemary

Preparation

Pour $4\frac{1}{3}$ to $5\frac{1}{3}$ cups of salt into a large oven dish.
Place the garlic, rosemary, and bay leaf inside the fish.
Place the fish on top of this bed of salt and cover with the remaining salt.
Place in the oven and cook at 390°F for 20 to 25 minutes.
When cooked, remove all the salt (above and below the fish), clean the fish, and serve.

Bromatological evaluation per portion

Kcal	110
Protein (%)	80.4
Fats (%)	16.4
Carbohydrates (%)	3.2
Fiber (g)	0
Cholesterol (mg)	0

Valuable contents for the eye: ★

Sea bass is low in fat, easily digested, high in protein, and rich in omega-3 fatty acids.

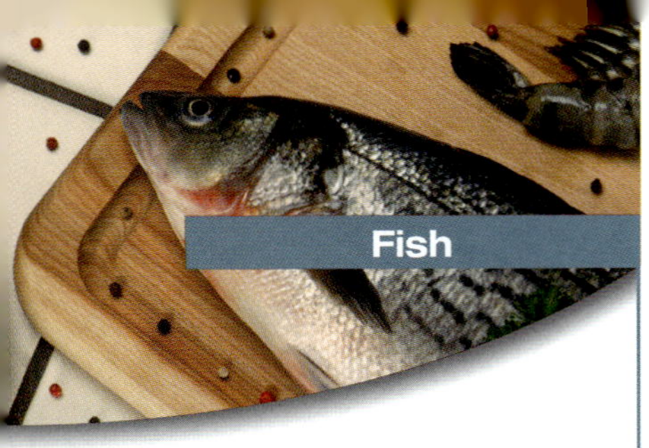

Bromatological evaluation per portion

Kcal	322
Protein (%)	43
Fats (%)	21.9
Carbohydrates (%)	35.1
Fiber (g)	2.6
Cholesterol (mg)	0

Valuable contents for the eye: ★ ★

Cod is low in fat and rich in omega-3 and selenium; its liver oil contains large quantities of vitamins A and D.

Olive oil is an excellent source of unsaturated fatty acids.

Parsley contains flavonoids and is also an apiol, an antispastic, and an antipyretic. It also stimulates uterine contractions.

Baked filet of cod

Ingredients and amounts for 4 people

✓ ¾ lb cod filets

✓ 6 potatoes

✓ 2 tablespoons extra virgin olive oil

✓ ½ teaspoon marjoram

✓ ½ teaspoon thyme

✓ 1 teaspoon parsley, finely chopped

✓ salt and pepper to taste

Preparation

Place the potatoes in water and bring to a boil for 10 minutes.

Slice the potatoes and arrange them to create a uniform layer in a wet oven dish.

Place the cod filets over the potatoes. Then add the marjoram, thyme, parsley, salt, and pepper.

Then add another layer of potatoes, this time sliced more thinly. Drizzle some olive oil over them.

Cook in the oven at 390°F for 20 to 25 minutes.

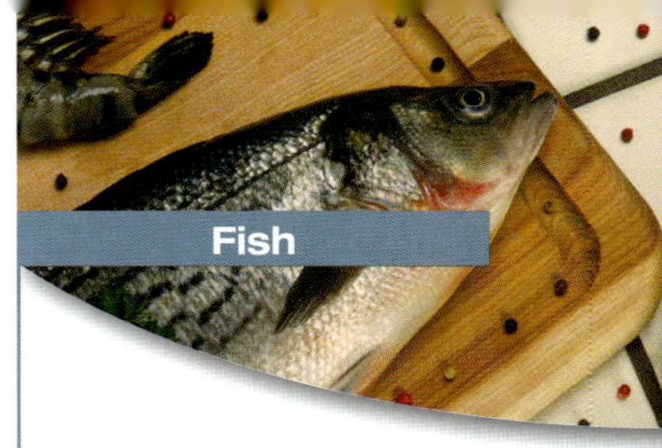

Swordfish: aromatic carpaccio (raw cured fish)

Ingredients and amounts for 4 people

✓ ¾ lb fresh swordfish thinly sliced

✓ juice of 1 lemon

✓ 3 tablespoons extra virgin olive oil

✓ 1 sprig of parsley

✓ 6 basil leaves

✓ 1 bunch of chives

✓ salt and pepper to taste

Preparation

Use the blender to emulsify the lemon juice with the oil, the chopped herbs (parsley, basil, chives), and a pinch of salt and pepper.
Place the slices of fish on a plate and pour the sauce over them.
Leave in the refrigerator to marinate for approximately 20 minutes, then serve.

Bromatological evaluation per portion

Kcal	232
Protein (%)	33.3
Fats (%)	66.5
Carbohydrates (%)	0.2
Fiber (g)	0
Cholesterol (mg)	0

Valuable contents for the eye: ★ ★

Swordfish is extremely low in fat and rich in protein and contains phosphorous and selenium.
Lemon contains high quantities of vitamin C and β-carotene. It also contains flavonoids (particularly in the pith or albedo underneath the peel).
Parsley contains flavonoids and is also an apiol, an antispastic, and an antipyretic. It also stimulates uterine contractions.
Olive oil is an excellent source of unsaturated fatty acids.
Chives have the same taste as onion, but are more digestible. They also contain flavonoids.
Basil owes its aroma to the numerous essential oils it contains. These stimulate salivary and gastric secretions.

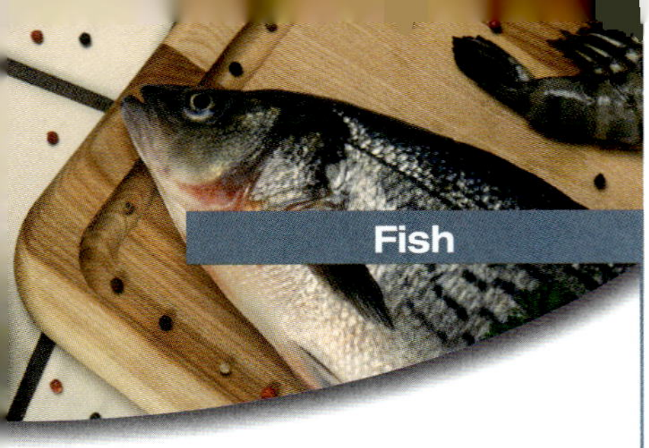

Fish

Steamed salmon

Bromatological evaluation per portion

Kcal	236
Protein (%)	40.4
Fats (%)	59.3
Carbohydrates (%)	0.3
Fiber (g)	0
Cholesterol (mg)	45.5

Valuable contents for the eye: ★

Salmon is rich in omega-3 and oligominerals, particularly astaxanthin, which it obtains from the crustaceans its eats.
Carrots are an excellent source of β-carotene; they also stimulate diuresis and intestinal motility.
Onion contains vitamin C and a good quantity of flavonoids (quercetin).
Parsley contains flavonoids and is also an apiol, an antispastic, and an antipyretic. It also stimulates uterine contractions.

Ingredients and amounts for 4 people

- ✓ 4 pieces of salmon
- ✓ 2 stalks of celery
- ✓ 1 carrot
- ✓ 1 onion
- ✓ 1 bunch of parsley
- ✓ 1 liter (33.8 oz) water
- ✓ salt to taste

Preparation

Heat a saucepan of water with the celery, carrot, onion, parsley, and a handful of salt.
Place the fish in a fish steamer on top of the pan; cook for approximately
15 minutes.
Remove the fish, clean, and place on a plate.
Season with a sauce suitable for fish (lemon sauce, tomato sauce, etc).

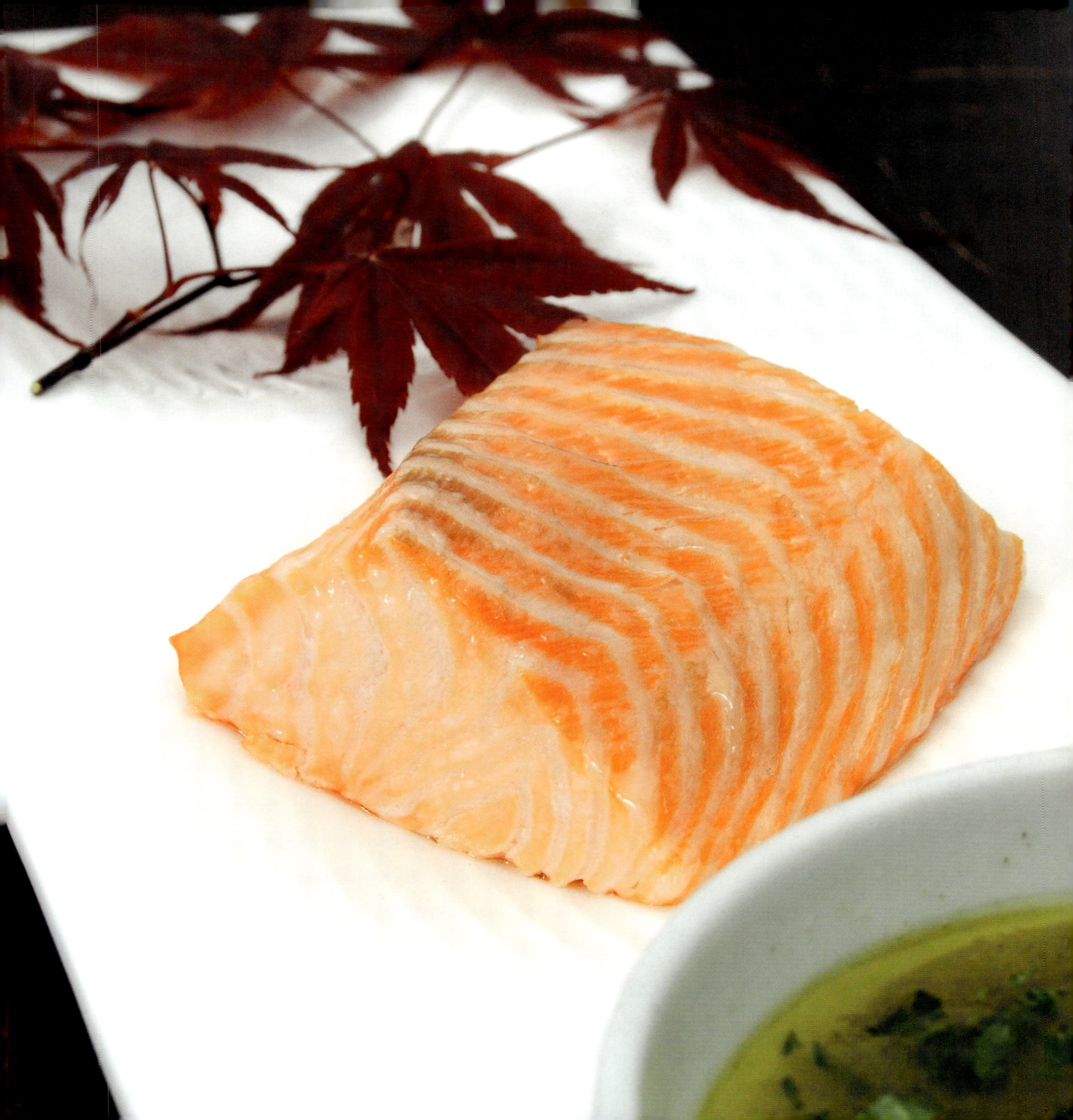

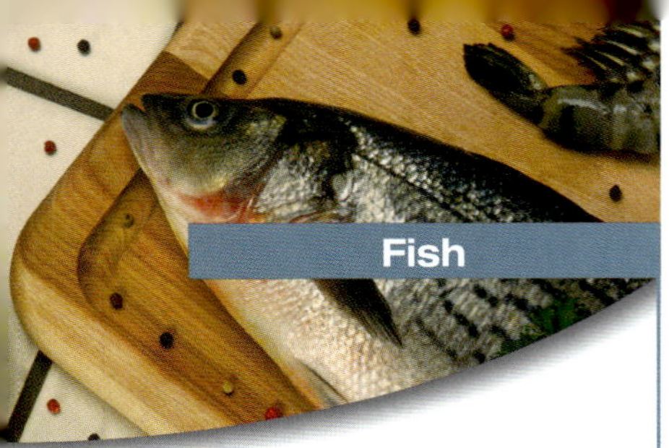

Fish

Bromatological evaluation per portion

Kcal	248
Protein (%)	32.8
Fats (%)	60.1
Carbohydrates (%)	7.1
Fiber (g)	0
Cholesterol (mg)	0

Valuable contents for the eye: ★★

Fish in general is rich in omega-3.
Olive oil is an excellent source of unsaturated fatty acids.
Like onion, **scallions** also contain flavonoids.
Chives have the same taste as onion but are more digestible. They also contain flavonoids.
The **orange** is rich in sucrose and contains high quantities of vitamin C and β-carotene.
Soy sauce is rich in isoflavons.

Swordfish, salmon, or tuna tartare

Ingredients and amounts for 4 people

- ✓ 10½ oz finely chopped, very fresh fish meat
- ✓ 1 scallion
- ✓ juice of 1 orange
- ✓ 4 tablespoons extra virgin olive oil
- ✓ 1 bunch chives
- ✓ 1 tablespoon soy sauce
- ✓ salt and pepper to taste

Preparation

Chop the chives and the scallion and place in a bowl with the fish and all the other ingredients.
Mix and let sit for 10 minutes.
Serve with a selection of raw vegetables.

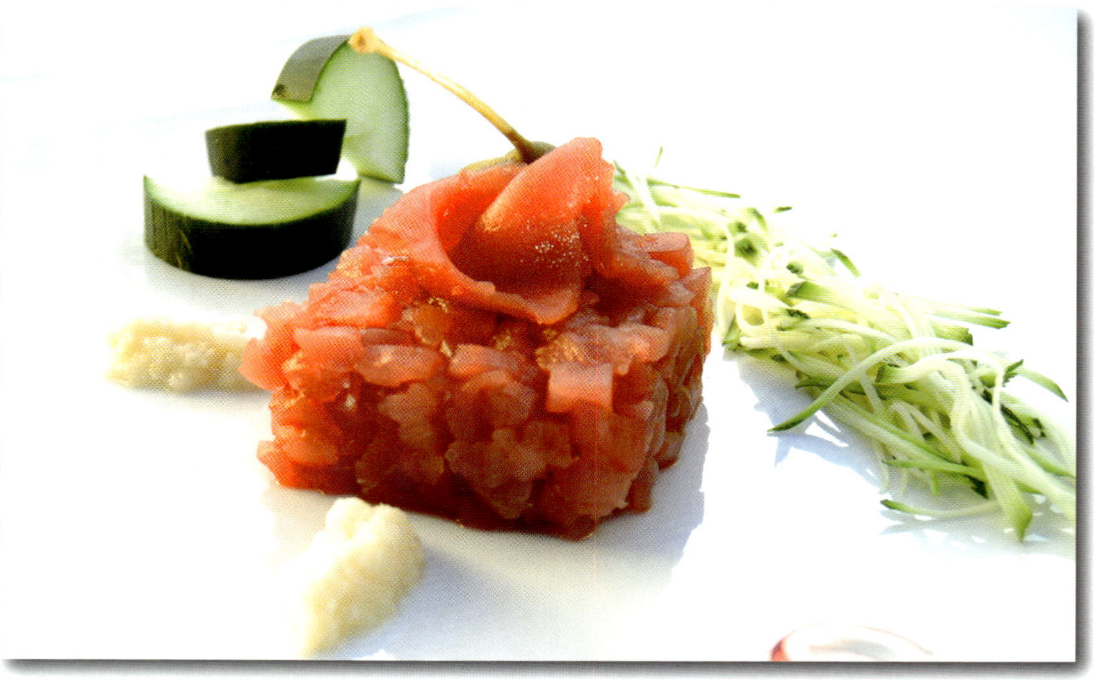

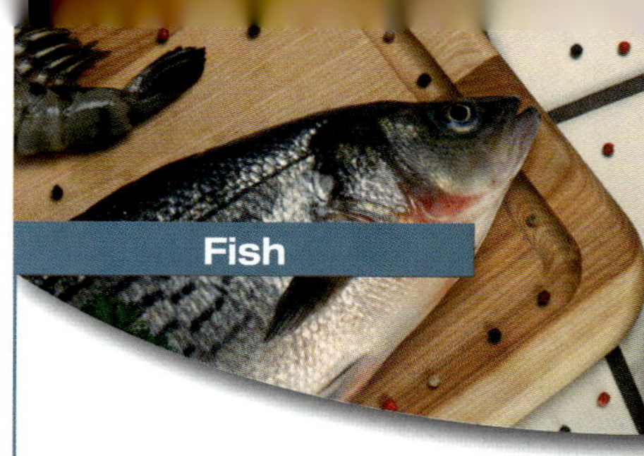

Swordfish in tomato sauce

Ingredients and amounts for 4 people

- ✓ 1⅓ lbs swordfish, sliced into 4 steaks
- ✓ 4 tablespoons extra virgin olive oil
- ✓ ½ clove of garlic
- ✓ 2 tablespoons desalted capers
- ✓ 4 tablespoons black olives
- ✓ 1¾ cups drained tomato pulp
- ✓ 1 tablespoon oregano
- ✓ salt and pepper to taste

Preparation

Heat the oil and brown the fish.
Add the tomato, capers, garlic, olives, and oregano.
Cook for 15 to 20 minutes and serve.

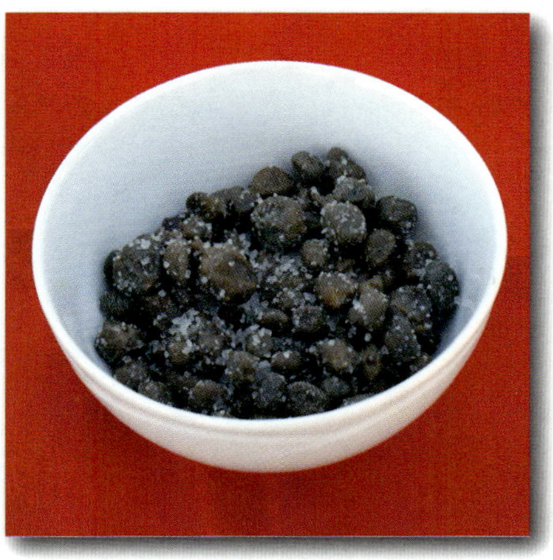

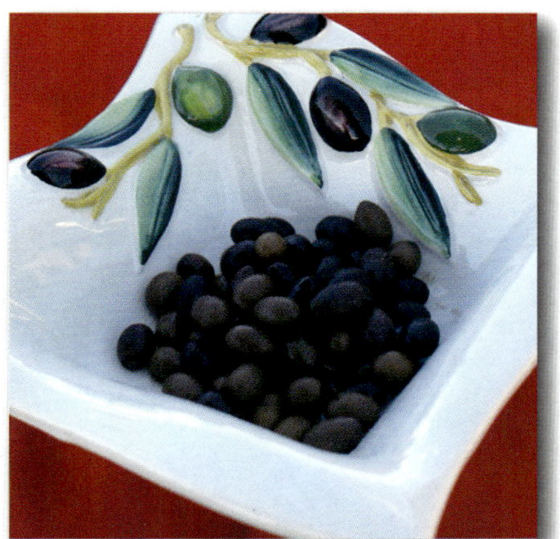

Bromatological evaluation per portion

Kcal	324
Protein (%)	26.2
Fats (%)	69.6
Carbohydrates (%)	4.2
Fiber (g)	1
Cholesterol (mg)	0

Valuable contents for the eye: ★★★

Swordfish is extremely low in fat and rich in protein and contains phosphorous and selenium.
Tomatoes are rich in vitamins and oligominerals, but particularly they contain carotenoids and are the most important source of lycopene.
Olives are rich in mono-unsaturated fats, vitamin E, and potassium.
Capers contain vitamins A, C, and E and also a considerable quantity of sodium.
Olive oil is an excellent source of unsaturated fatty acids.
Oregano is rich in essential oils.

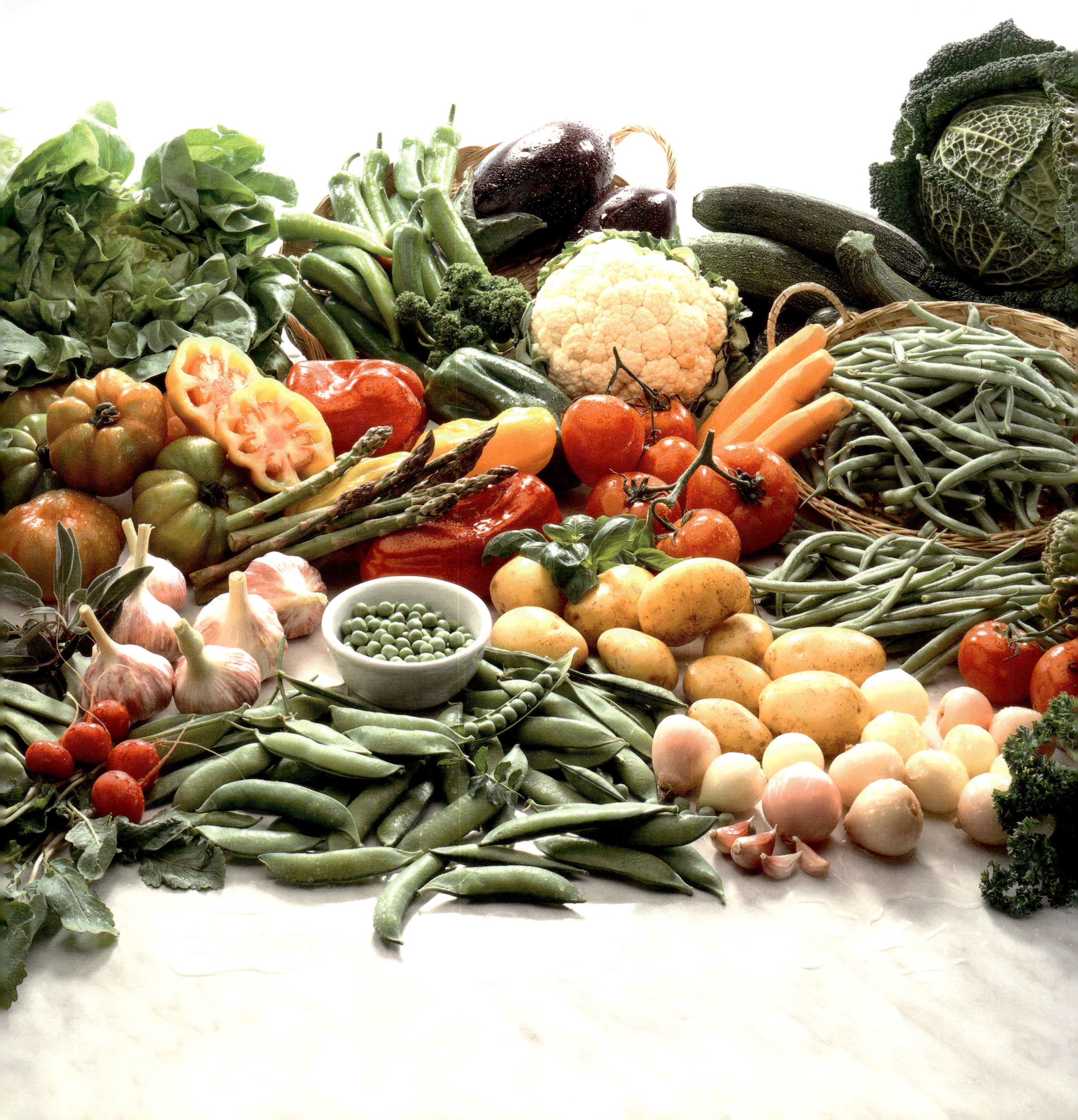

Vegetables

A slogan very close to the hearts of nutritionists summarized the way of satisfying the daily vitamin requirements by an aphorism, "Eat something red, green, and yellow every day."

A single vegetable will never contain the complete vitamin spectrum because the content varies considerably from one vegetable to another. The red of the tomatoes hides a large quantity of vitamin C, some vitamin P and B2, but also lycopene. The same applies to the intense green of certain vegetables, rich in antioxidants and protective agents (leading the way, the huge cabbage family) but poor in the vitamin B complex. Not even the orange carrot can supply us with the vitamin B complex or vitamin A, whereas there is a large quantity of carotenoids, the progenitors of vitamin A.

It is best therefore to stick to the old straightforward rule of alternating the vegetables according to the seasons; this rotation will provide most of the vitamin-mineral and anti-oxidant requirements of the human body. At one time, the seasonal changes obliged the alternation of the various species; now, the technological progress of the canning industry, the greenhouse cultivations, and air transport make an important contribution to supplying our tables with every type of fruit and vegetable at any time of the year. The benefits and drawbacks of globalization!

We can now satisfy our taste buds and personal preference for a specific type of vegetable; however, alternating our selection will guarantee not only a greater quantity of vitamins and minerals but also the right proportions of fibers and an excess of antioxidants that can attenuate the cell damage caused by the free radicals.

All vegetables have a mineral content, primarily potassium and to a lesser degree magnesium; modern dietology assigns an important role to these substances in the organic balances.

Finally, a slight preference should be given to the consumption of carefully washed raw vegetables, although we must put aside any worries that cooked vegetables will have lost all of their beneficial properties.

Vitamin C is rapidly denatured by high temperatures; however, even prolonged exposure to sunlight can have the same effect. The opposite is true for carotenes, which have the advantage of resisting heat. Fibers lose none of their protective qualities for the digestive apparatus with cooking.

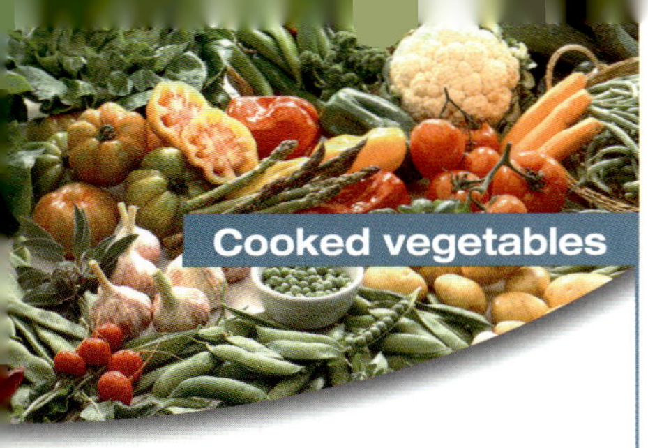

Bromatological evaluation per portion

Kcal	44
Protein (%)	28.9
Fats (%)	9.2
Carbohydrates (%)	61.9
Fiber (g)	3.1
Cholesterol (mg)	0

Valuable contents for the eye: ★★★

Asparagus is rich in fiber and contains vitamin B6, vitamin C, folic acid, carotenoids, and flavonoids.
Strawberries are a good source of vitamin C and anthocyanosides.
Balsamic vinegar is low in calories but has a very intense taste.

Asparagus with strawberries

Ingredients and amounts for 4 people

✓ 1 lb asparagus tips (white asparagus tips are preferred)
✓ 3 to 4 large strawberries
✓ 2 tablespoons balsamic vinegar
✓ salt and black pepper to taste

Preparation

Peel the ends of the asparagus and remove the more fibrous parts. Boil in abundant salty water for 12 to 13 minutes.
Blend the strawberries with the balsamic vinegar, salt, and pepper.
Pour the blended mixture over the boiled asparagus and serve.

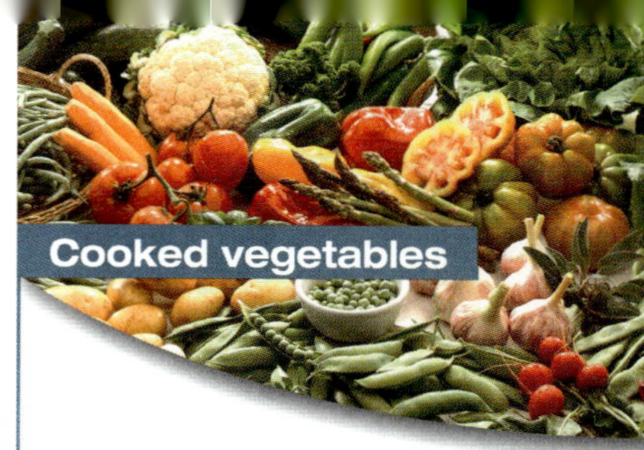

Classical-style lentils

Ingredients and amounts for 4 people

✓ ½ lb (8 oz) lentils
✓ 3½ tablespoons lard or finely sliced smoky bacon
✓ 1 bay leaf
✓ 2 basil leaves
✓ 2 tablespoons extra virgin olive oil
✓ 1 onion
✓ 1 carrot
✓ 1 stalk of celery
✓ 3½ oz canned tomatoes
✓ ½ liter (16.9 oz) vegetable stock
✓ salt and pepper to taste

Preparation

Soak the lentils in cold water for at least 6 hours; drain.
In a casserole dish, brown the lard and the vegetables (finely chopped onion, celery, carrot) in the oil. Add the lentils.
When the lentils have been seasoned, add the canned tomatoes, some stock, salt, pepper, and the herbs (bay leaf and basil).
Cover and cook very slowly for at least 1 hour, adding hot stock at intervals.
At the end of the cooking period, the sauce should be fairly dense.

Bromatological evaluation per portion

Kcal	380
Protein (%)	12.6
Fats (%)	61.2
Carbohydrates (%)	26.2
Fiber (g)	7.1
Cholesterol (mg)	14.2

Valuable contents for the eye: ★★★

Lentils are a good source of zinc.
Onion contains vitamin C and a good quantity of flavonoids (quercetin).
Tomatoes are rich in vitamins and oligominerals, but particularly they contain carotenoids and are the most important source of lycopene.
Carrots are an excellent source of β-carotene. Moreover, they stimulate diuresis and intestinal motility.
Olive oil is an excellent source of unsaturated fatty acids.

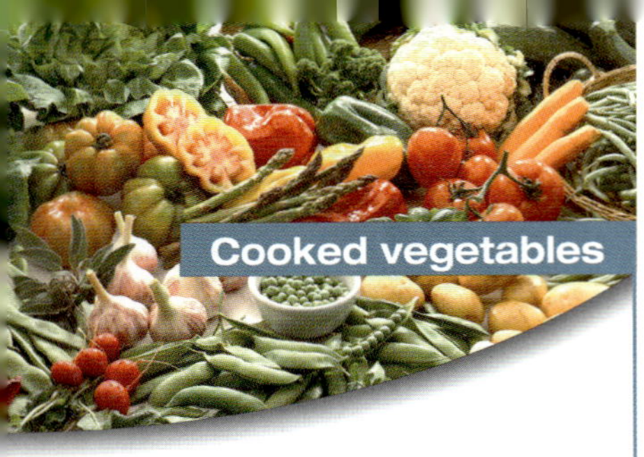

Zucchini flowers fried in peanut oil

Bromatological evaluation per portion

Kcal	376
Protein (%)	4.2
Fats (%)	72.5
Carbohydrates (%)	23.3
Fiber (g)	0
Cholesterol (mg)	0

Valuable contents for the eye: ★★

Zucchini flowers are low in calories and very rich in carotenoids and vitamins C and E.

Peanut oil contains monounsaturated fatty acids, which makes it very stable during the frying process.

Ingredients and amounts for 4 people

- ✓ 8 zucchini flowers
- ✓ 7 tablespoons plain white flour
- ✓ ½ teaspoon beer yeast or 2 tablespoons beer
- ✓ 1 pinch of salt
- ✓ 10½ oz peanut oil

Preparation of the batter

Gently mix the flour with the beer yeast, 2 to 3 spoons of warm water, and a pinch of salt. Let sit for 30 minutes in a warm environment.

Preparation of the flowers

Clean the flowers, cut them in half, wash them, and dry thoroughly.
Dip the flowers in the batter and transfer to the boiling peanut oil; cook at approximately 350°F; turn them over when the batter assumes a pinkish hue.
For best results, fry one flower at a time.
Serve hot after having dried the excess oil on absorbent paper towels.

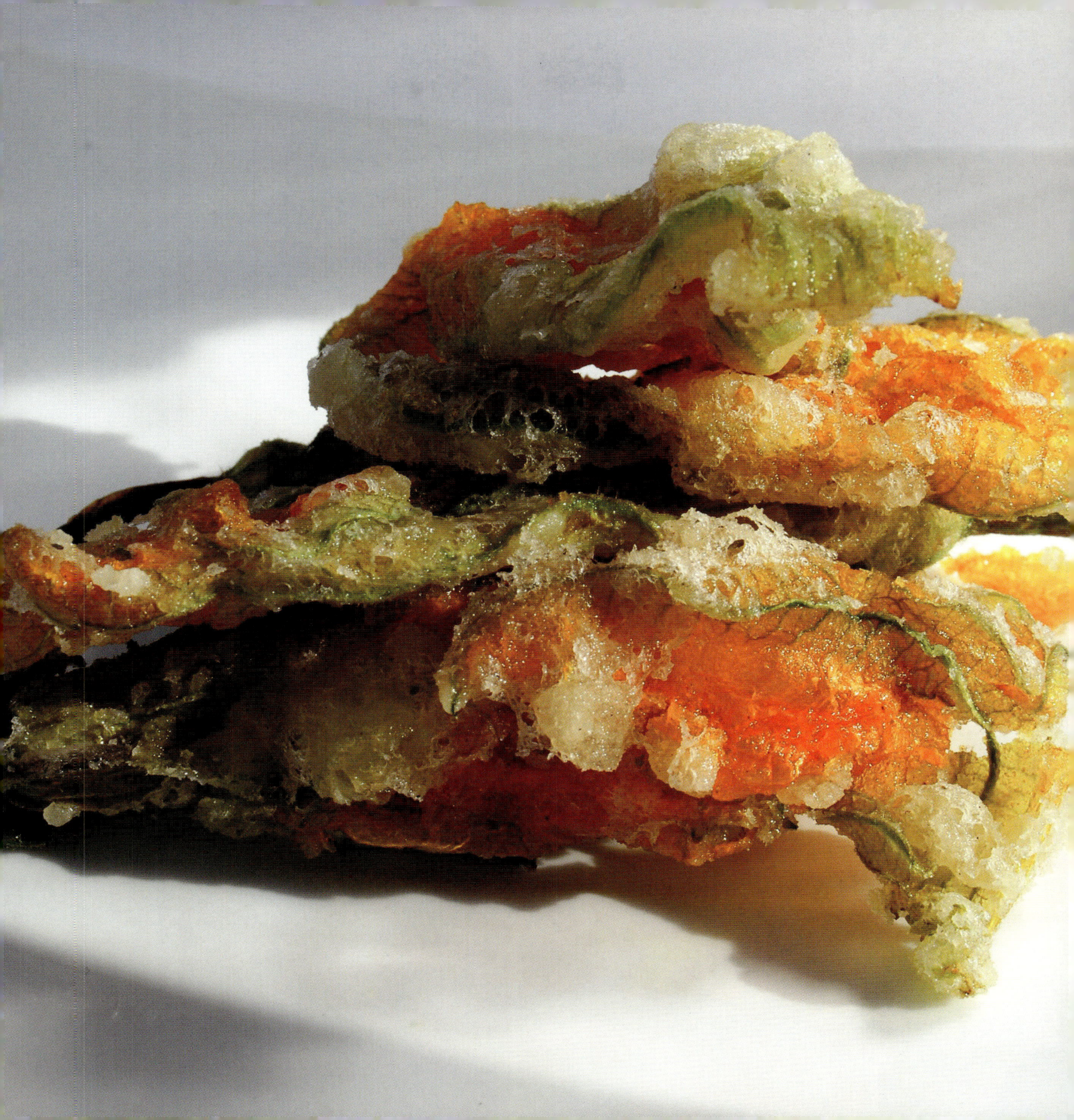

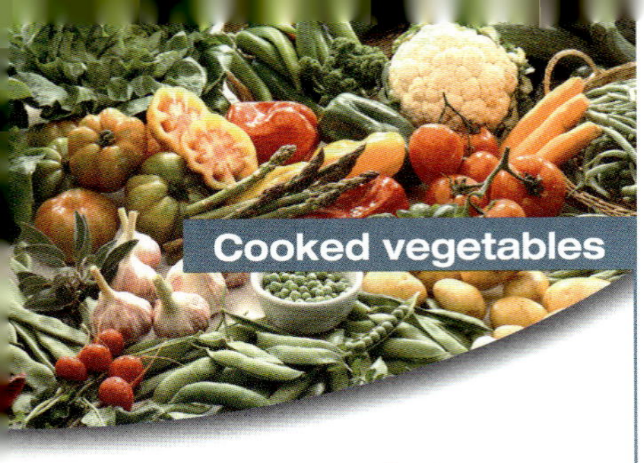

Bromatological evaluation per portion

Kcal	283
Protein (%)	8.7
Fats (%)	37
Carbohydrates (%)	54.3
Fiber (g)	5
Cholesterol (mg)	0

Valuable contents for the eye: ★★

Tomatoes are rich in vitamins and oligominerals, but particularly they contain carotenoids and are the most important source of lycopene.
The **potato** is rich in starch and contains potassium and vitamins C and B5.
Olive oil is an excellent source of unsaturated fatty acids.
Onion contains vitamin C and a good quantity of flavonoids (quercetin).
Garlic contains selenium, zinc and alline, which is responsible for the taste and the penetrating, persistent odor of garlic. When alline is transformed into allicine, it has an antibacterial action and it lowers cholesterol and blood pressure levels.

Potatoes and tomatoes (Pugliese style)

Ingredients and amounts for 4 people

✓ ¾ lb ripe tomatoes
✓ 1 lb potatoes
✓ 2 onions
✓ 1 bunch of parsley
✓ 1 clove of garlic
✓ ½ teaspoon oregano
✓ 3 tablespoons extra virgin olive oil
✓ 2 tablespoons breadcrumbs
✓ salt and pepper to taste

Preparation

Peel the potatoes, cut them into slices approximately 1-cm thick, and boil them in water for 5 minutes.
Wash the tomatoes, cut them in half, and turn them upside-down to drain off the water.
Remove the external layer of the onions and cut them into slices approximately 2-cm thick.
Finely chop the garlic, parsley, and oregano; add the salt and pepper.
Heat the oil in an oven-safe dish.
Spread the slices of onion in the dish and sprinkle some of the chopped garlic mix on top.
Add the slices of potatoes and some more of the chopped garlic mixture.
Cover with the half tomatoes, with the cut side facing upward.
Sprinkle with the remaining chopped garlic mixture and then the breadcrumbs.
Drizzle with the residual oil.
Cook in the oven at 390°F to 425°F for 30 to 35 minutes.

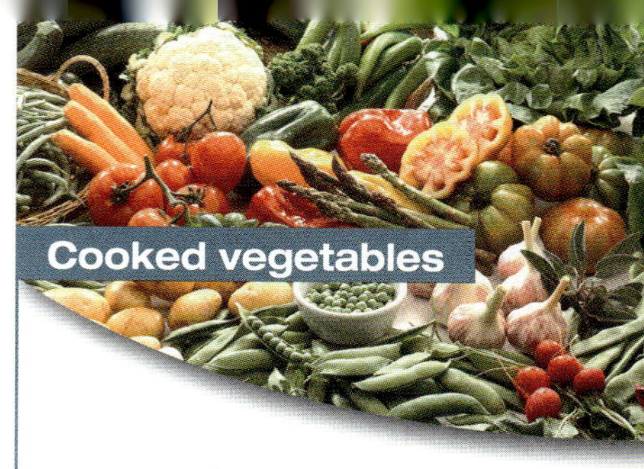

Rostì potatoes

Ingredients and amounts for 4 people

- ✓ 6 potatoes
- ✓ 3 tablespoons sunflower seed oil
- ✓ 1 teaspoon butter
- ✓ salt to taste

Preparation

Cut the potatoes into thin sticks (1-in long and $^{1}/_{10}$-in thick) and dry them well.
In a pan, heat the sunflower seed oil.
Add the potatoes and compress them; cook over moderate heat.
A few minutes later, add the butter, and with the help of a flat lid, turn the potatoes over to allow the other side to cook.
Continue cooking until both surfaces are browned.
Salt to taste prior to serving.

Bromatological evaluation per portion

Kcal	253
Protein (%)	5.5
Fats (%)	50.2
Carbohydrates (%)	44.3
Fiber (g)	2.6
Cholesterol (mg)	7.5

Valuable contents for the eye: ★

The **potato** is rich in starch and contains potassium and vitamins C and B5.
Butter is a milk product consisting of saturated fatty acids.
Sunflower seed oil contains omega-6 and vitamin E, even though part of this is lost during the extraction process.

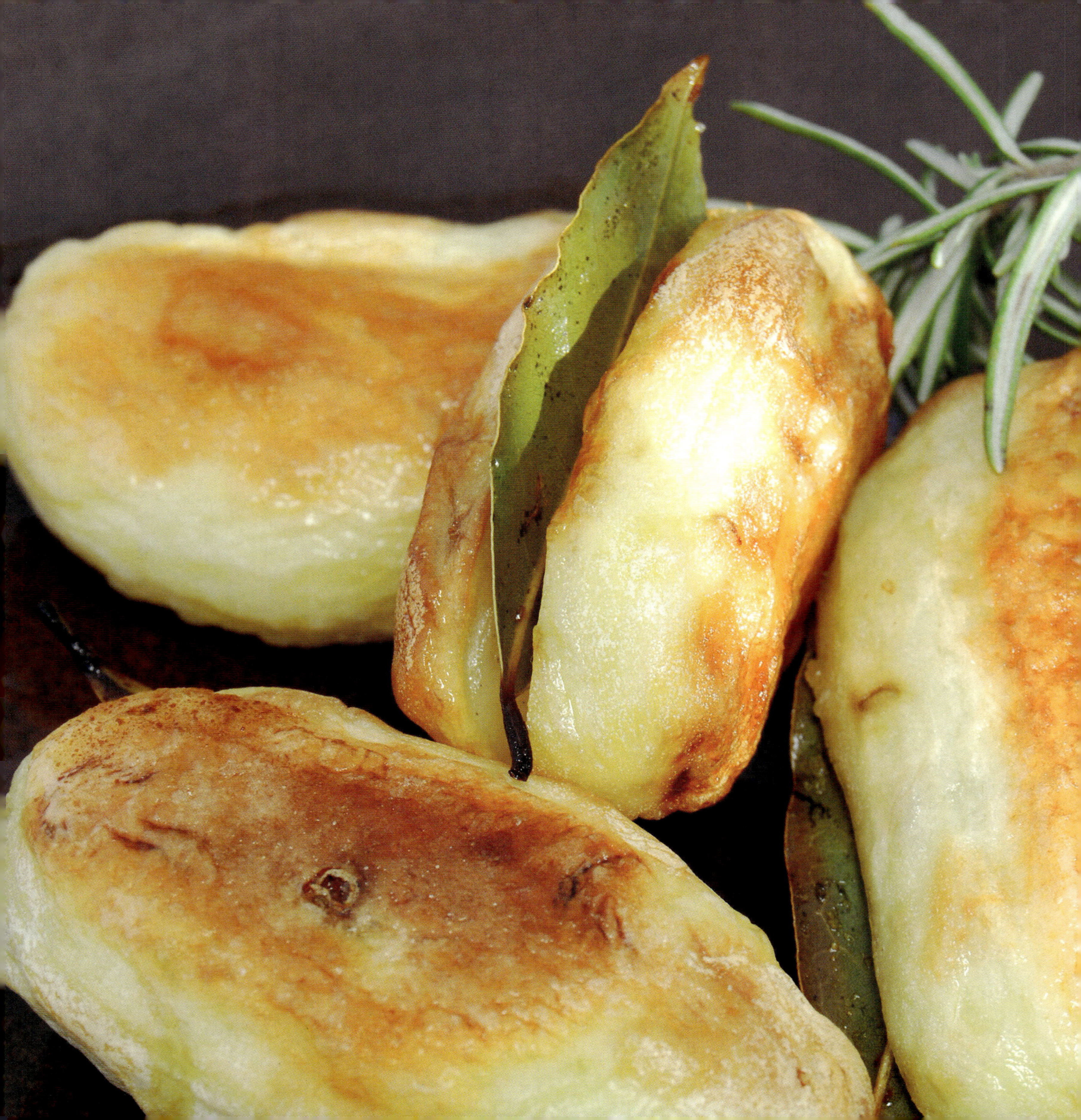

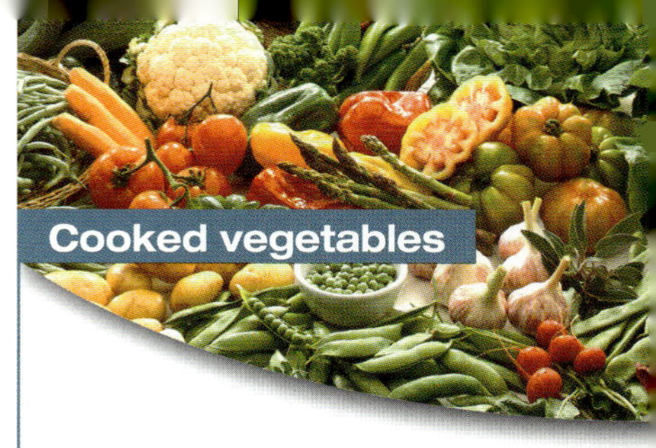

Potatoes baked with bay leaf

Ingredients and amounts for 4 people

- ✓ 6 potatoes
- ✓ 6 bay leaves
- ✓ 3 tablespoons peanut oil
- ✓ 1 teaspoon butter
- ✓ salt to taste

Preparation

Wash and peel the potatoes, and boil in water for 10 minutes. Cut a slit in the surface without splitting the potato completely.

In the slit, place a bay leaf dipped in salt and half a teaspoon of oil.

Pour more oil onto the surface of the potato.

Place in the oven at 390°F, and cook for 25 to 30 minutes; at the end of the cooking add a teaspoon of butter.

Bromatological evaluation per portion

Kcal	226
Protein (%)	5.7
Fats (%)	50
Carbohydrates (%)	44.3
Fiber (g)	2.6
Cholesterol (mg)	12.5

Valuable contents for the eye: ★

The **potato** is rich in starch and contains potassium and vitamins C and B5.

Butter is a milk product consisting of saturated fatty acids.

Peanut oil contains monounsaturated fatty acids that makes it stable during the frying process.

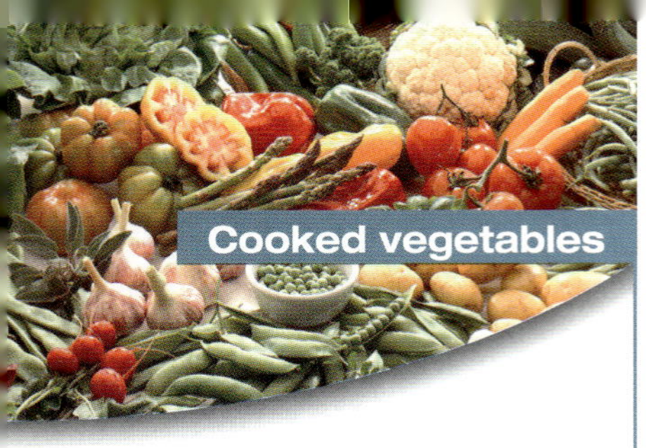

Potato-rosemary bake

Bromatological evaluation per portion

Kcal	226
Protein (%)	5.7
Fats (%)	50
Carbohydrates (%)	44.3
Fiber (g)	2.6
Cholesterol (mg)	12.5

Valuable contents for the eye: ★

The **potato** is rich in starch and contains potassium and vitamins C and B5.

Olive oil is an excellent source of unsaturated fatty acids.

Butter is a milk product consisting of saturated fatty acids.

Ingredients and amounts for 4 people

✓ 6 potatoes
✓ 1 sprig of rosemary
✓ 2 cloves of garlic
✓ 3 tablespoons extra virgin olive oil
✓ 1 teaspoon butter
✓ salt to taste

Preparation

Clean and cut the potatoes into ½-in slices; parboil them in salty water. Pour the oil into an oven-safe dish, add the potatoes and the rosemary, and stir the potatoes in oil until coated.
Cook in the oven at 390°F for 30 minutes. Mix well every 10 minutes.
Add salt, diced garlic, and butter when cooked and grill for 2 to 3 minutes.

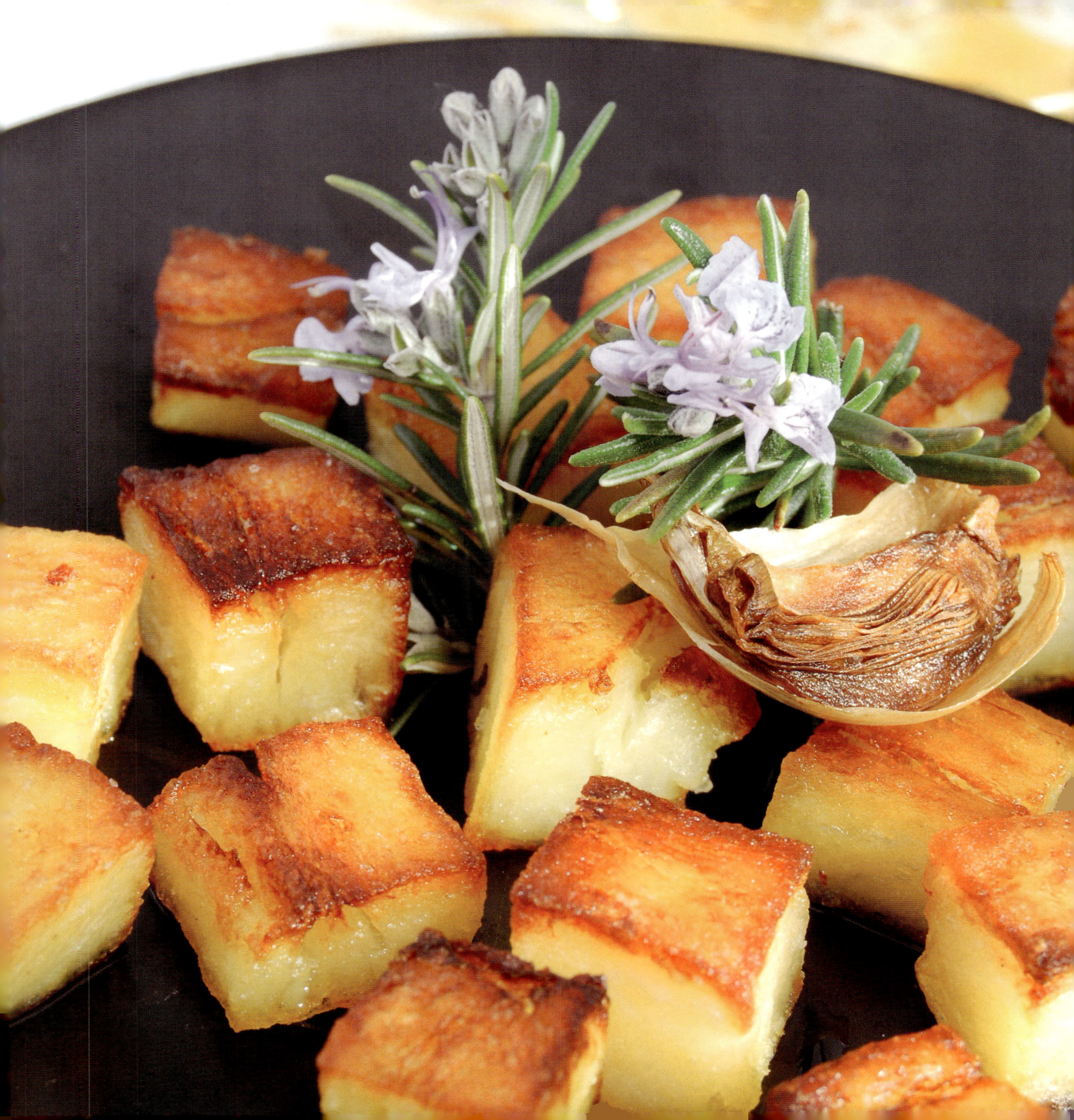

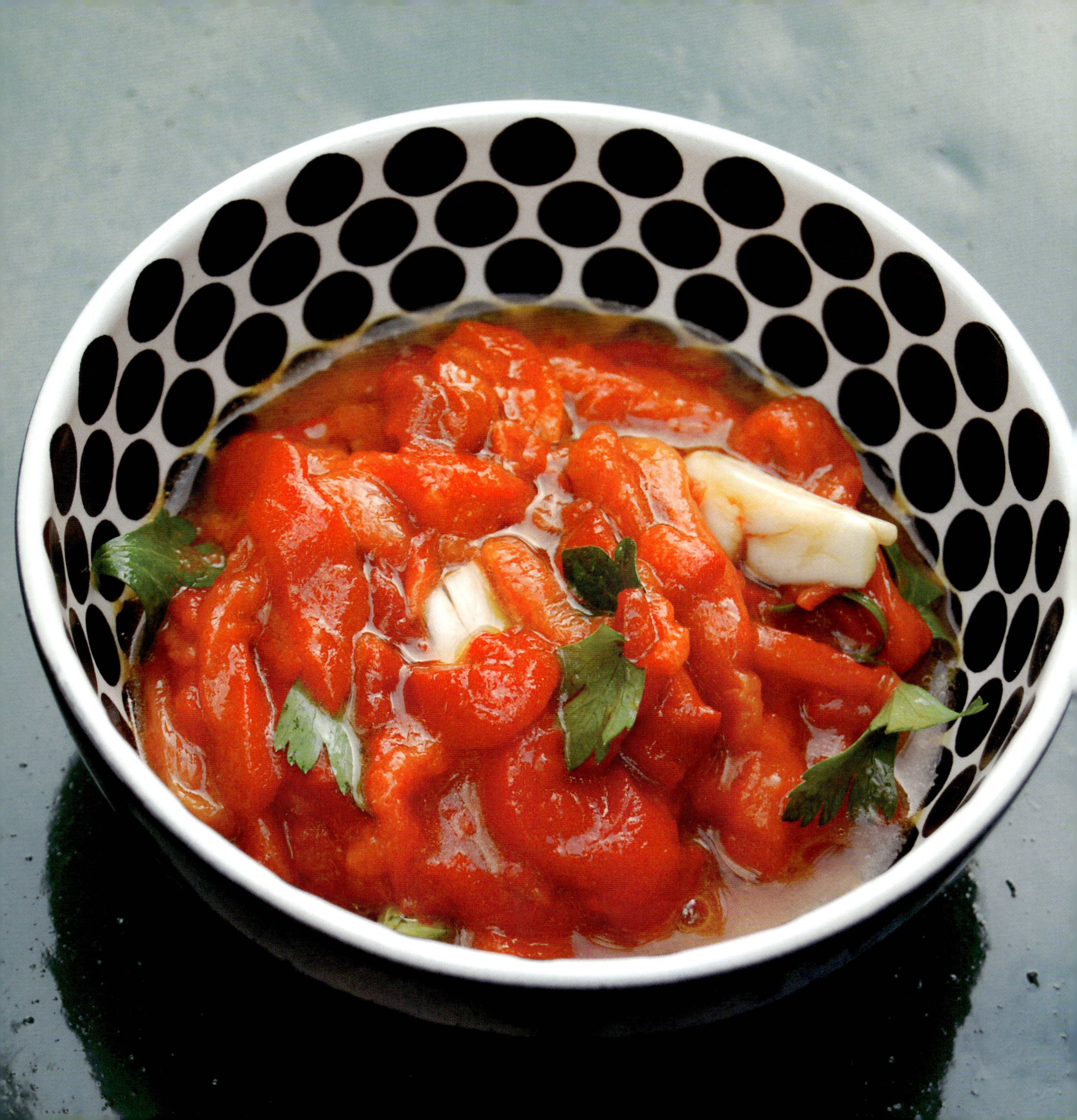

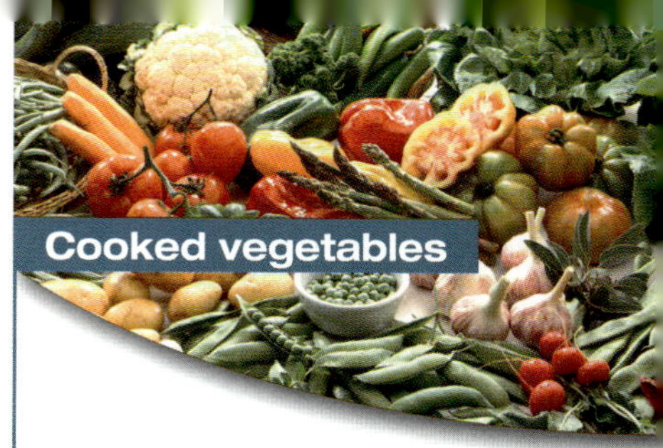

Sweet peppers

Ingredients and amounts for 4 people

- ✓ 1 red pepper
- ✓ 1 yellow pepper
- ✓ 2 tablespoons extra virgin olive oil
- ✓ 3 basil leaves
- ✓ 1 clove of garlic
- ✓ salt to taste

Preparation

Place the peppers in the oven at 425°F.
After a few minutes, when they are well roasted, remove from the oven and dry on absorbent paper towels. When they have cooled, remove the skins, and cut into strips. Season with oil, basil, chopped garlic, and salt.

Bromatological evaluation per portion

Kcal	117
Protein (%)	2.9
Fats (%)	78.7
Carbohydrates (%)	18.4
Fiber (g)	2.1
Cholesterol (mg)	0

Valuable contents for the eye: ★★

Sweet peppers are a good source of carotenoids, in particular lutein.
Olive oil is an excellent source of unsaturated fatty acids.

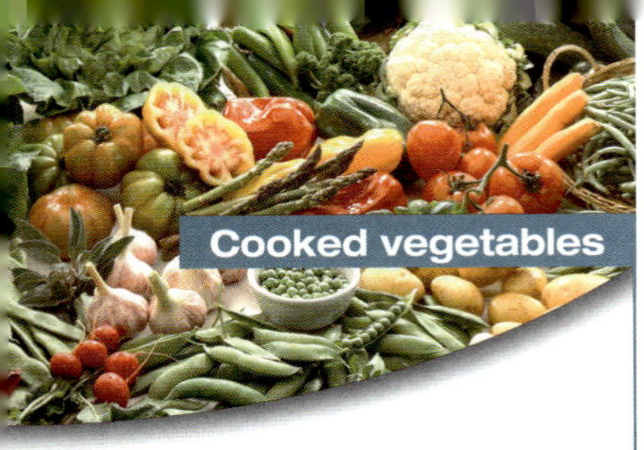

Caponata primavera (springtime caponata)

Bromatological evaluation per portion

Kcal	227
Protein (%)	7.8
Fats (%)	45.7
Carbohydrates (%)	46.5
Fiber (g)	3.9
Cholesterol (mg)	0

Valuable contents for the eye: ★★★

The **eggplant** is low in calories and high in carotenoids, flavonoids, and vitamin C.

Sweet peppers are a good source of carotenoids, particularly lutein.

The **potato** is rich in starch and contains potassium and vitamins C and B5.

Zucchini is low in calories and rich in carotenoids and vitamins C and E.

Olive oil is an excellent source of unsaturated fatty acids.

Onion contains vitamin C and a good quantity of flavonoids (quercetin).

Ingredients and amounts for 4 people

- ✓ 1 eggplant
- ✓ 1 sweet red pepper
- ✓ 1 sweet yellow pepper
- ✓ 2 potatoes
- ✓ 2 zucchinis
- ✓ 1 clove of garlic
- ✓ 1 onion
- ✓ 4 tablespoons extra virgin olive oil
- ✓ salt and pepper to taste

Preparation

Dice the eggplant; salt and drain for approximately 30 minutes in a colander.

Place the peppers in the oven at 390°F. When they are slightly roasted, remove them and peel when cooled.

Peel and slice the potatoes, and slice the zucchini.

Pour oil into a pan; heat and brown the garlic and onion. Remove the garlic and add the other vegetables.

Cook, adding a small quantity of water when required.

Add salt and pepper.

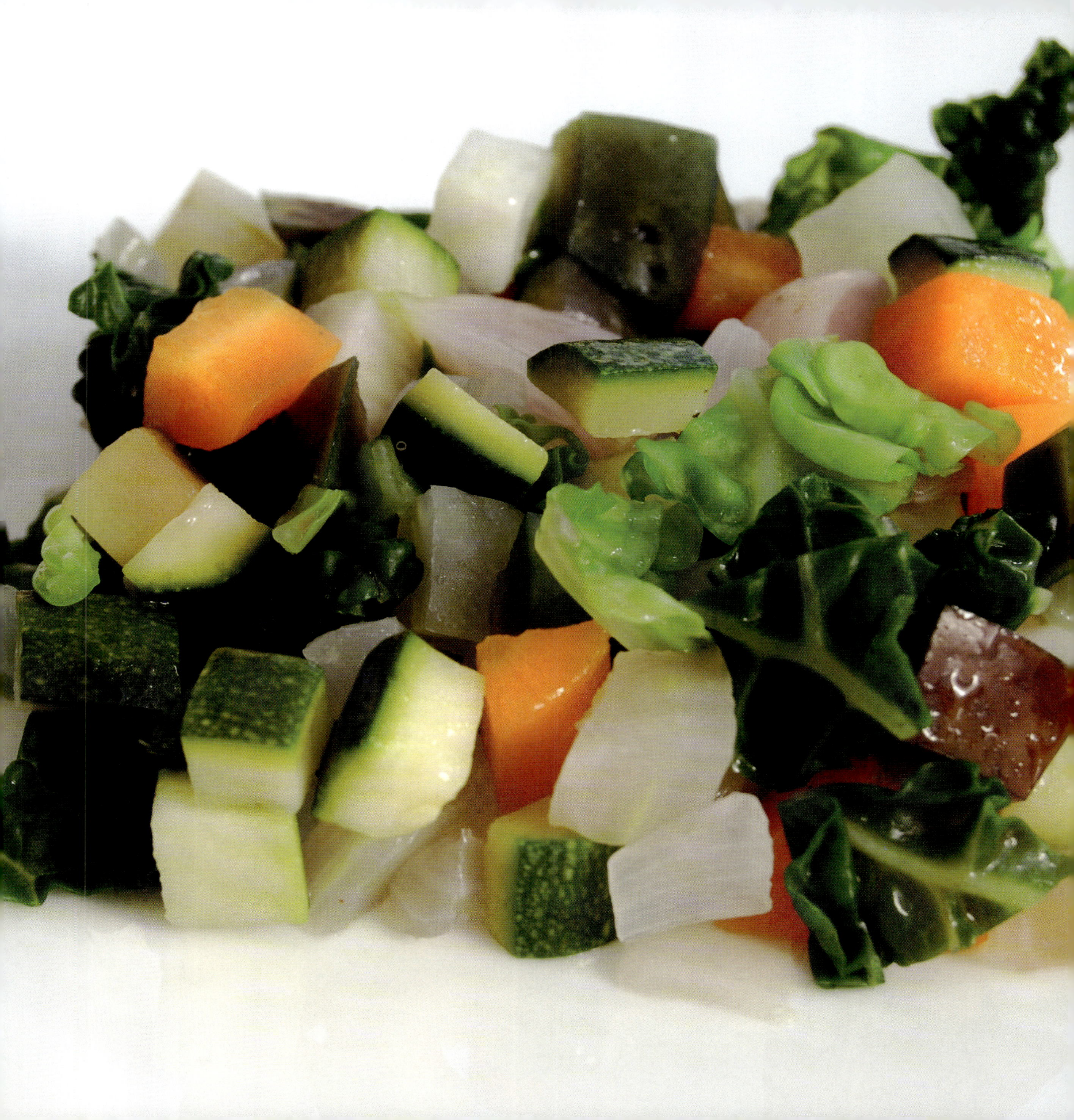

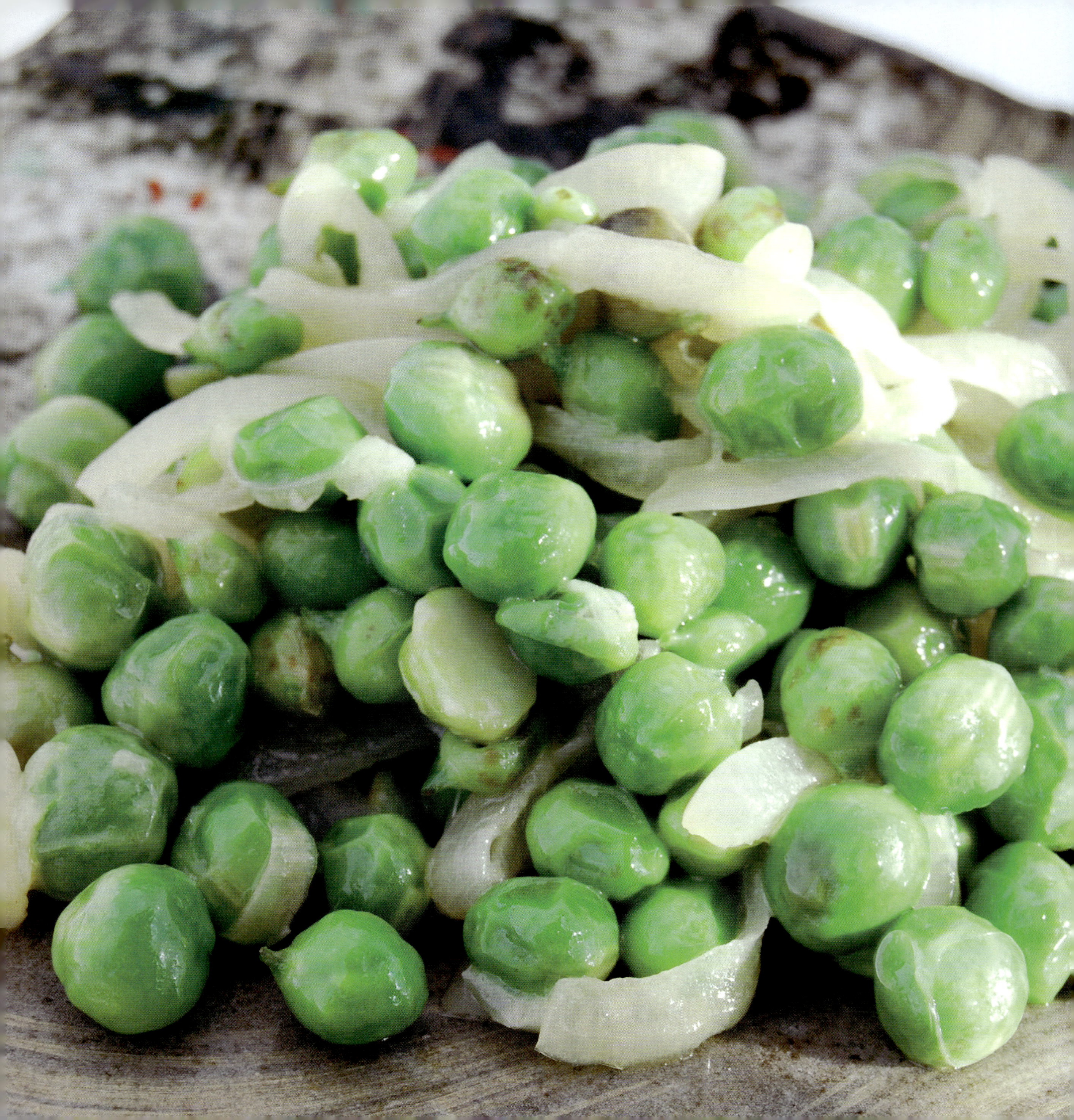

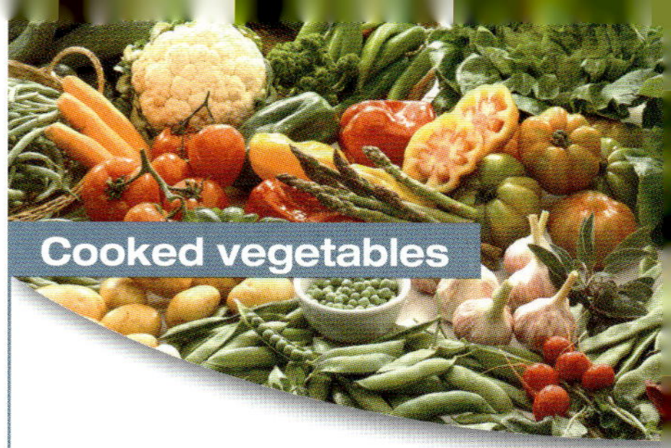

Fresh peas in the pan

Ingredients and amounts for 4 people

- ✓ 1⅓ cups fresh peas
- ✓ ½ scallion
- ✓ 2 tablespoons butter
- ✓ 2 tablespoons extra virgin olive oil

Preparation

Brown the scallion in the butter and the oil.
Add the fresh peas and cook in a small quantity of water.
Cook for approximately 10 minutes to enhance the fresh flavor.
At the end of cooking, a teaspoon of sugar can be added to sweeten the peas.

Bromatological evaluation per portion

Kcal	140
Protein (%)	12.4
Fats (%)	60.2
Carbohydrates (%)	27.4
Fiber (g)	2.5
Cholesterol (mg)	12.5

Valuable contents for the eye: ★★★

Peas are rich in vitamin C, carotenoids, and phytosterols (which lower the cholesterol levels).
Scallions contain vitamin C and a good quantity of flavonoids (quercetin).
Olive oil is an excellent source of unsaturated fatty acids.
Butter is a milk product consisting of saturated fatty acids.

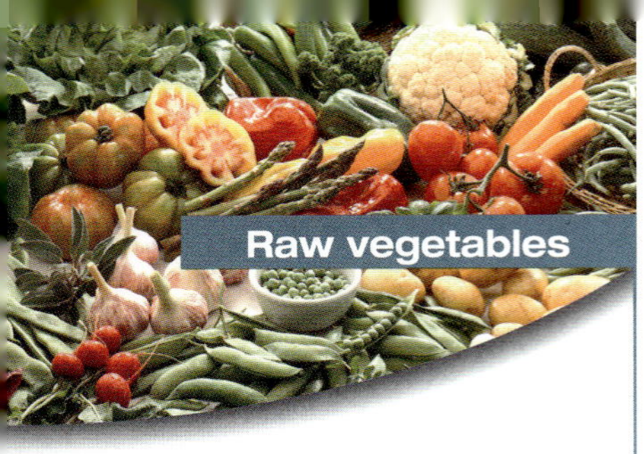

Bromatological evaluation per portion

Kcal	157
Protein (%)	15.6
Fats (%)	81.9
Carbohydrates (%)	2.5
Fiber (g)	2.3
Cholesterol (mg)	13.6

Valuable contents for the eye: ★★

The **artichoke** is rich in fiber, mineral salts, and folic acid.
Parmesan cheese is rich in easily digestible protein, is low in fat, and contains vitamin A and some vitamins of the B group.
Olive oil is an excellent source of unsaturated fatty acids.

Raw sliced artichokes with Parmesan cheese shavings

Ingredients and amounts for 4 people

✓ 4 fresh tender artichokes
✓ 3½ tablespoons Parmesan cheese shavings
✓ 4 tablespoons extra virgin olive oil
✓ 8 Roman mint leaves
✓ 1 teaspoon balsamic vinegar
✓ salt and pepper to taste

Preparation

Remove the tough external leaves of the artichokes and the upper half and keep the tender hearts.
Cut the artichokes into 4 pieces and eliminate the internal tufts and any thorns.
Dip into water mixed with the juice of ½ lemon for a few minutes. Dry.
Cut the artichokes into thin slices and place on 4 plates.
Slice the Parmesan cheese with a truffle shaver and place the shavings on top of the artichokes.
Season with some extra virgin olive oil, balsamic vinegar, salt, pepper and some mint leaves.

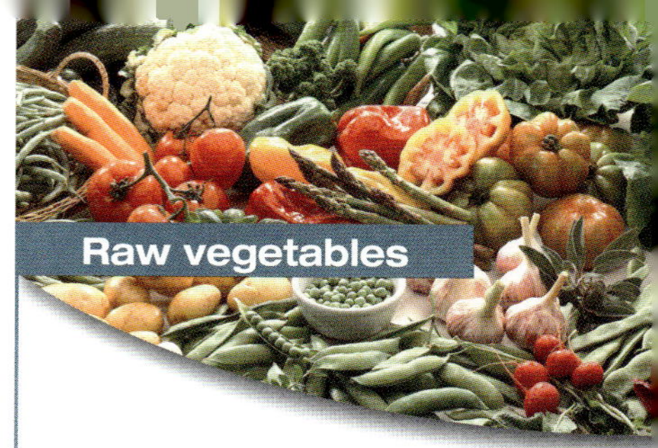

Artichoke salad

Ingredients and amounts for 4 people

- ✓ 4 fresh tender artichokes
- ✓ juice of 2 lemons
- ✓ 1 bunch of fresh parsley
- ✓ 4 mint leaves
- ✓ 4 tablespoons extra virgin olive oil
- ✓ salt and pepper to taste

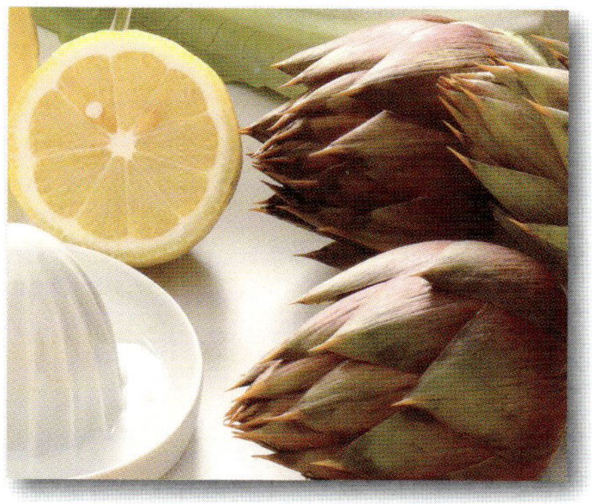

Preparation

Remove the tough external leaves, the upper half, and the stalks of the artichokes.
Cut the artichokes into 4 pieces and eliminate the internal tufts and any thorns.
Dip into water mixed with the juice of half a lemon for a few minutes.
Dry, cut into thin slices, and season with the sauce.

Sauce

Dissolve salt and pepper in the lemon juice and mix well.
Add the mint, finely chopped parsley, and the oil. Mix well to obtain a smooth liquid.

Bromatological evaluation per portion

Kcal	102
Protein (%)	6
Fats (%)	89.2
Carbohydrates (%)	4.8
Fiber (g)	2.7
Cholesterol (mg)	0

Valuable contents for the eye: ★★

The **artichoke** is rich in fiber, mineral salts, and folic acid.
Lemons contain high amounts of vitamin C, β-carotene, and flavonoids (particularly in the pith or albedo underneath the peel).
Mint contains flavonoids and essential oils, including menthol.
Olive oil is an excellent source of unsaturated fatty acids.

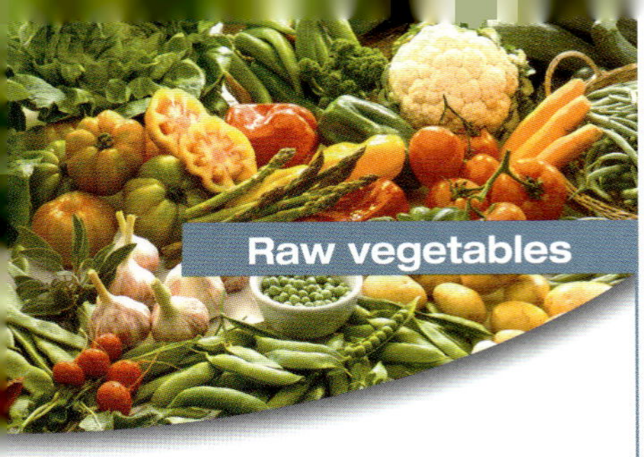

Valerian lettuce **with** walnuts

Bromatological evaluation per portion

Kcal	164
Protein (%)	6.8
Fats (%)	88
Carbohydrates (%)	5.2
Fiber (g)	2.2
Cholesterol (mg)	0

Valuable contents for the eye: ★★★

Valerian lettuce is an excellent source of fiber and carotenoids (lutein).
Walnuts are extremely high in calories and contain omega-3 fatty acids.
Celery has diuretic properties and is also an aphrodisiac; it contains minerals, water-soluble vitamins, and flavonoids.
Parsley contains flavonoids and apiol, a substance that is antispasmodic, antipyretic, and a stimulant of uterine contractions.
Olive oil is an excellent source of unsaturated fatty acids.

Ingredients and amounts for 4 people

- ✓ 14 oz valerian lettuce
- ✓ 2/3 cup walnuts
- ✓ 3 tablespoons extra virgin olive oil
- ✓ 1 tablespoon young balsamic vinegar
- ✓ 1 sprig of finely chopped parsley
- ✓ 6 basil leaves
- ✓ 1 stalk of celery
- ✓ salt and pepper

Preparation

Tail and wash the lettuce, and dry well. Add the walnuts and season with the dressing.

Dressing

Place the balsamic vinegar, oil, basil, finely chopped celery, parsley, salt and pepper in a bowl.
Mix all the ingredients.

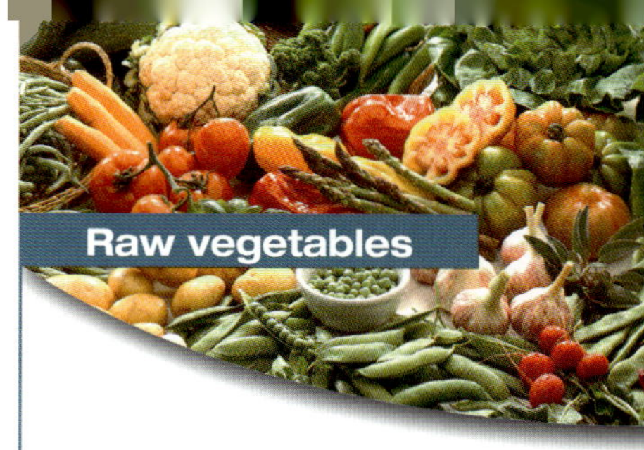

Cucumber, melon, and strawberry salad

Ingredients and amounts for 4 people

- ✓ 1 medium cucumber
- ✓ ½ melon
- ✓ ⅔ cup strawberries
- ✓ juice of 1 lemon
- ✓ 1 tablespoon of extra virgin olive oil
- ✓ 1 teaspoon ground chili pepper
- ✓ 2 tablespoons chopped fresh parsley
- ✓ salt to taste

Preparation

Remove the seeds and threads from the melon; use a melon scoop to create melon balls with the flesh.

Peel the cucumber, remove the seeds, and slice.

Top the strawberries and cut them into slices.

Mix the melon balls, strawberries, and cucumber.

Add the lemon juice, oil, salt, chili pepper, and parsley and mix.

Bromatological evaluation per portion

Kcal	51
Protein (%)	8.3
Fats (%)	59.3
Carbohydrates (%)	32.4
Fiber (g)	1.5
Cholesterol (mg)	0

Valuable contents for the eye: ★★★

Cucumber is low in calories and contains a large amount of water. It also contains vitamin C, potassium, and carotenoids.

Melon is rich in vitamin C and carotenoids.

Strawberries are a good source of vitamin C and anthocyanosides.

Lemons contain large quantities of vitamin C and β-carotene and also flavonoids (particularly in the pith, beneath the peel).

Chili pepper contains capsaicin, which makes it spicy. It also contains carotenoids and flavonoids.

Olive oil is an excellent source of unsaturated fatty acids.

Parsley contains flavonoids and apiol, a substance that is antispasmodic, antipyretic, and a stimulant of uterine contractions.

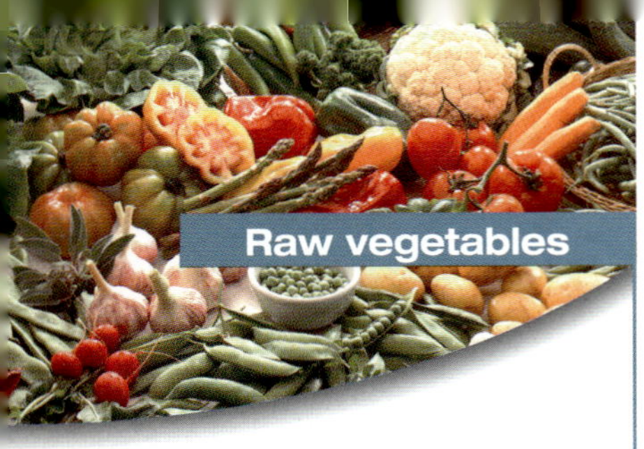

Cucumber and tomato salad

Bromatological evaluation per portion

Kcal	114
Protein (%)	4.5
Fats (%)	81.6
Carbohydrates (%)	13.9
Fiber (g)	2.5
Cholesterol (mg)	0

Valuable contents for the eye: ★★★

Tomatoes are rich in vitamins and oligominerals, but particularly they contain carotenoids and are the most important source of lycopene.
Cucumber is low in calories and contains a large amount of water. It also contains vitamin C, potassium, and carotenoids.
Olive oil is an excellent source of unsaturated fatty acids.
Red wine vinegar has a sharp taste and is rich in flavonoids.
Oregano is rich in essential oils.

Ingredients and amounts for 4 people

- ✓ 4 ripe tomatoes
- ✓ 2 tender cucumbers
- ✓ 2 tablespoons red wine vinegar
- ✓ 4 tablespoons extra virgin olive oil
- ✓ ½ teaspoon oregano
- ✓ 1 clove of garlic
- ✓ salt and pepper to taste

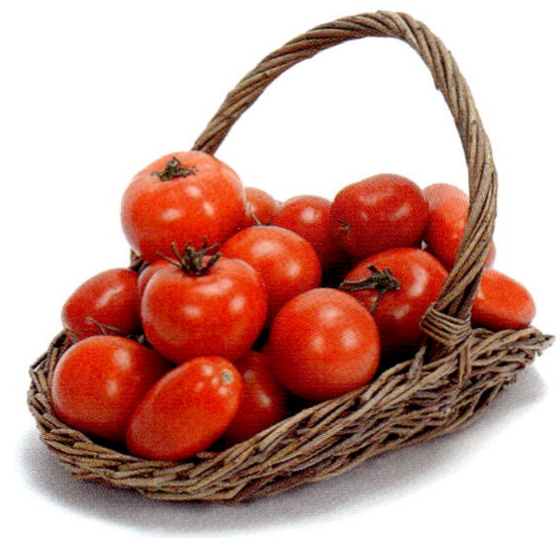

Preparation

Wash the tomatoes, cut into segments, and remove the seeds.
Sprinkle with salt and place in a colander for 5 to 6 minutes to drain the water.
Peel the cucumbers, top and tail, and cut into thin slices.
Cut the garlic clove in half.
Mix the tomatoes and the cucumber in a bowl and season with the dressing.

Dressing

Place the oregano, salt, pepper, vinegar, oil, and garlic into a bowl.
Mix all the ingredients; let sit for a few moments to enhance the flavor.
Remove the garlic before pouring over the tomatoes and cucumber.

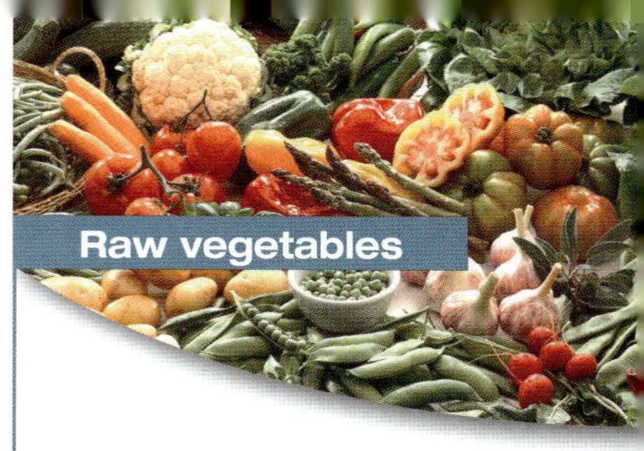

Tomato and basil salad

Ingredients and amounts for 4 people

- ✓ 8 ripe tomatoes
- ✓ 18 fresh basil leaves
- ✓ ¼ teaspoon oregano
- ✓ 1 clove of garlic
- ✓ 6 tablespoons extra virgin olive oil
- ✓ 1 teaspoon wine vinegar
- ✓ salt and black pepper to taste

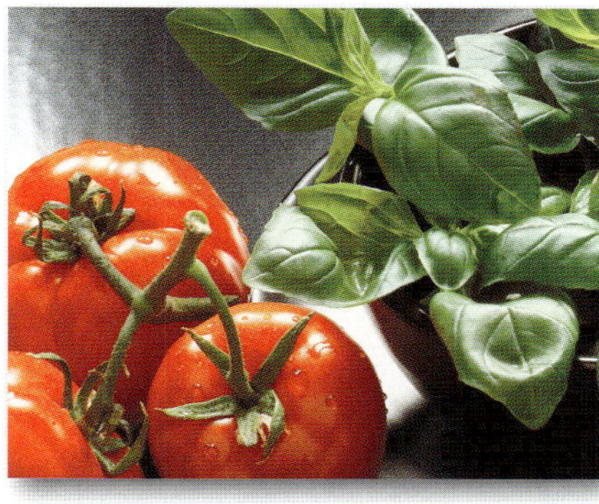

Preparation

Wash the tomatoes, cut into segments, and remove the seeds.
Sprinkle with salt and place in a colander for 5 to 6 minutes to drain the water.
Place in a salad bowl and add the washed, dried basil leaves.
Add the dressing and serve.

Dressing

Place the oregano, salt, pepper, vinegar, oil, and garlic into a bowl.
Mix all the ingredients and let sit for a few moments to enhance the flavor.
Remove the garlic.
Use to season the tomatoes.

Bromatological evaluation per portion

Kcal	129
Protein (%)	6.5
Fats (%)	72.6
Carbohydrates (%)	20.9
Fiber (g)	4
Cholesterol (mg)	0

Valuable contents for the eye: ★★★

Tomatoes are rich in vitamins and oligominerals, but particularly they contain carotenoids and are the most important source of lycopene.
Olive oil is an excellent source of unsaturated fatty acids.
Basil owes its aroma to the numerous essential oils it contains; these stimulate salivary and gastric secretions.
Wine vinegar has a sharp taste and is rich in flavonoids, particularly the red wine variety.

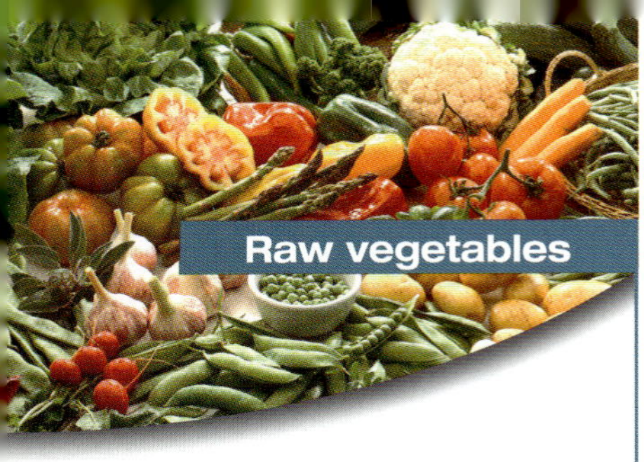

Mixed salad

Bromatological evaluation per portion

Kcal	119
Protein (%)	9.5
Fats (%)	79.1
Carbohydrates (%)	11.4
Fiber (g)	2
Cholesterol (mg)	0

Valuable contents for the eye: ★

Lettuce is an excellent source of fiber and carotenoids (lutein).

Arugula has a spicy flavor and contains carotenoids and flavonoids.

Soy bean shoots are extremely rich in isoflavons.

Olive oil is an excellent source of unsaturated fatty acids.

Ingredients and amounts for 4 people

- ✓ 1 bunch of arugula
- ✓ 2 heads red radicchio
- ✓ 1 bunch of curly endive lettuce
- ✓ 3½ tablespoons fresh soy bean shoots
- ✓ 1 clove of garlic
- ✓ 1 tablespoon white wine vinegar
- ✓ 4 tablespoons extra virgin olive oil
- ✓ 1 teaspoon Dijon mustard
- ✓ salt and pepper to taste

Preparation

Tail, wash, and gently dry the vegetables.
Cut the lettuces into generous strips; leave the soy bean shoots intact.
Place all the ingredients in a salad bowl and add the dressing.

Dressing

Place the mustard, salt, crushed garlic, and vinegar in a bowl.
Mix well to dissolve the salt.
Add the pepper and oil and stir well to mix all the ingredients.

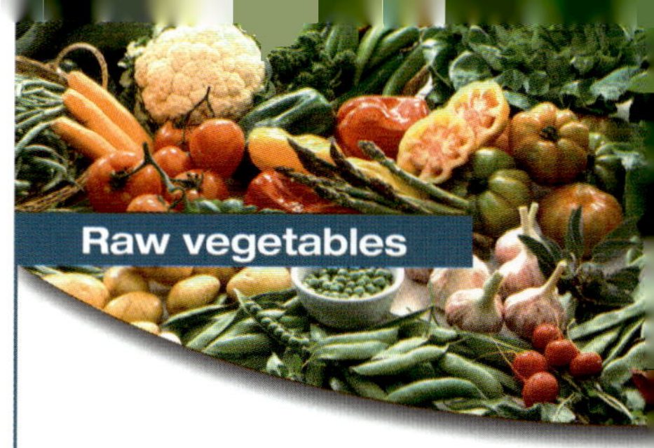

Spinach salad

Ingredients and amounts for 4 people

✓ 2⅔ cups young spinach leaves
✓ ⅔ cup Parmesan cheese shavings
✓ 4 tablespoons extra virgin olive oil
✓ 2 tablespoons balsamic vinegar
✓ salt and pepper to taste

Preparation

Place the salt, pepper, and balsamic vinegar in a bowl and mix well; add the oil and mix again.
Place the spinach leaves in a salad bowl and add the dressing.
Add the Parmesan cheese shavings. Mix again and serve immediately.

Bromatological evaluation per portion

Kcal	264
Protein (%)	24.2
Fats (%)	70.5
Carbohydrates (%)	5.3
Fiber (g)	2.4
Cholesterol (mg)	31.8

Valuable contents for the eye: ★ ★ ★

Spinach leaves are rich in vitamin C and lutein. They are also rich in iron; however, they contain oxalate, which reduces the absorption.
Parmesan cheese is rich in easily digestible protein, is low in fat, and contains vitamin A and some vitamins of the B group.
Olive oil is an excellent source of unsaturated fatty acids.
Balsamic vinegar has a low calorie content but an extremely intense flavor.

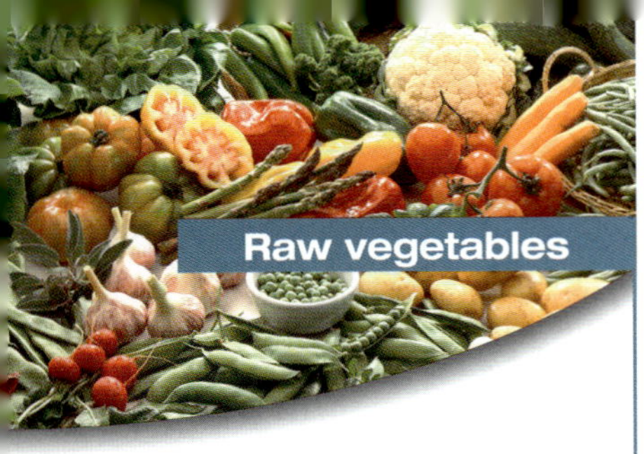

Mixed green salad

Bromatological evaluation per portion

Kcal	189
Protein (%)	7
Fats (%)	73.4
Carbohydrates (%)	19.6
Fiber (g)	5.5
Cholesterol (mg)	0

Valuable contents for the eye: ★

Lettuce is an excellent source of fiber and carotenoids (lutein).

Red wine vinegar has a sharp taste and is rich in flavonoids.

Olive oil is an excellent source of unsaturated fatty acids.

Ingredients and amounts for 4 people

- ✓ 2 cups various types of lettuce (cos, cabbage lettuce, chicory, arugula, valerian, etc)
- ✓ 4 tablespoons red wine vinegar
- ✓ 8 tablespoons extra virgin olive oil
- ✓ ¼ tablespoon salt
- ✓ Black pepper to taste

Preparation

Tail, wash, and dry the lettuce leaves well.

Place the leaves in a salad bowl, drizzle the dressing, and mix carefully.

Serve immediately.

Dressing

Place the salt, pepper, and vinegar in a bowl and mix well until the salt has dissolved.

Add the oil and mix well.

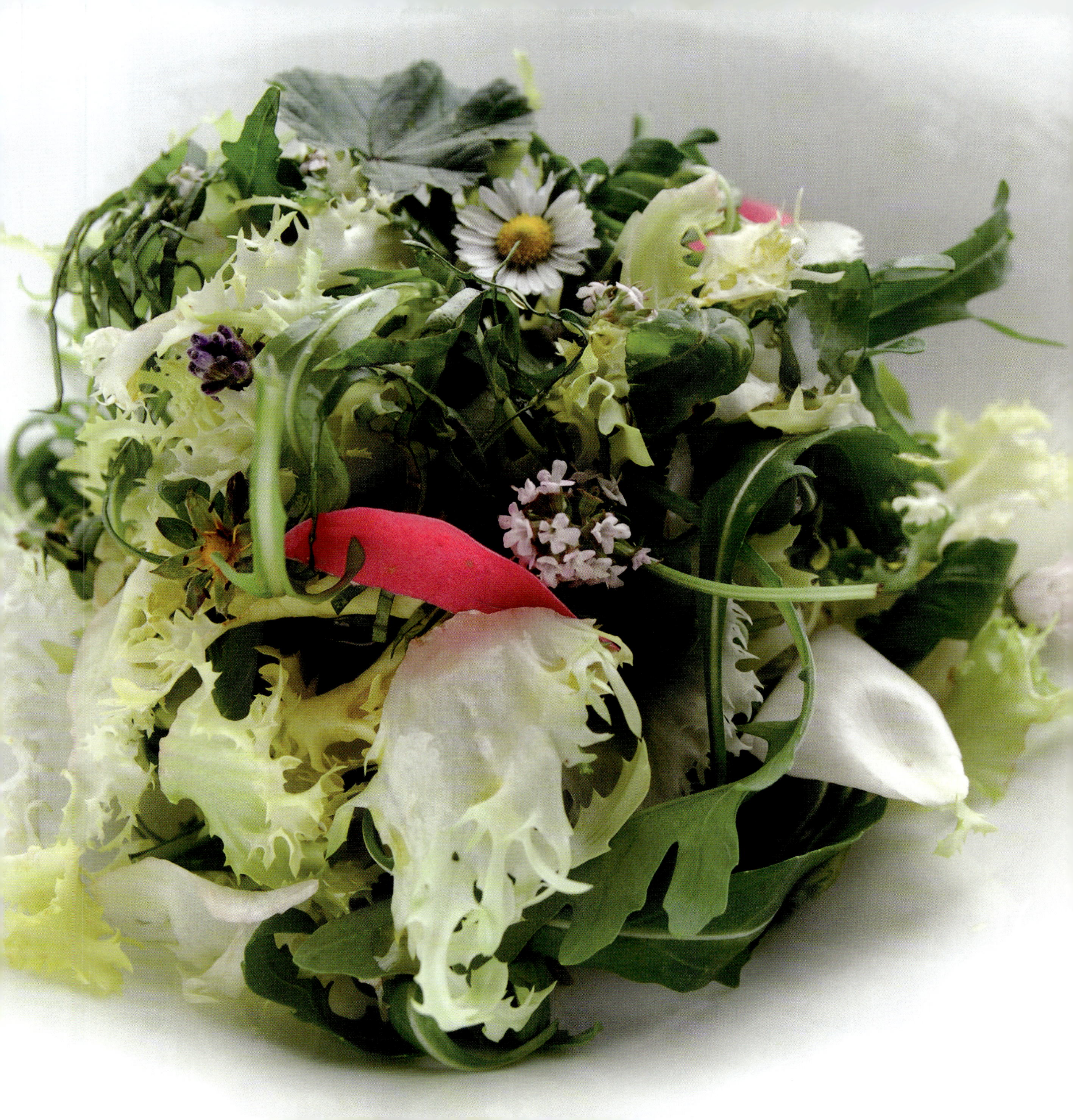

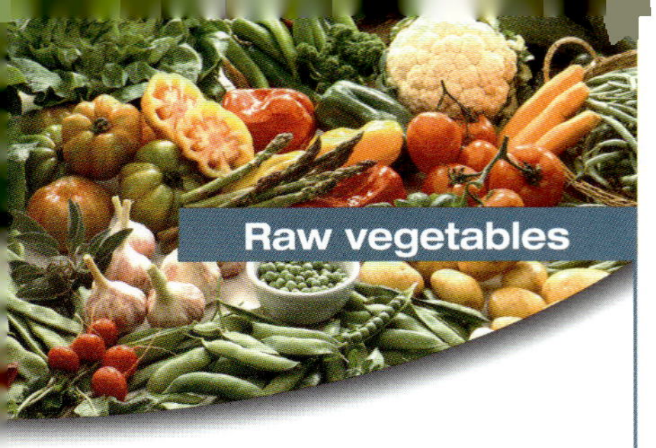

Mixed salad of carrots, fennel, tomatoes, and chicory lettuce

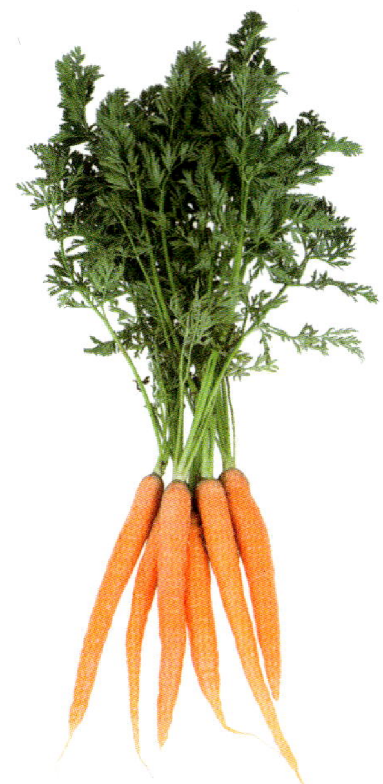

Bromatological evaluation per portion

Kcal	119
Protein (%)	4.7
Fats (%)	72.4
Carbohydrates (%)	22.9
Fiber (g)	3.5
Cholesterol (mg)	0

Valuable contents for the eye: ★★★

Carrots are an excellent source of β-carotene; they stimulate diuresis and intestinal motility.

Fennel contains flavonoids, anethol in particular, which is an antispasmodic substance.

Tomatoes are rich in vitamins and oligominerals, but particularly they contain carotenoids and are the most important source of lycopene.

Limes contain high quantities of vitamin C and β-carotene; they also contain flavonoids (particularly in the pith or albedo underneath the peel).

Olive oil is an excellent source of unsaturated fatty acids.

Ingredients and amounts for 4 people

- ✓ 2 carrots
- ✓ 2 ripe tomatoes
- ✓ 1 fennel
- ✓ 1 bunch of chickory lettuce
- ✓ 1 teaspoon Dijon mustard
- ✓ 1 teaspoon lemon juice
- ✓ 4 tablespoons extra virgin olive oil
- ✓ salt and pepper to taste

Preparation

Clean and cut the carrots à la Julienne (ie, cut them into sticks 1 inch long by 1/10 inch wide).

Remove the tougher layers of the fennel and cut the remainder into fine slices.

Peel the tomatoes, cut them in half, remove the seeds, and let them drain.

Place the various vegetables in a salad bowl, starting with the chicory lettuce.

Drizzle the dressing over the vegetables. Mix and serve immediately.

Dressing

Place the salt, pepper, lemon juice, and mustard in a bowl and mix well until the salt has dissolved; add the oil and mix the dressing until creamy.

Salad of papaya, avocado pear, and walnut

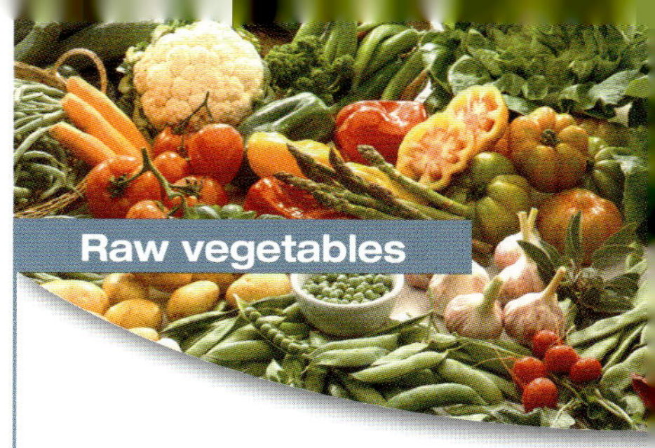

Ingredients and amounts for 4 people

- ✓ 1 very ripe medium-sized papaya
- ✓ 2 ripe avocado pears
- ✓ 30 walnuts
- ✓ 2 lemons
- ✓ 1 teaspoon balsamic vinegar
- ✓ 4 tablespoons extra virgin olive oil
- ✓ salt and pepper to taste

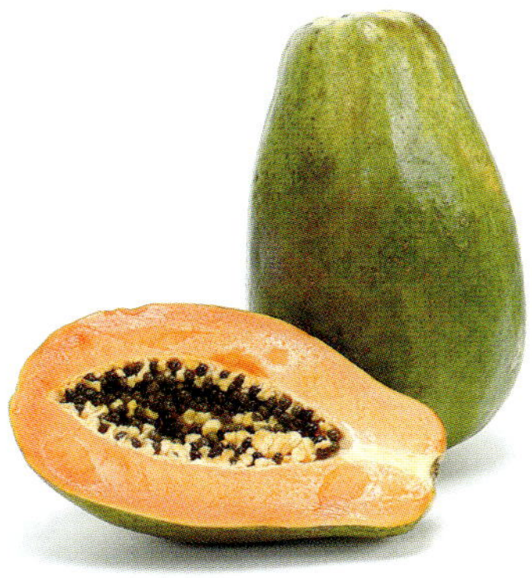

Preparation

Crush the walnuts.
Squeeze the juice from the 2 lemons.
Peel the avocados and extract the stone; cut into slices and cover with lemon juice to stop them from turning black.
Remove the skin and seeds of the papaya, and cut into slices.
Place slices of papaya and avocado pear on a plate and sprinkle the crushed walnuts over the top.
Coat with the well-stirred dressing.

Dressing

Place the salt and the balsamic vinegar in a bowl, and mix until the salt is dissolved. Add the juice of 1 lemon, pepper, and oil. Mix well until emulsified.

Bromatological evaluation per portion

Kcal	347
Protein (%)	5.6
Fats (%)	87.3
Carbohydrates (%)	7.1
Fiber (g)	5
Cholesterol (mg)	0

Valuable contents for the eye: ★★★

Papaya is very rich in vitamin C, selenium, flavonoids, and carotenoids.
Avocado pears are extremely high in calories and rich in monounsaturated fats but contain vitamin E and glutathione, a vitamin of the B complex, potassium, and β-sitosterol (a substance that can lower cholesterol levels).
Walnuts are high in calories and contain large quantities of omega-3 fatty acids.
Lemons contain high quantities of vitamin C and β-carotene; they also contain flavonoids (particularly in the pith or albedo underneath the peel).
Olive oil is an excellent source of unsaturated fatty acids.

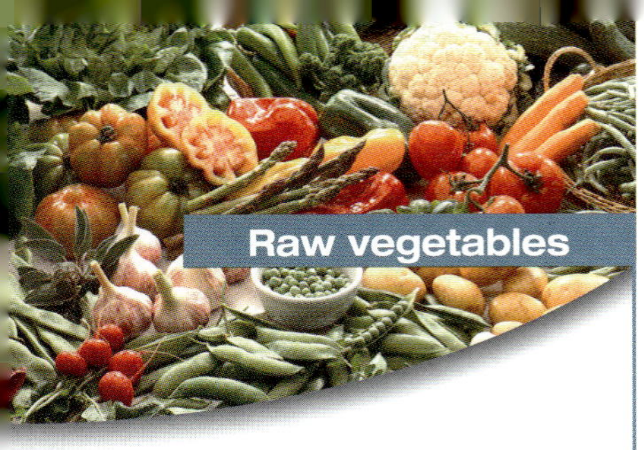

Cabbage and carrot salad

Bromatological evaluation per portion

Kcal	118
Protein (%)	6.4
Fats (%)	76.7
Carbohydrates (%)	16.9
Fiber (g)	3.2
Cholesterol (mg)	0

Valuable contents for the eye: ★ ★

Carrots are an excellent source of β-carotene; they stimulate diuresis and intestinal motility.

Savoy cabbage is rich in vitamin C, in particular carotenoids such as lutein.

Olive oil is an excellent source of unsaturated fatty acids.

Wine vinegar has a sharp taste and is rich in flavonoids, particularly the red wine variety.

Ingredients and amounts for 4 people

✓ 4 fresh carrots
✓ 1 cup cabbage (savoy)
✓ 2 tablespoons red wine vinegar
✓ 6 tablespoons extra virgin olive oil
✓ salt and pepper to taste

Preparation

Wash, dry, and thinly slice the cabbage.
Wash, dry, and peel the carrots, cutting them à la Julienne.
Mix the carrots and the cabbage in a salad bowl and add the vinegar-based dressing.

Dressing

Place the salt, pepper, and vinegar in a bowl and mix well.
Add the oil and mix to create a smooth emulsion.

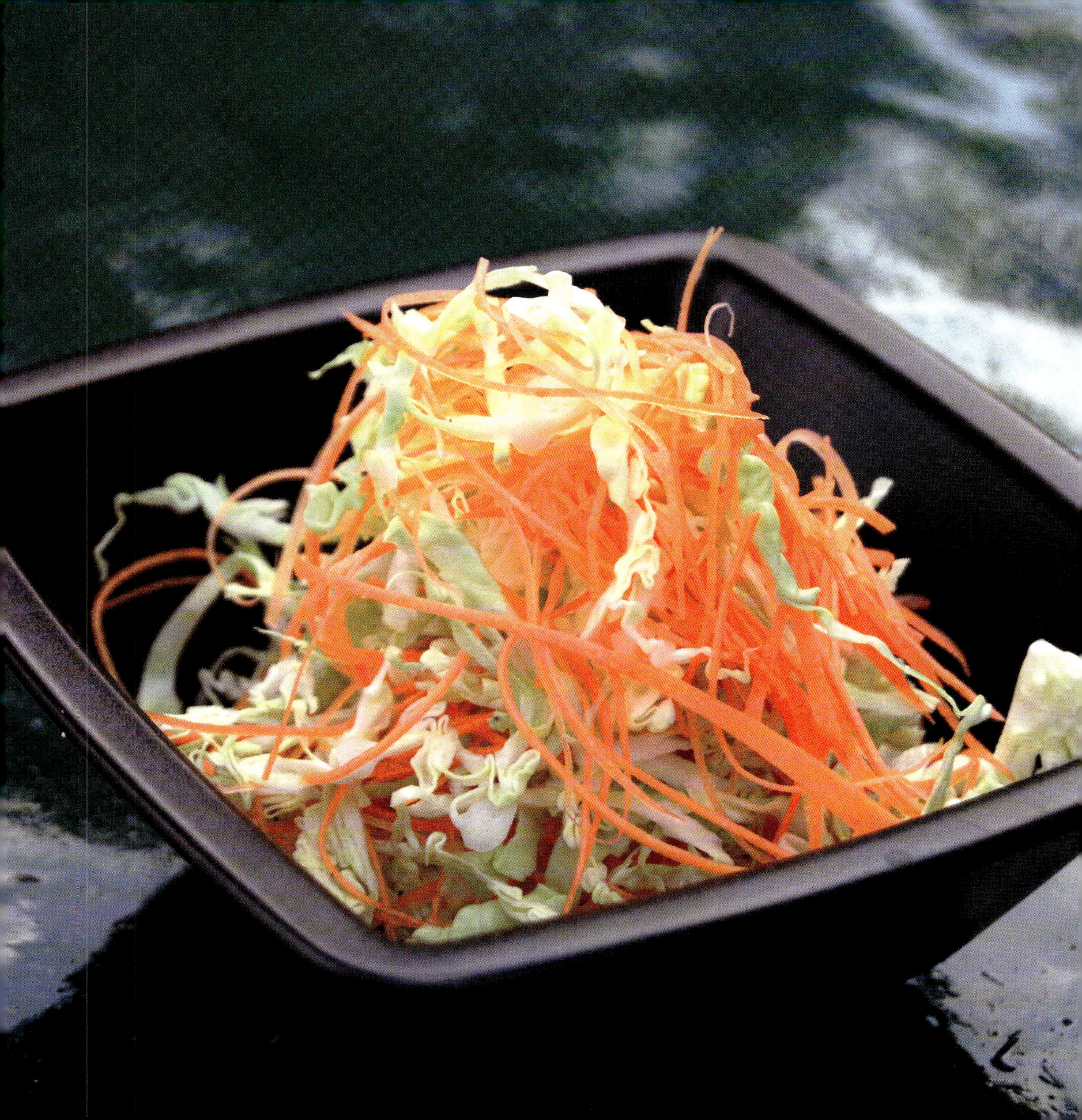

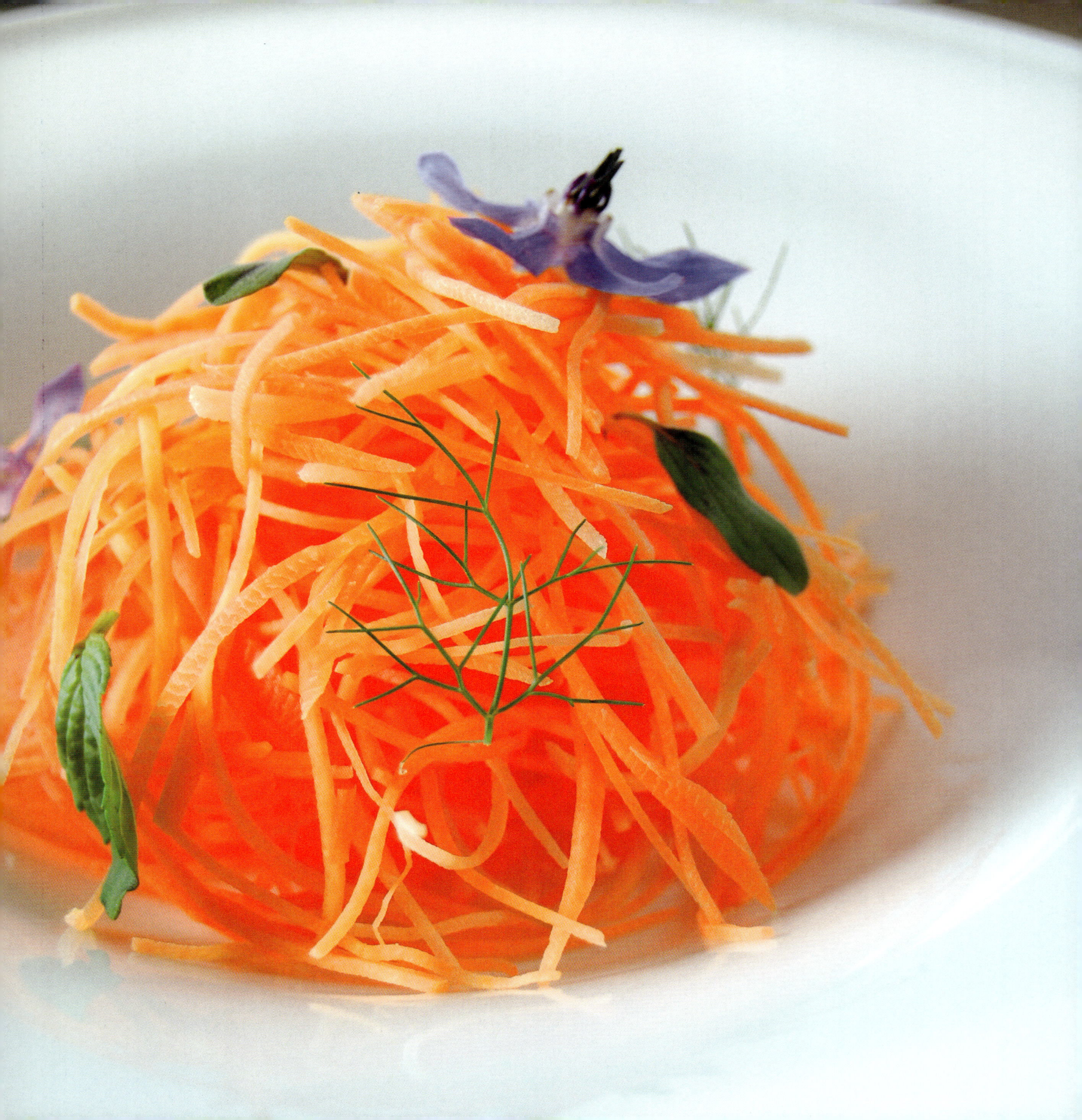

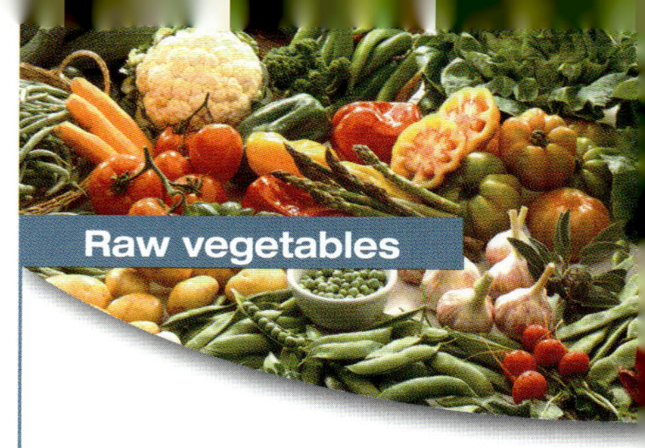

Carrots à la Julienne

Ingredients and amounts for 4 people

- ✓ 10½ oz carrots
- ✓ juice of 1 lemon
- ✓ 3 tablespoons extra virgin olive oil
- ✓ salt to taste

Preparation

Wash the carrots and top, tail, and peel them. Cut them into sticks 1-in long for a thickness of 1/10 in. Soak them in cold water for a few minutes for them to become crunchy.

Season with salt, lemon, and oil and serve garnished with herbs and flowers.

Bromatological evaluation per portion

Kcal	102
Protein (%)	3.7
Fats (%)	71.7
Carbohydrates (%)	24.6
Fiber (g)	3.6
Cholesterol (mg)	0

Valuable contents for the eye: ★★★

Carrots are an excellent source of β-carotene; they stimulate diuresis and intestinal motility.

Lemons contain high quantities of vitamin C and β-carotene; they also contain flavonoids (particularly in the pith or albedo underneath the peel).

Olive oil is an excellent source of unsaturated fatty acids.

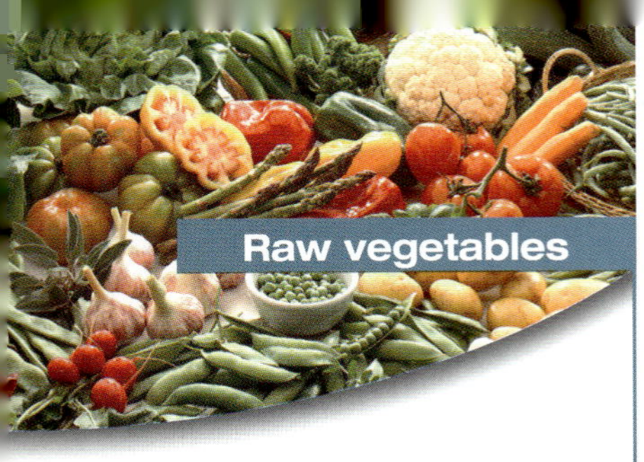

Cruditè

Bromatological evaluation per portion

Kcal	189
Protein (%)	7.1
Fats (%)	74
Carbohydrates (%)	18.9
Fiber (g)	6.4
Cholesterol (mg)	0

Valuable contents for the eye: ★★

Carrots are an excellent source of β-carotene; they stimulate diuresis and intestinal motility.

Fennel contains flavonoids, in particolar anethol, which has an antispasmodic effect.

In addition to being rich in fiber and mineral salts, **artichokes** are rich in folic acid.

All the **broad leaf vegetables** in general (lettuce, prickly lettuce, etc.) contain carotenoids and flavonoids; their green color is given by the chlorophyll, which covers the yellow color of the carotenes.

Onion contains vitamin C and a good quantity of flavonoids (quercetin).

Radishes have a strong flavor and they contain mineral salts, vitamins B and C, and flavonoids.

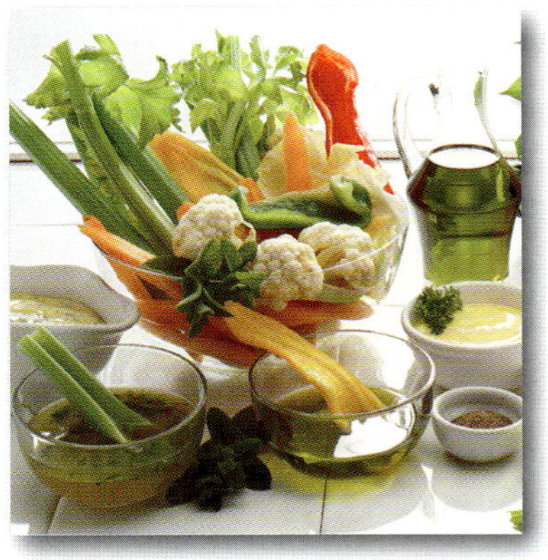

Ingredients and amounts for 4 people

- ✓ Seasonal vegetables: carrots, celery hearts, fennel, artichokes, radishes, Belgian endive lettuce, red radicchio, cos, fresh scallions
- ✓ juice of 2 lemons
- ✓ 1 cup extra virgin olive oil
- ✓ salt and pepper to taste

Preparation

Carefully wash every vegetable and cut into slices, sticks, or segments, removing any tough or woody part (when the artichokes and carrots have been prepared, soak in separate bowls of water and lemon until served).

Place the different vegetables in groups in a large salad bowl at the center of a table, easily accessible to guests.

Dressing

Place 1 teaspoon salt and ¼ teaspoon pepper in a bowl and dissolve with the juice of one lemon. Mix well, add the oil, and mix again.

Pour the dressing into 4 small, fairly deep bowls and use as dips for the vegetables.

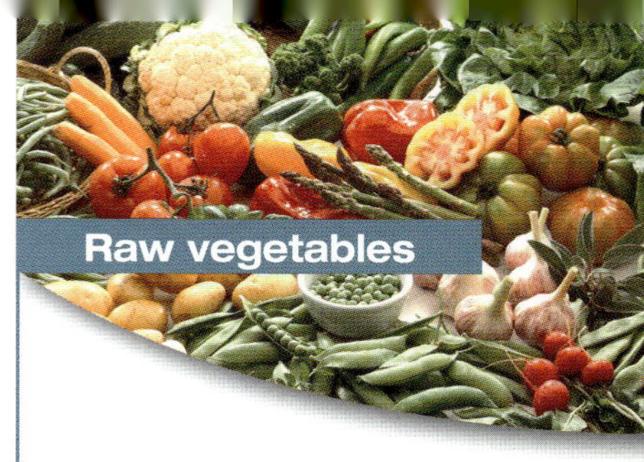

Tzatziki

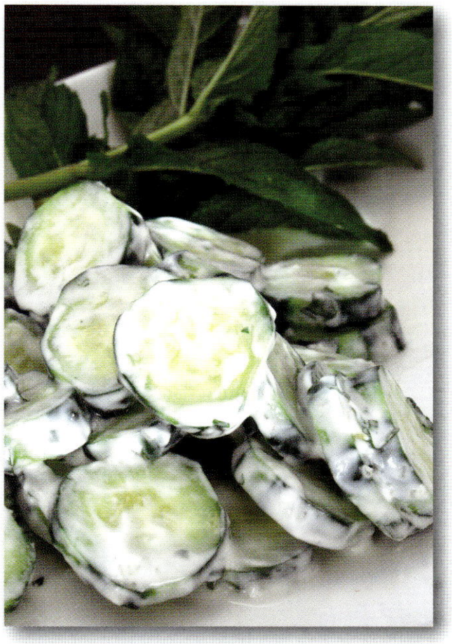

Ingredients and amounts for 4 people

- ✓ 24½ oz (3.5 cups) natural white yogurt
- ✓ 1 cucumber
- ✓ ½ onion
- ✓ 1 clove of garlic
- ✓ 1 sprig of parsley
- ✓ 4 basil leaves
- ✓ 4 mint leaves

Preparation

Finely hand-chop the onion, parsley, garlic, mint, and basil (do not use a blender).

Peel and thinly slice the cucumber, salt the surfaces, and drain for 15 minutes.

Mix the chopped vegetables and the cucumber with the yogurt and place in the refrigerator.

Serve cold.

Bromatological evaluation per portion

Kcal	117
Protein (%)	23.7
Fats (%)	47
Carbohydrates (%)	29.3
Fiber (g)	0.8
Cholesterol (mg)	17.6

Valuable contents for the eye: ★★

Yogurt has a high repletion index; in addition to the live milk enzymes, it contains vitamins of the B group and folic acid.

Cucumber is low in calories and contains a large amount of water. It also contains vitamin C, potassium, and carotenoids.

Onion contains vitamin C and a good quantity of flavonoids (quercetin).

Garlic contains selenium, zinc and alline, which is responsible for the taste and the penetrating, persistent odor of garlic. When alline is transformed into allicine, it has an antibacterial action and it lowers cholesterol and blood pressure levels.

Parsley contains flavonoids and apiol, a substance that is antispasmodic, antipyretic, and a stimulant of uterine contractions.

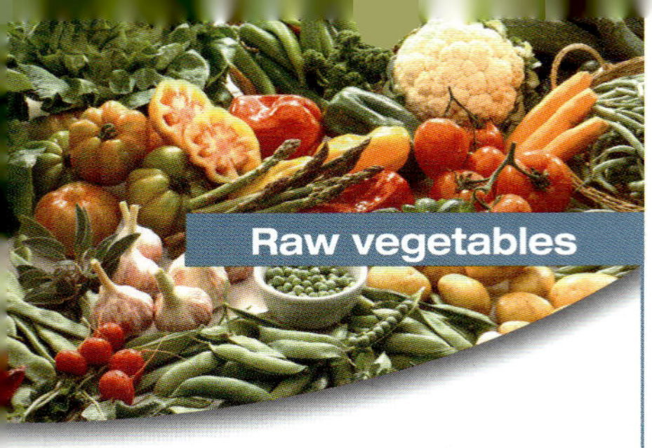

Raw vegetables

Fresh zucchini carpaccio

Bromatological evaluation per portion

Kcal	201
Protein (%)	19.5
Fats (%)	78.8
Carbohydrates (%)	1.7
Fiber (g)	0.9
Cholesterol (mg)	26.3

Valuable contents for the eye: ★

Zucchini is low in calories and very rich in carotenoids and vitamins C and E.

Parmesan cheese is rich in easily digestible protein, is low in fat, and contains vitamin A and some vitamins of the B group.

Lemons contain high quantities of vitamin C and β-carotene; they also contain flavonoids (particularly in the pith or albedo underneath the peel).

Olive oil is an excellent source of unsaturated fatty acids.

Ingredients and amounts for 4 people

- ✓ 10½ oz (1⅓ cups) very fresh zucchini
- ✓ 7 tablespoons grated Parmesan cheese
- ✓ 4 tablespoons extra virgin olive oil
- ✓ juice of 1 lemon
- ✓ salt and pepper to taste

Preparation

Thinly slice the zucchini and arrange as a single layer on each plate. Just before serving, pour the dressing over the zucchini and sprinkle with the Parmesan cheese.

Dressing

Combine salt, pepper, and the lemon juice. Mix well.
Add the oil and mix well.

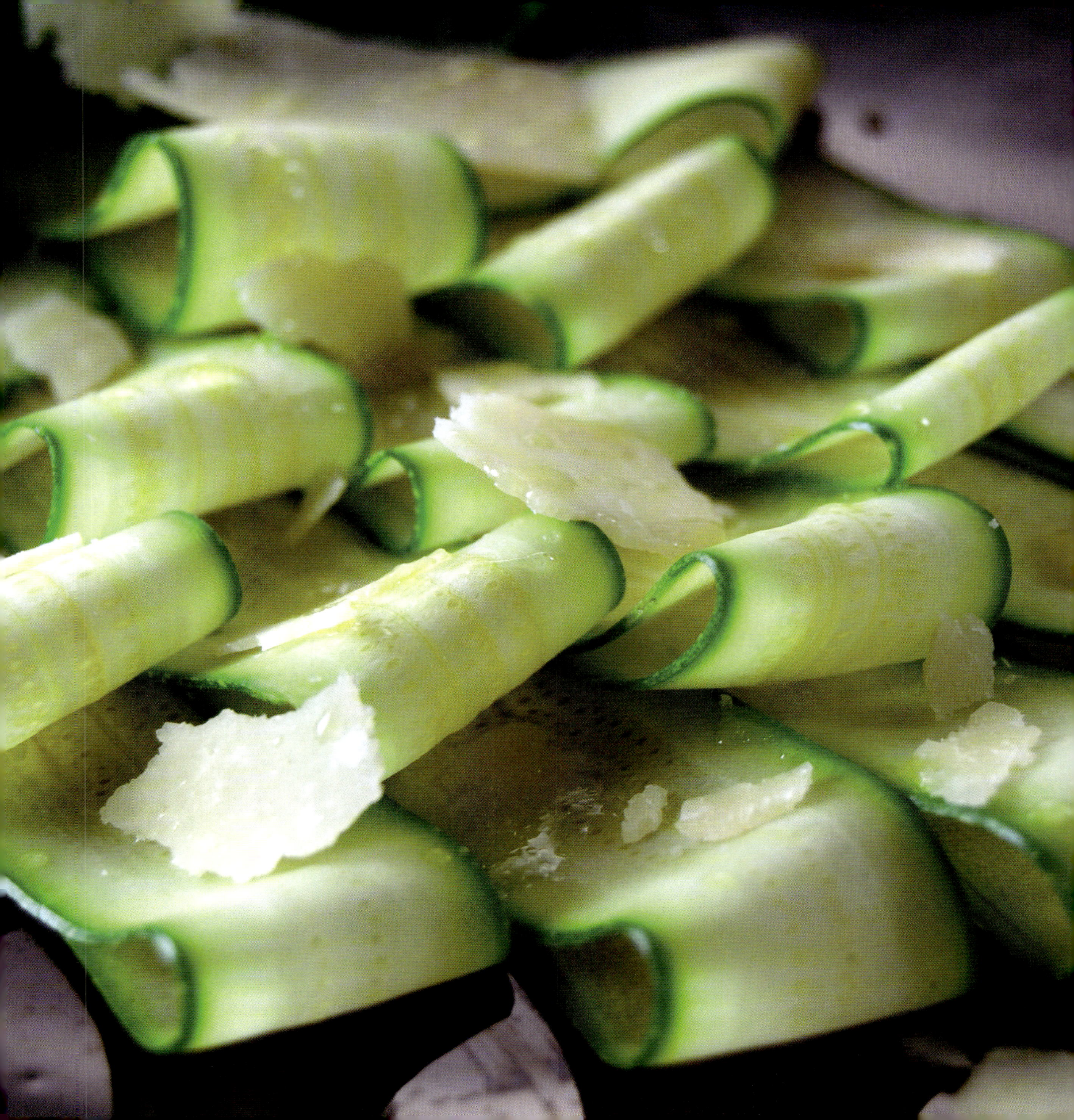

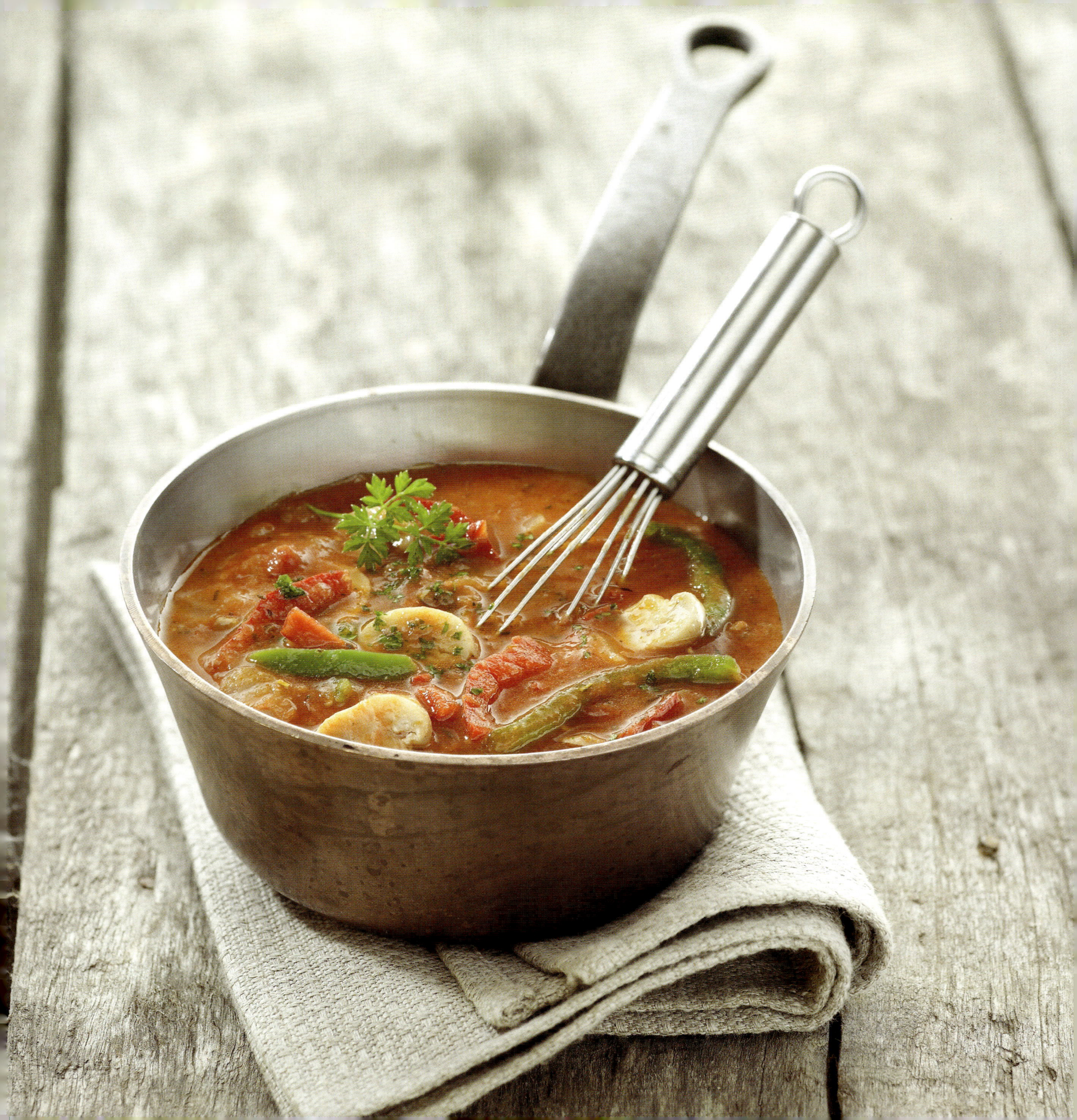

Meat sauces and pasta condiments

The Romans frequently used sauces to hide bad tastes in foods that tended to naturally deteriorate rapidly. However, there is no doubt that, of all the recipes, the preparation of sauces is the most varied—it ranges from apparent simplicity to the strange to sauces of unexpected complexity.

By their very nature, sauces are fairly complicated chemical and physical systems and are therefore influenced by the quality of the ingredients and by how they are heated, in addition to the secrets and skills of the master chefs. It is possible that the personal touch that characterizes them makes the sauces something of an unknown entity for nutritionists, who are unable to give a precise calculation of the caloric intake or the degree of digestibility.

At the beginning of the 20th century, the cooking guidebooks written by the great Escoffier, an expert in classical French cuisine, listed almost 200 different sauces. According to Escoffier, "The sauces are a fundamental part of the French cuisine; they create and maintain the universal supremacy of our cuisine."

Quite rightly, Italian chefs preferred the purées of fresh vegetables, particularly tomato sauce or basil pesto, or more simply a mixture of oil and wine—even though mayonnaise and white sauce are used frequently. In other words, Italian chefs prefer to highlight the taste of good quality meat or fresh vegetables rather than characterize it or camouflage it with sauces.

Sauces can be split into 2 main groups—those based on starch (white sauce, Spanish sauce, or velouté) and those based on eggs and butter (mayonnaise, Hollandaise, Bérnaise).

It stands to reason that those with an egg and butter base are less suitable for people with cholesterol problems! By the same measure, the spicier sauces such as Tabasco or Worchestershire can cause problems with digestion.

Lastly, it will not be a totally useless exercise if we underline the dietetic benefits and the appetizing value of a sauce prepared with fresh or canned tomatoes, onion, olive oil, and garlic—sauces that can be enriched from time to time with other vegetables rich in carotenoids, such as sweet peppers, eggplants, zucchinis, capers, and olives.

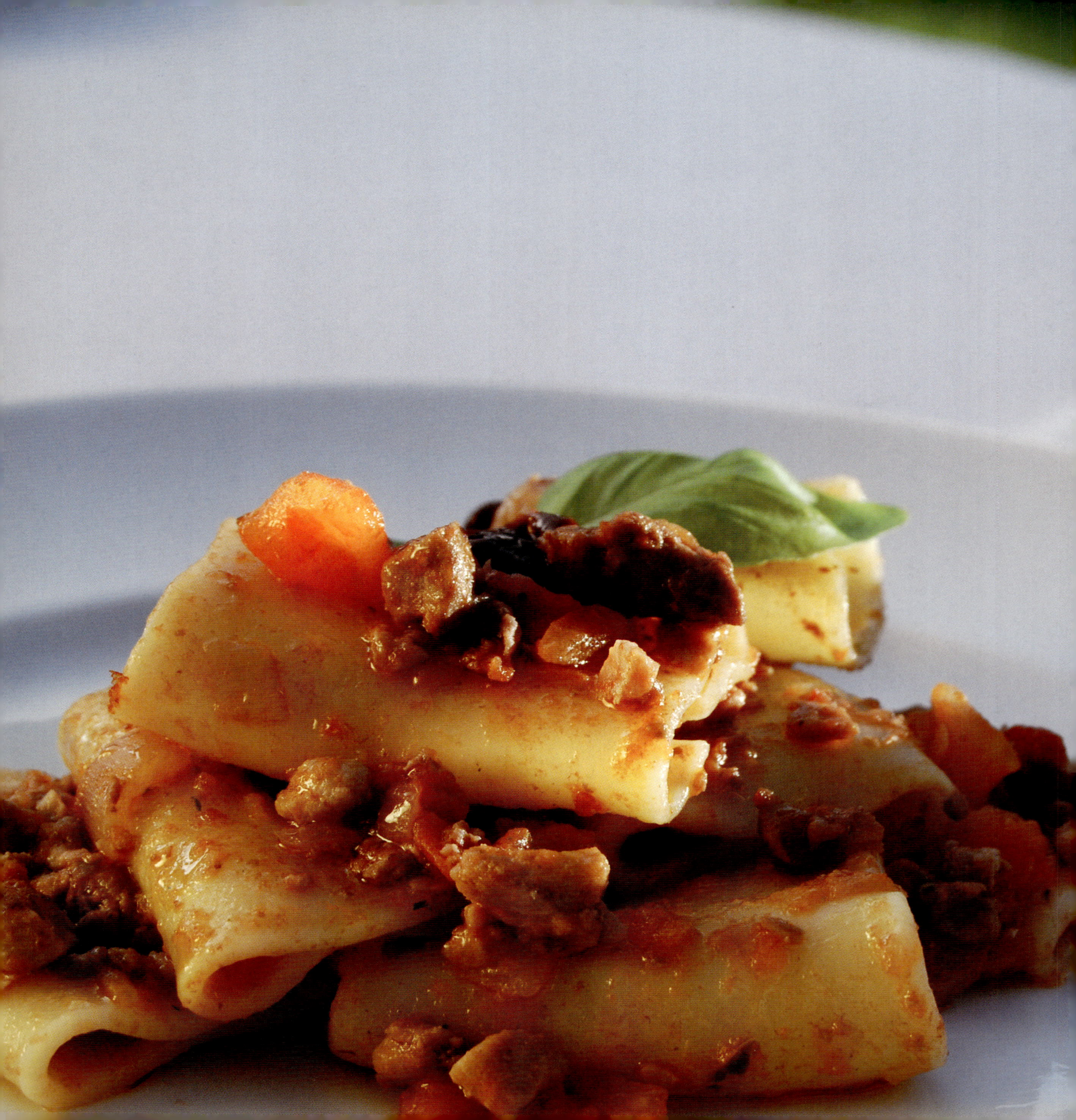

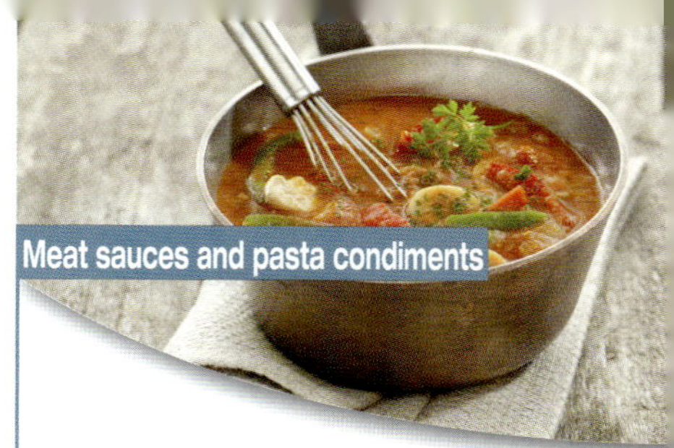

Beef and tomato pasta sauce

Ingredients and amounts for 4 people

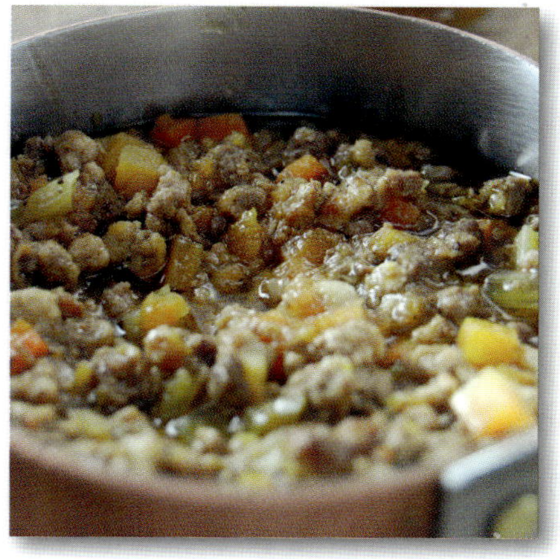

- ✓ 10½ oz (1⅓ cups) lean minced beef
- ✓ 3½ tablespoons minced pork belly
- ✓ 14 oz canned tomatoes
- ✓ 1 onion
- ✓ 1 carrot
- ✓ 1 stalk of celery
- ✓ 1 glass white wine
- ✓ 2 tablespoons butter
- ✓ 6 tablespoons extra virgin olive oil
- ✓ 1 bunch of aromatic herbs
- ✓ salt and pepper to taste

Preparation

Heat the butter, oil, and minced pork in a pan; add the onion, celery, and finely chopped carrot. Cook for 15 minutes.
Add the beef and cook for 2 to 3 minutes over high heat while stirring.
Add the wine and allow it to evaporate.
Add the tomato, herbs, salt, and pepper and simmer for 40 minutes very slowly until the sauce has thickened.
Serve on freshly boiled pasta and top with freshly grated Parmesan cheese.

Bromatological evaluation per portion

Kcal	348
Protein (%)	23.9
Fats (%)	68.2
Carbohydrates (%)	7.9
Fiber (g)	2.4
Cholesterol (mg)	73

Valuable contents for the eye: ★

Beef is rich in iron and fairly high in fat.
Lean pork is an excellent source of protein and is rich in vitamins of the B group.
Tomatoes are rich in vitamins and oligominerals, but particularly they contain carotenoids and are the most important source of lycopene.
Onion contains vitamin C and a good quantity of flavonoids (quercetin).
Carrots are an excellent source of β-carotene; they also stimulate diuresis and intestinal motility.
Olive oil is an excellent source of unsaturated fatty acids.
Parmesan cheese is rich in easily digestible protein, is low in fat, and contains vitamin A and some vitamins of the B group.

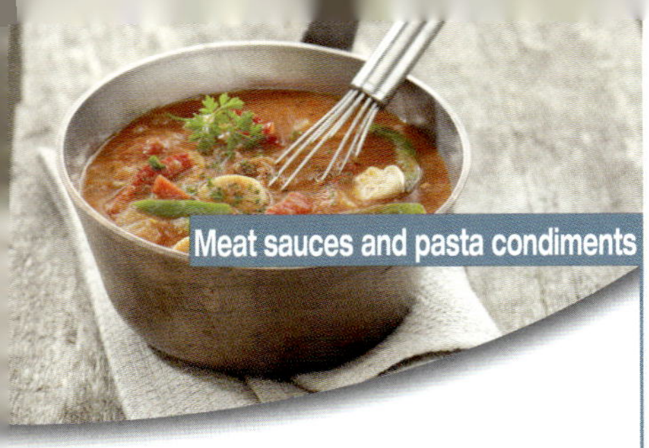

Pesto alla **Genovese** for **pasta** (**basil pesto**)

Bromatological evaluation per portion

Kcal	306
Protein (%)	9.5
Fats (%)	87.9
Carbohydrates (%)	2.6
Fiber (g)	0.4
Cholesterol (mg)	10.4

Valuable contents for the eye: ★

Basil owes its aroma to the numerous essential oils it contains; these stimulate salivary and gastric secretions.

Olive oil is an excellent source of unsaturated fatty acids.

Pine nuts are very small but rich in flavonoids and omega-6.

Pecorino cheese (sheep's milk) cheese has a strong taste and is rich in calcium

Parmesan cheese is rich in easily digestible protein, is low in fat, and contains vitamin A and some vitamins of the B group.

Garlic contains selenium, zinc, and alline, which is responsible for the taste and the penetrating, persistent odor of garlic. When alline is transformed into allicine, it has an antibacterial action, it lowers the cholesterol levels and the blood pressure.

Ingredients and amounts for 4 people

- ✓ ⅓ cup basil leaves
- ✓ ⅓ cup of extra virgin olive oil
- ✓ 2 tablespoons pine nuts
- ✓ 2 tablespoons grated pecorino (sheep's milk) cheese
- ✓ 2¾ tablespoons grated Parmesan cheese
- ✓ 2 cloves of fresh garlic
- ✓ ½ teaspoon salt

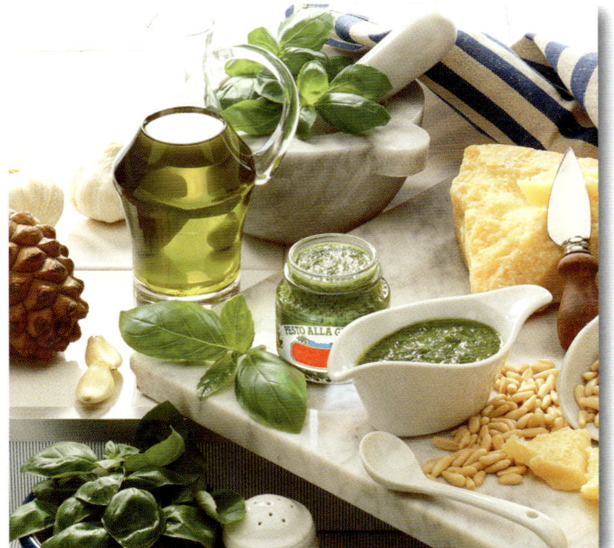

Preparation

Pour the oil into the blender and place in the freezer until it becomes very cold and viscous.

Remove the basil leaves from the plant. Wash and dry them carefully with a cloth or kitchen towel, taking care not to fold or compress them (this is very important).

Place the dry leaves in the blender and add the pine nuts, the whole cloves of topped and tailed garlic, oil, and salt. Blend at a low speed to obtain a smooth paste. It should be repeated several times.

The preparation must be fairly rapid to prevent the basil from oxidizing (turning black); blending must be brief (10 seconds approximately) to avoid the paste from over heating and oxidizing; add the cheeses and blend, again at a low speed, and again for a short time.

Add a tablespoon of hot water (used to boil the pasta) to the pesto prior to mixing it with the drained pasta.

Rabbit meat sauce for pasta

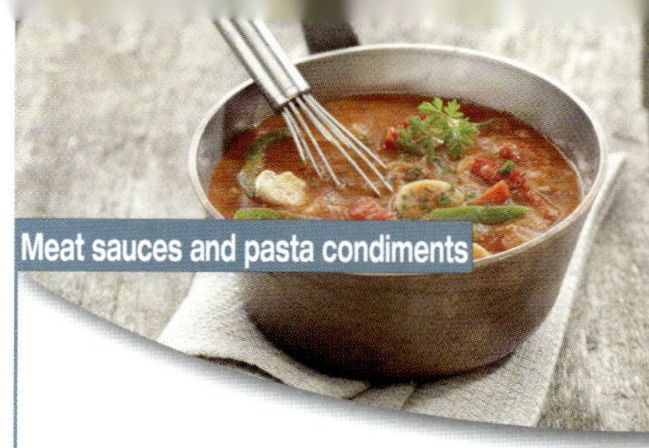

Meat sauces and pasta condiments

Ingredients and amounts for 4 people

✓ 10½ oz rabbit meat
✓ 3½ oz pork sausage
✓ 1 glass dry white wine
✓ 1 bunch of parsley
✓ 1 sprig of sage
✓ 3 cloves of garlic, with skin
✓ 1 shallot, chopped
✓ 3 tablespoons extra virgin olive oil
✓ salt and pepper to taste

Preparation

Cut the rabbit meat into pieces, making sure it is free from bones and other inedible parts; place the meat in a casserole dish with the oil, shallot, sausage, garlic, wine, salt, pepper, and herbs (sage and parsley).
Cover and leave on low heat until the meat is cooked (30 to 40 minutes).
If the sauce condenses too much, dilute with a ladleful of water.
Remove the garlic before serving.

Bromatological evaluation per portion

Kcal	353
Protein (%)	37.6
Fats (%)	61
Carbohydrates (%)	1.4
Fiber (g)	0
Cholesterol (mg)	73.8

Valuable contents for the eye: ★

Rabbit meat is a very lean white meat.
Lean pork is an excellent source of protein and is rich in vitamins of the B group.
Olive oil is an excellent source of unsaturated fatty acids.
Like onion, **shallots** also contain flavonoids.
Garlic contains selenium, zinc, and alline, which is responsible for the taste and the penetrating, persistent odor of garlic. When alline is transformed into allicine, it has an antibacterial action, it lowers the cholesterol levels and the blood pressure.

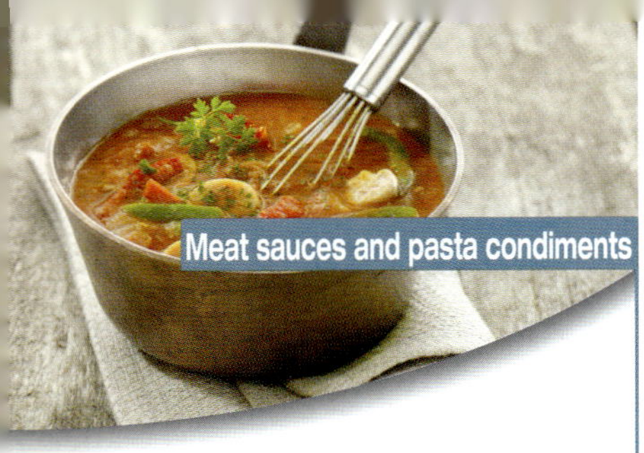

Tuna fish sauce for pasta

Bromatological evaluation per portion

Kcal	264
Protein (%)	17.4
Fats (%)	76.8
Carbohydrates (%)	5.8
Fiber (g)	2.7
Cholesterol (mg)	0

Valuable contents for the eye: ★ ★ ★

Tuna fish is rich in protein and contains good quantities of omega-3.

Tomatoes are rich in vitamins and oligominerals, but particularly they contain carotenoids and are the most important source of lycopene.

Olive oil is an excellent source of unsaturated fatty acids.

Olives are rich in monounsaturated fats, vitamin E, and potassium.

Capers contain vitamins A, C, and E and also a considerable quantity of sodium.

Garlic contains selenium, zinc, and alline, which is responsible for the taste and the penetrating, persistent odor of garlic. When alline is transformed into allicine, it has an antibacterial action, it lowers the cholesterol levels and the blood pressure.

Ingredients and amounts for 4 people

- ✓ 7 oz fresh tuna fish (diced)
- ✓ 6 ripe tomatoes
- ✓ 8 tablespoons extra virgin olive oil
- ✓ 16 stoned olives
- ✓ 2 tablespoons desalted capers
- ✓ 2 cloves of garlic
- ✓ 1 sprig of parsley
- ✓ salt to taste

Preparation

Heat the oil and add the garlic, tomatoes and parsley. Cook for 4 to 5 minutes. Remove the garlic.

Add the tuna fish, capers, and sliced olives. Cook for 5 to 6 minutes.

In the meantime, cook the pasta, drain, pour into a serving dish, and pour the sauce on top.

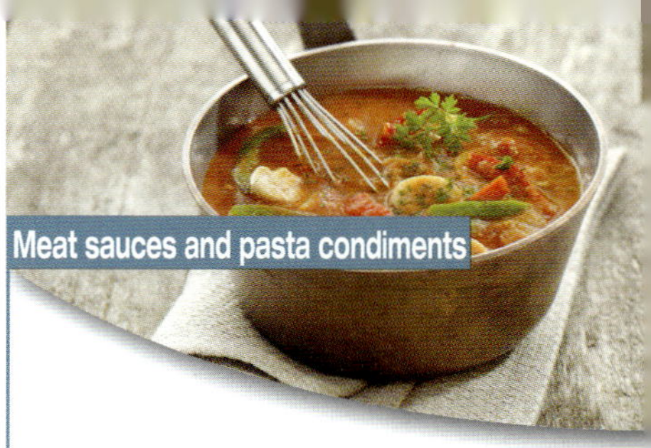

Vegetarian pasta sauce

Ingredients and amounts for 4 people

- ✓ 10½ oz (1⅓ cups) tomatoes
- ✓ 7 oz zucchini
- ✓ 5¼ oz (⅔ cup) eggplant
- ✓ 1 clove of garlic
- ✓ 1 sprig of parsley
- ✓ 1 sprig of basil
- ✓ 2 tablespoons extra virgin olive oil
- ✓ 2 tablespoons butter
- ✓ salt to taste

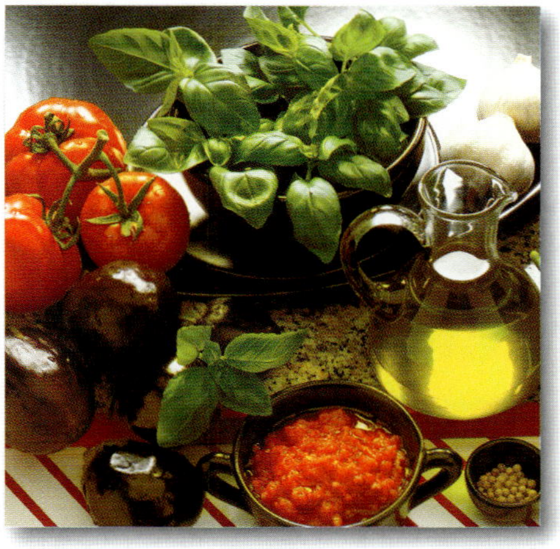

Preparation

Cut the clove of garlic into 2 to 3 pieces. Warm the oil in a pan; brown the garlic.

Peel and dice the eggplant, brown in the pan, and add salt and the sliced zucchini.

Scald the tomatoes in hot water, remove the skin and the seeds, and add to the sauce.

Add the pasta (previously cooked in a large quantity of salty water); add the butter, chopped parsley, and cut basil.

Bromatological evaluation per portion

Kcal	128
Protein (%)	7
Fats (%)	78.8
Carbohydrates (%)	14.2
Fiber (g)	4.6
Cholesterol (mg)	17.5

Valuable contents for the eye: ★ ★ ★

Tomatoes are rich in vitamins and oligominerals, but particularly they contain carotenoids and are the most important source of lycopene.

Zucchini is low in calories and rich in carotenoids and vitamins C and E.

Eggplant is low in calories and are rich in carotenoids, flavonoids, and vitamin C.

Olive oil is an excellent source of unsaturated fatty acids.

Basil owes its aroma to the numerous essential oils it contains; these stimulate salivary and gastric secretions.

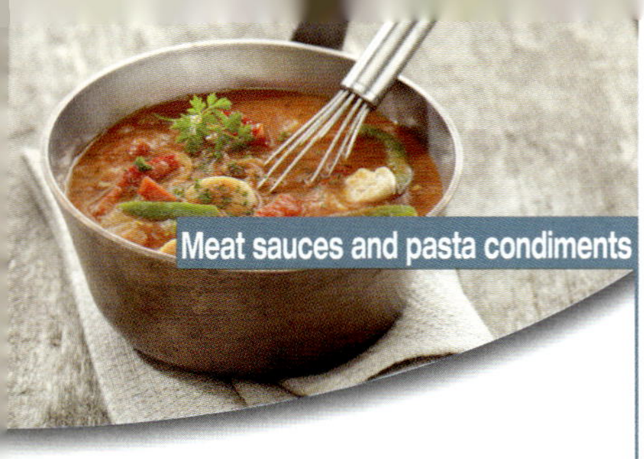

Fish sauce for pasta

Bromatological evaluation per portion

Kcal	202
Protein (%)	48.5
Fats (%)	48
Carbohydrates (%)	3.5
Fiber (g)	0
Cholesterol (mg)	0

Ingredients and amounts for 4 people

✓ 1 10½ to 14 oz scorpion fish
✓ 2 to 3 fish (each 7 to 10½ oz (grouper, monkfish, sea bass)
✓ 1 clove of garlic
✓ 3½ oz canned tomato
✓ 4 tablespoons extra virgin olive oil
✓ salt and pepper to taste

Preparation

Carefully clean the fish, removing the scales, skin, interiors, and bones and cut into filets or pieces.
Brown the clove of garlic in olive oil, then remove it from the oil.
Brown the fish in the oil.
Add the canned tomato or 4 to 5 small Pachino cherry tomatoes, cut into 4 pieces.
Add a small amount of water, enough to cook the fish; add salt and pepper to taste.
Cook for 15 to 20 minutes and then dry.
Use to season the pasta (spaghetti or linguine pasta).
The excellence of the sauce depends largely on the freshness and type of fish and the degree of sweetness of the tomatoes.

Valuable contents for the eye: ★★

Fish is generally rich in omega-3.
Tomatoes are rich in vitamins and oligominerals, but particularly they contain carotenoids and are the most important source of lycopene.
Olive oil is an excellent source of unsaturated fatty acids.
Garlic contains selenium, zinc, and alline, which is responsible for the taste and the penetrating, persistent odor of garlic. When alline is transformed into allicine, it has an antibacterial action, it lowers the cholesterol levels and the blood pressure.

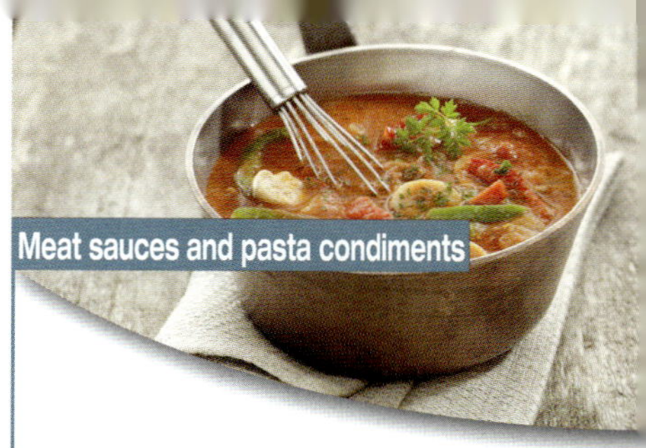

Bavarese pasta sauce

Ingredients and amounts for 4 people

- ✓ 1 lb small sweet Pachino tomatoes
- ✓ 7 tablespoons grated Parmesan cheese
- ✓ 2 tablespoons breadcrumbs
- ✓ 1 sprig of parsley
- ✓ 1 sprig of basil (chopped)
- ✓ 4 tablespoons extra virgin olive oil
- ✓ salt and black pepper to taste

Preparation

Line an oven dish with parchment paper.

Cut the tomatoes in half, leaving the seeds. Season the tomatoes with extra virgin olive oil.

Place them in the dish and sprinkle with salt, black pepper, parsley, basil, Parmesan, and a dusting of breadcrumbs.

Place in the oven to cook.

Use this sauce to season spaghetti boiled in hot salty water.

Bromatological evaluation per portion

Kcal	220
Protein (%)	18.6
Fats (%)	70.5
Carbohydrates (%)	10.9
Fiber (g)	1.5
Cholesterol (mg)	22.7

Valuable contents for the eye: ★ ★

Tomatoes are rich in vitamins and oligominerals, but particularly they contain carotenoids and are the most important source of lycopene.

Parmesan cheese is rich in easily digestible protein, is low in fat, and contains vitamin A and some vitamins of the B group.

Parsley contains flavonoids and is also an apiol, an antispasmodic, and an antipyretic. It also stimulates uterine contractions.

Basil owes its aroma to the numerous essential oils it contains; these stimulate salivary and gastric secretions.

Olive oil is an excellent source of unsaturated fatty acids.

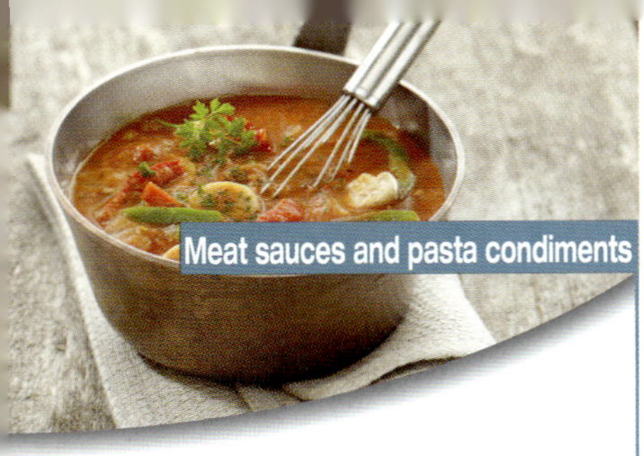

Orange sauce for grilled fish

Bromatological evaluation per portion

Kcal	210
Protein (%)	6.3
Fats (%)	83.9
Carbohydrates (%)	9.8
Fiber (g)	0.7
Cholesterol (mg)	8

Valuable contents for the eye: ★★

Oranges are rich in sucrose, vitamin C, and β-carotene. They also contain flavonoids (particularly in the pith or albedo underneath the peel).
Capers contain vitamins A, C, and E and also a considerable quantity of sodium.
Olives are rich in monounsaturated fats, vitamin E, and potassium.
Olive oil is an excellent source of unsaturated fatty acids.
Leeks contain flavonoids.

Ingredients and amounts for 4 people

- ✓ juice of 1 orange
- ✓ 1 finely sliced leek
- ✓ 1½ oz thinly sliced bacon
- ✓ 2 tablespoons desalted capers
- ✓ 20 stoned black olives
- ✓ 4 tablespoons extra virgin olive oil

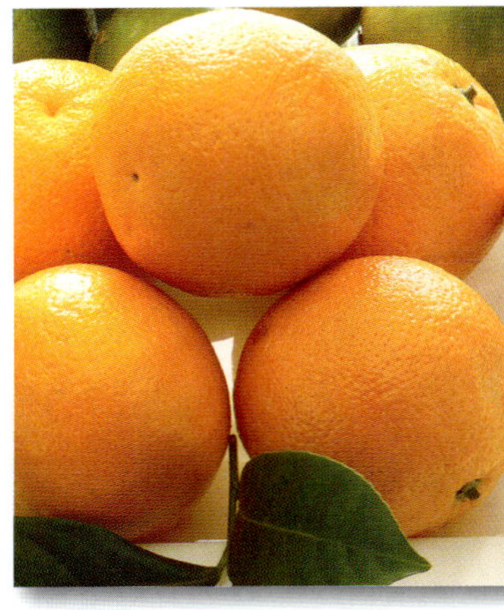

Preparation

Gently fry the leek and bacon in a small amount of oil. Add the capers and the olives; cook for 2 minutes.
Remove from the heat, add the orange juice, mix, and pour over grilled fish.

Caper and anchovy sauce for grilled fish

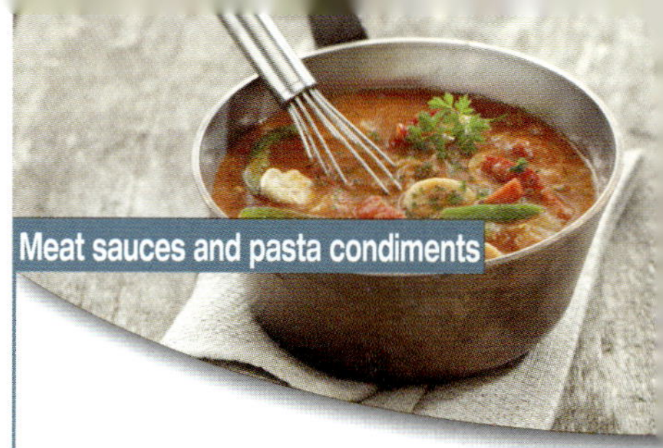

Ingredients and amounts for 4 people

✓ 4 tablespoons well-drained pickled capers
✓ 4 anchovy filets
✓ 1 clove of garlic
✓ 8 tablespoons extra virgin olive oil
✓ yellow zest of 1 lemon

Preparation

Place the lemon zest, capers, anchovies, garlic, and oil in the blender to produce a homogenous mixture.
Pour over grilled fish.

Bromatological evaluation per portion

Kcal	117
Protein (%)	10
Fats (%)	85.7
Carbohydrates (%)	4.3
Fiber (g)	0.5
Cholesterol (mg)	0

Valuable contents for the eye: ★★

Capers contain vitamins A, C, and E and also a considerable quantity of sodium.
Anchovies are lean fish and contain omega-3 fatty acids.
Garlic contains selenium, zinc, and alline, which is responsible for the taste and the penetrating, persistent odor of garlic. When alline is transformed into allicine, it has an antibacterial action, it lowers the cholesterol levels and the blood pressure.
Olive oil is an excellent source of unsaturated fatty acids.

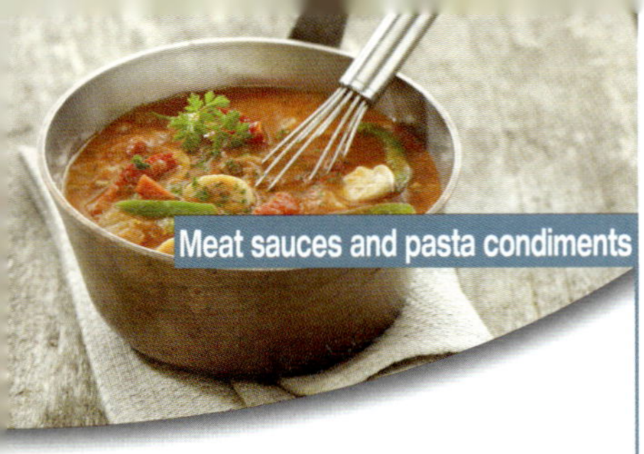

Olive sauce for grilled fish

Bromatological evaluation per portion

Kcal	198
Protein (%)	3.9
Fats (%)	94.6
Carbohydrates (%)	1.5
Fiber (g)	0.7
Cholesterol (mg)	66.8

Valuable contents for the eye: ★★★

Olives are rich in monounsaturated fats, vitamin E, and potassium.
Capers contain vitamins A, C, and E and also a considerable quantity of sodium.
Eggs are rich in saturated fatty acids but also contain a good quantity of mono- and polyunsaturated fats. Unfortunately, they contain cholesterol but they are also an important source of lutein.
Olive oil is an excellent source of unsaturated fatty acids.
Garlic contains selenium, zinc, and alline, which is responsible for the taste and the penetrating, persistent odor of garlic. When alline is transformed into allicine, it has an antibacterial action, it lowers the cholesterol levels and the blood pressure.

Ingredients and amounts for 4 people

- ✓ 24 stoned black olives
- ✓ 12 desalted capers
- ✓ 1 sprig of parsley
- ✓ 1 clove of garlic
- ✓ yolk of 1 hard-boiled egg
- ✓ 1 teaspoon white-wine or light-red vinegar
- ✓ 4 tablespoons extra virgin olive oil
- ✓ salt and pepper to taste

Preparation

Place the olives, capers, garlic, parsley, vinegar, and oil in the blender; pour the blended mixture into a bowl and add the egg yolk, salt, and pepper and mix to a smooth cream.
Pour over the grilled fish.

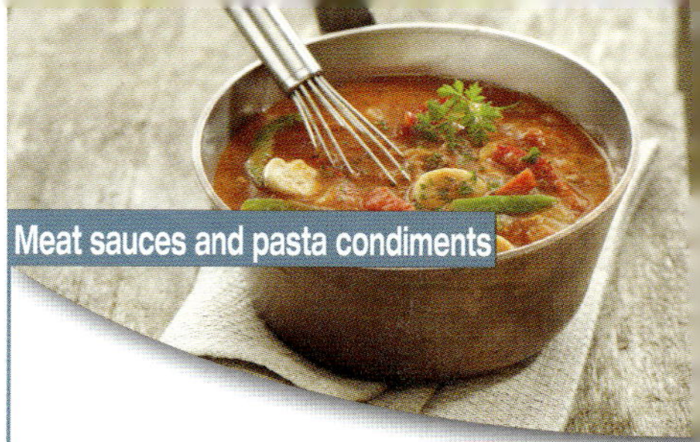

Lemon sauce for poached fish

Ingredients and amounts for 4 people

✓ juice of 2 lemons
✓ 4 tablespoons extra virgin olive oil
✓ 1 bunch of fresh parsley (chopped)
✓ salt to taste

Preparation

Place the salt and the lemon juice in a cup and mix well until the salt dissolves; add the oil and blend well. Add the parsley and mix.
Pour over the poached fish.

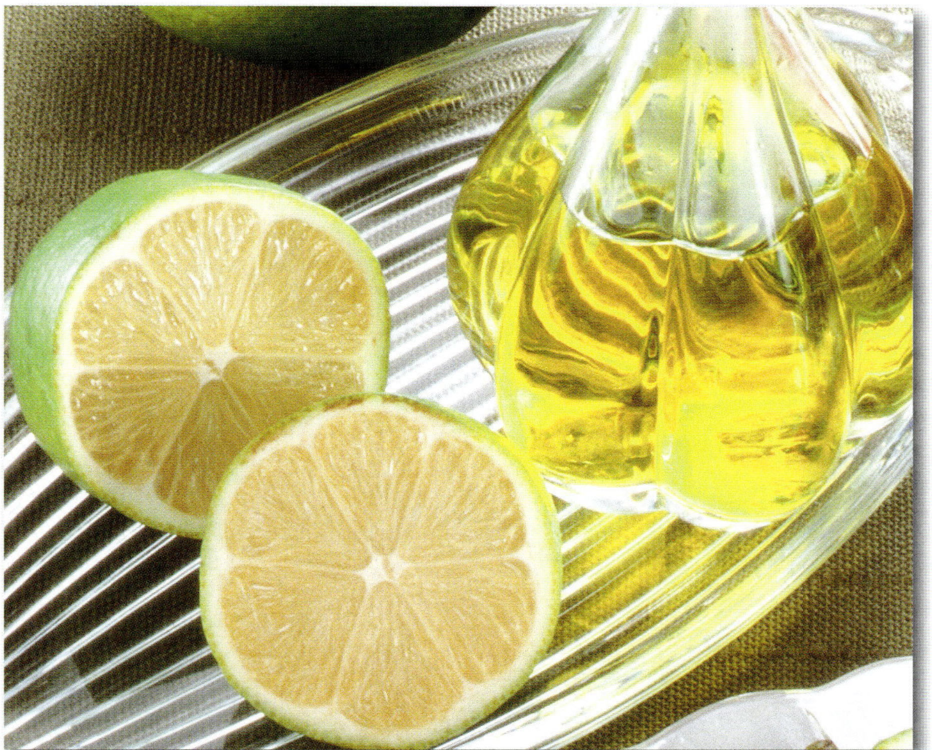

Bromatological evaluation per portion

Kcal	92
Protein (%)	1.4
Fats (%)	97.5
Carbohydrates (%)	1.1
Fiber (g)	0
Cholesterol (mg)	0

Valuable contents for the eye: ★

Lemon contains high quantities of vitamin C and β-carotene. It also contains flavonoids (particularly in the pith or albedo underneath the peel).
Olive oil is an excellent source of unsaturated fatty acids.
Parsley contains flavonoids and is also an apiol, an antispasmodic, and an antipyretic. It also stimulates uterine contractions.

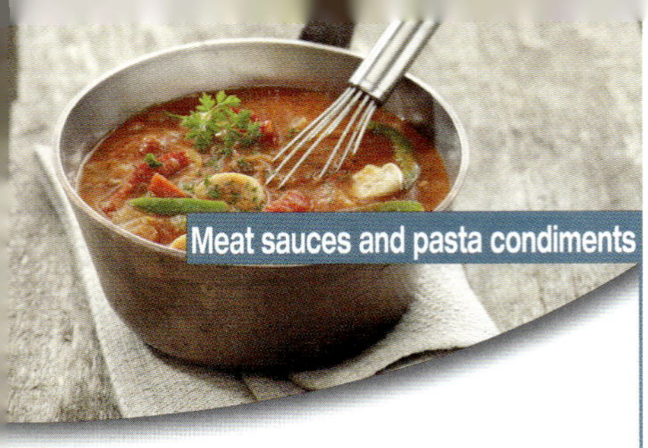

Spicy herb sauce for grilled fish

Bromatological evaluation per portion

Kcal	138
Protein (%)	0.9
Fats (%)	98.5
Carbohydrates (%)	0.6
Fiber (g)	5
Cholesterol (mg)	0

Valuable contents for the eye: ★

Olive oil is an excellent source of unsaturated fatty acids.

Chili pepper contains capsaicin, which makes it spicy; it also contains carotenoids and flavonoids.

Garlic contains selenium, zinc, and alline, which is responsible for the taste and the penetrating, persistent odor of garlic. When alline is transformed into allicine, it has an antibacterial action, it lowers the cholesterol levels and the blood pressure.

Oregano is rich in essential oils.

Ingredients and amounts for 4 people

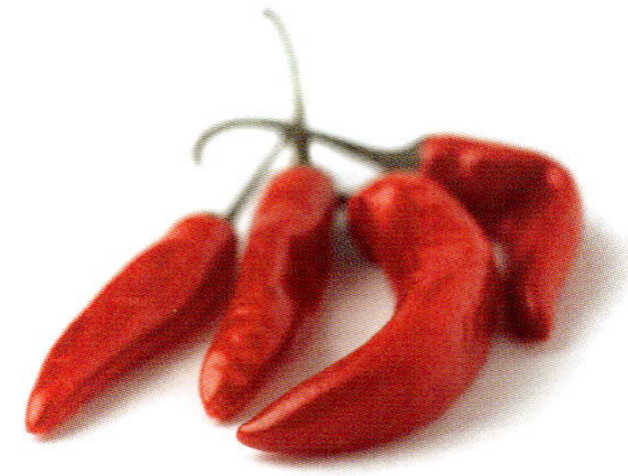

- ✓ 6 tablespoons extra virgin olive oil
- ✓ 1 clove of garlic (chopped)
- ✓ 1 small fresh chili pepper (chopped)
- ✓ ½ teaspoon oregano
- ✓ 1 sprig of fresh parsley (chopped)
- ✓ salt and pepper to taste

Preparation

Heat the oil in a pan; turn off the heat and add all the ingredients, which should be fried gently for just a few seconds.
Pour over grilled fish.

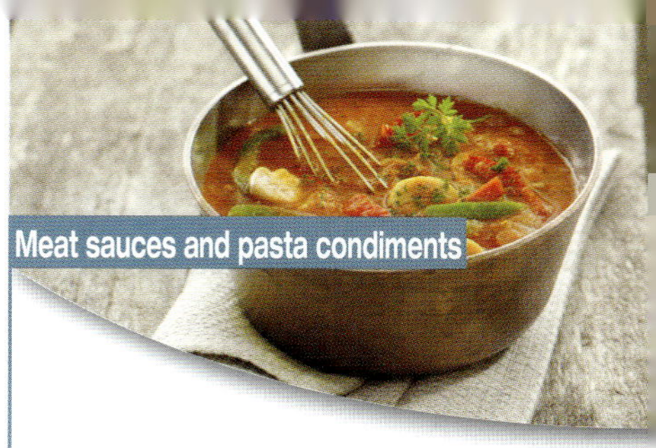

Tomato sauce for grilled fish

Ingredients and amounts for 4 people

- ✓ 4 very ripe tomatoes
- ✓ 2 cloves of garlic
- ✓ 1 sprig of parsley
- ✓ 2 tablespoons extra virgin olive oil
- ✓ salt and pepper to taste

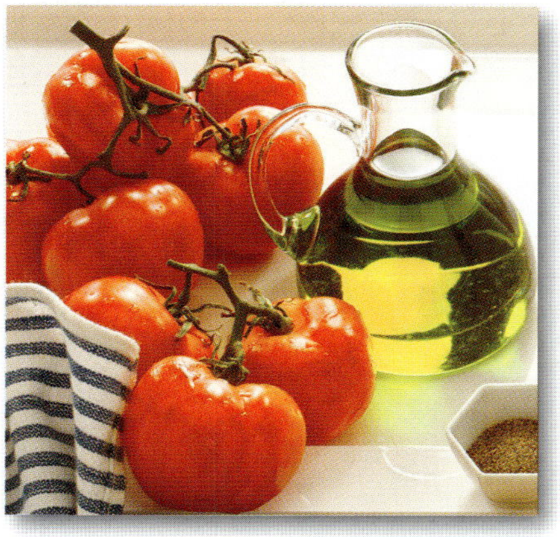

Preparation

Peel the tomatoes and remove the seeds; cut them into pieces and sprinkle with salt. Allow the water to drain.
Cut the garlic in half and mix with the tomatoes.
Let sit for 30 minutes.
Season with oil, salt, pepper, and finely chopped parsley.
Remove garlic before serving.
Use only fresh products.

Bromatological evaluation per portion

Kcal	67
Protein (%)	7.9
Fats (%)	70.9
Carbohydrates (%)	21.2
Fiber (g)	2.5
Cholesterol (mg)	0

Valuable contents for the eye: ★

Tomatoes are rich in vitamins and oligominerals, but particularly they contain carotenoids and are the most important source of lycopene.
Garlic contains selenium, zinc, and alline, which is responsible for the taste and the penetrating, persistent odor of garlic. When alline is transformed into allicine, it has an antibacterial action, it lowers the cholesterol levels and the blood pressure.
Parsley contains flavonoids and is also an apiol, an antispasmodic, and an antipyretic. It also stimulates uterine contractions.
Olive oil is an excellent source of unsaturated fatty acids.

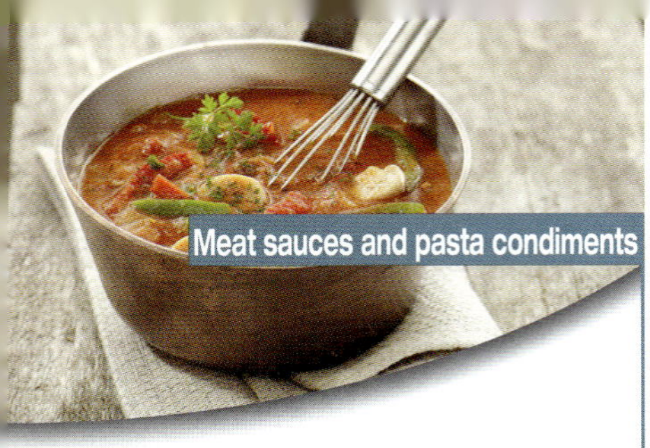

Arugula sauce for grilled fish

Bromatological evaluation per portion

Kcal	102
Protein (%)	4.8
Fats (%)	88.9
Carbohydrates (%)	6.3
Fiber (g)	0.7
Cholesterol (mg)	0

Valuable contents for the eye: ★

Olive oil is an excellent source of unsaturated fatty acids.
Lemon contains high quantities of vitamin C and β-carotene. It also contains flavonoids (particularly in the pith or albedo, underneath the peel).
Arugula has a spicy flavor and contains carotenoids and flavonoids.
Parsley contains flavonoids and is also an apiol, an antispasmodic, and an antipyretic. It also stimulates uterine contractions.
Basil owes its aroma to the numerous essential oils it contains; these stimulate salivary and gastric secretions.

Ingredients and amounts for 4 people

✓ 4 tablespoons extra virgin olive oil
✓ 1 clove of garlic
✓ 12 fresh basil leaves
✓ 1 teaspoon parsley
✓ 1 bunch of arugula
✓ juice of 1 lemon
✓ salt and pepper to taste

Preparation

Place all the ingredients in a blender for a few seconds; allow pieces of arugula to be visible.
Pour over the grilled fish.

Green sauce for boiled fish or potatoes

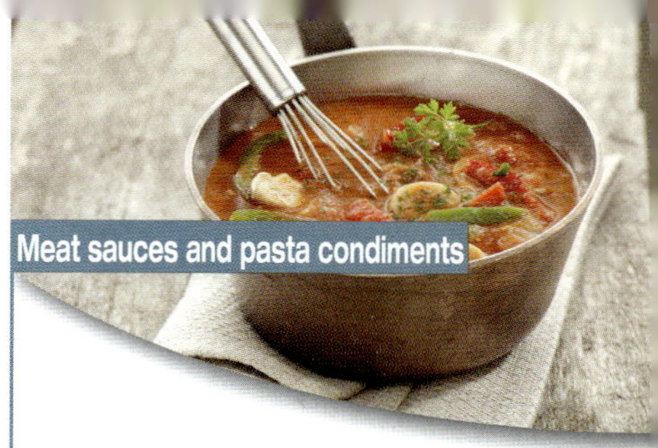

Ingredients and amounts for 4 people

- ✓ 3½ oz bread (the soft part or inside)
- ✓ 3 tablespoons vinegar
- ✓ 1 shallot
- ✓ 2 anchovy filets
- ✓ 2 tablespoons desalted capers
- ✓ yolk of 1 hard-boiled egg
- ✓ 6 basil leaves, chopped
- ✓ 1 sprig of parsley, chopped
- ✓ 8 tablespoons extra virgin olive oil
- ✓ salt and pepper to taste

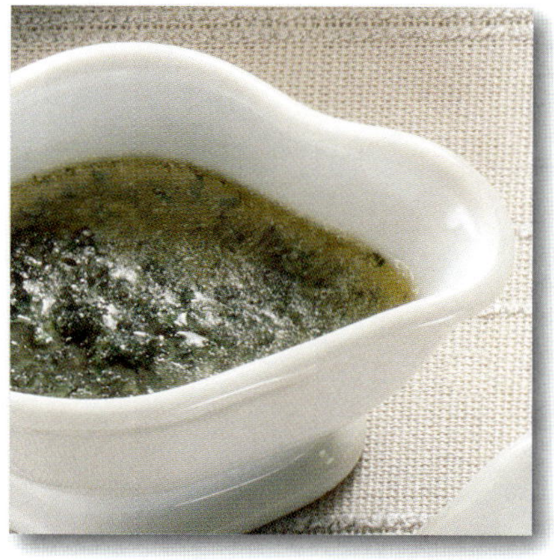

Preparation

Soak the soft part of the bread in vinegar.

Place the chopped shallot, anchovies, capers, basil, and parsley in the blender. Blend.

Squeeze the excess vinegar from the bread and add to the blender with the egg yolk.

Add salt, pepper, and oil and blend once again.

Keep cool until served.

Bromatological evaluation per portion

Kcal	318
Protein (%)	4.6
Fats (%)	88.9
Carbohydrates (%)	6.5
Fiber (g)	1
Cholesterol (mg)	38.7

Valuable contents for the eye: ★★

The greater the "wholemeal" content, the richer the **bread** will be in vitamins and fiber.

Anchovies are fish low in fat and contain omega-3 fatty acids.

Capers contain vitamins A, C, and E and also a considerable quantity of sodium.

Basil owes its aroma to the numerous essential oils it contains; these stimulate salivary and gastric secretions.

Parsley contains flavonoids and is also an apiol, an antispasmodic, and an antipyretic. It also stimulates uterine contractions.

Like onion, **shallots** also contain flavonoids.

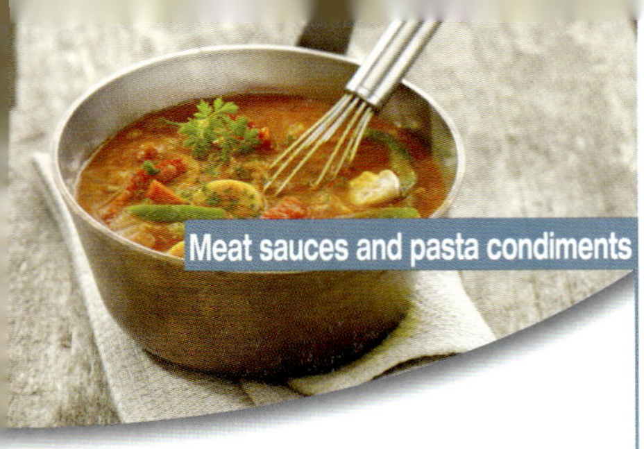

Garlic sauce for fresh vegetables

Bromatological evaluation per portion

Kcal	246
Protein (%)	6.5
Fats (%)	89.3
Carbohydrates (%)	4.2
Fiber (g)	0
Cholesterol (mg)	0

Valuable contents for the eye: ★

This is a very tasty way for consuming **vegetables**, ensuring an excellent intake of vitamins, micronutrients, and fibers.

Ingredients and amounts for 4 people

- ✓ 2 cloves of garlic
- ✓ white of 1 hard-boiled egg
- ✓ 10 tablespoons extra virgin olive oil
- ✓ 3 tablespoons milk
- ✓ salt to taste

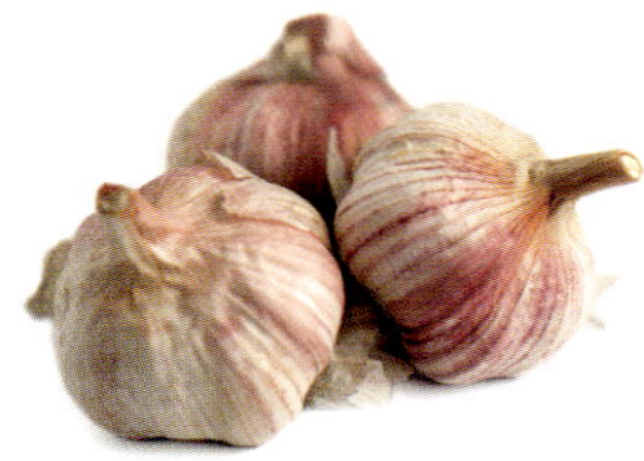

Preparation

Place all the ingredients in the blender. Blend for a few seconds. Use as a vegetable dip or to season salads.

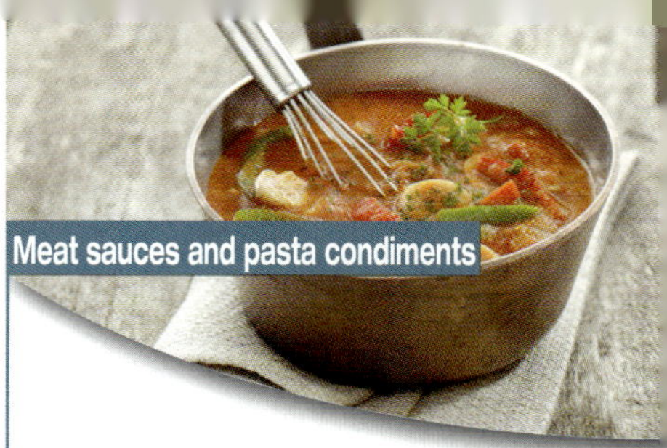

Mayonnaise

Ingredients and amounts for 4 people

- ✓ 1 whole egg at room temperature
- ✓ 1 small amount of mustard (tip of a spoon)
- ✓ 3½ oz sunflower seed oil
- ✓ juice of ½ lemon
- ✓ pinch of salt

Preparation

It is essential that the egg is at room temperature and not used straight from the refrigerator.
Place all the ingredients in the blender. Blend slowly (speed 1 or 2) for 1 to 2 minutes until creamy.

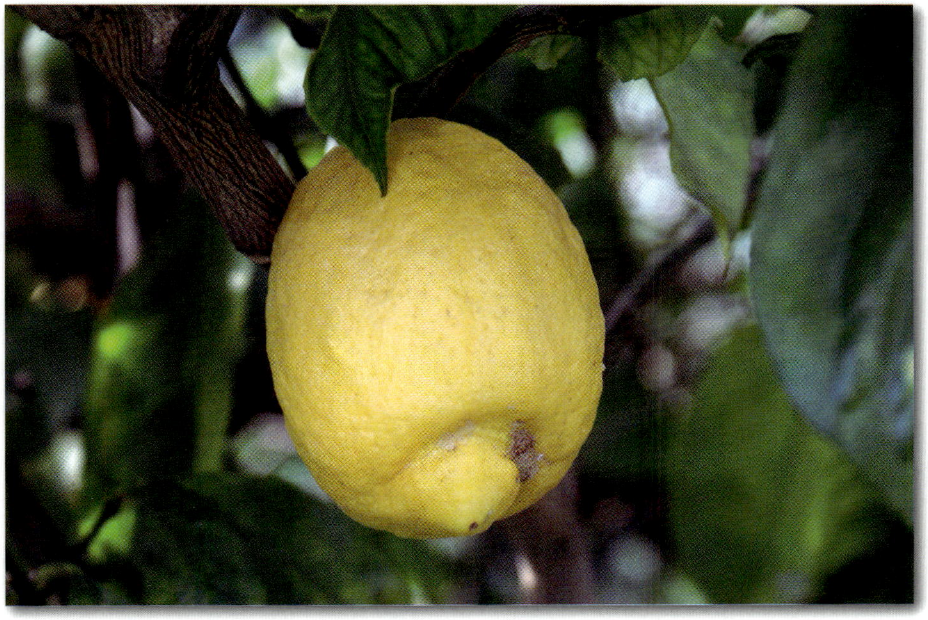

Bromatological evaluation per portion

Kcal	164
Protein (%)	2.6
Fats (%)	96.2
Carbohydrates (%)	1.2
Fiber (g)	0
Cholesterol (mg)	17.5

Valuable contents for the eye: ★

Eggs are rich in saturated fatty acids but also contain a good quantity of mono- and polyunsaturated fats. Unfortunately, they contain cholesterol but they are also an important source of lutein.
Sunflower seed oil contains omega-6 and vitamin E, even though part of this vitamin is lost during the industrial processing.

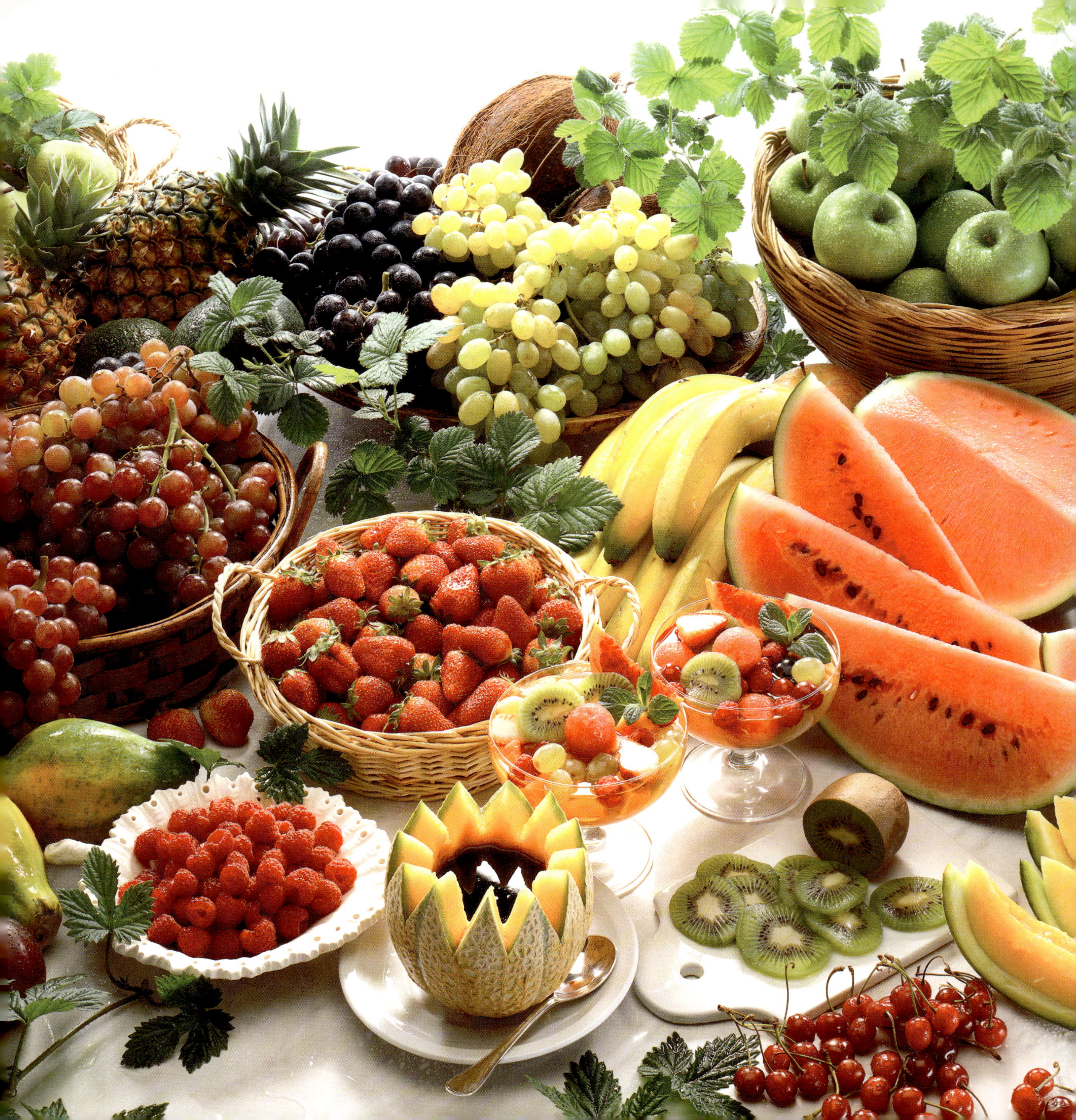

Fruit

Fruit must be given its rightful dignity as a food; it is particularly useful for people who have problems satisfying their appetites and limits the tendency to overload with calories and fat. But that is not all.
The most interesting contents of fresh fruit range from the high vitamin C content of the citrus fruits to the carotenoids (precursors of vitamin A) found in the cucumber family and apricots; or the polyphenols (flavonoids) found in apples, peaches, plums, and cherries. Consequently, rotating the quality of fruit is highly recommended, with a preference for seasonal produce, which has the additional advantage of avoiding fruit grown in hothouses or those given some form of preservative treatment.
Unfortunately, fresh fruit is somewhat of a rarity in coffee bars, in sandwich bars, or in fast food outlets; fruit is usually only found in limited quantities in some imaginative drink and rarely as a fresh fruit juice. The 2 preparations are very different, both in terms of the number of calories and in terms of the origin (the sugar added to the imaginative drinks as opposed to the pulp in the fruit juices); moreover, in the drinks, a large part of the fruit's original fiber is missing, as these preparations are for drinking not chewing.
It is a well-known fact that the energy provided by fruit originates almost exclusively from the simple sugars. This is not a problem for people who are not suffering from diabetes or an excess of triglycerides in the blood. People who avoid taking even one spoonful of sugar in coffee should be reminded that there is the equivalent of 3 spoonfuls of sugar in a medium-sized apple or orange.
The younger generation who prefers sugary, fizzy drinks over fruit juices should be reminded that a 12 oz can of a typical sweetened drink (the sweetener is often glucose syrup) contains approximately 7 teaspoons of sugar (the equivalent of 140 calories), a considerable amount of caffeine, no vitamins, and none of the other natural protective agents.
Summer fruits are at least 90% water and, therefore, they contain just a few grams of sugar: cucumber 3.4%, melon 7.4%, strawberries and raspberries 5.3%, black currants 8%, blackberries 10%. Moreover, fruit is rich in protective elements (from anti-oxidants to fibers). It is no coincidence that the World Health Organization (WHO) and the more important scientific societies recommend a substantial daily consumption of fruit and vegetables.
One piece of advice: fruit, particularly when fresh, is normally eaten at the end of a meal; ideally, it should not be eaten with the main meals but at breakfast or as a snack between meals.

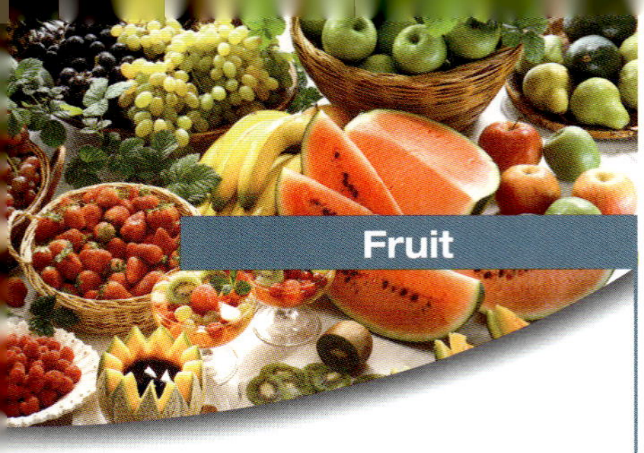

Baked cherries

Bromatological evaluation per portion

Kcal	200
Protein (%)	2.1
Fats (%)	19.3
Carbohydrates (%)	78.6
Fiber (g)	1.7
Cholesterol (mg)	12.5

Valuable contents for the eye: ★★

Cherries are rich in simple sugars; they have a moderate content of carotenoids, vitamin C, and flavonoids. **Sugar** is a pure form of rapidly available energy. **Butter** is a milk product consisting of saturated fatty acids.

Ingredients and amounts for 4 people

✓ 1 1/3 lbs cherries

✓ 7 tablespoons sugar

✓ 1½ tablespoons butter

✓ 1½ tablespoons cherry brandy

Preparation

Wash, dry, and stone the cherries.

Place the butter, cherries, and sugar in a pan and cook over strong heat for 5 minutes; pour the cherry brandy over the fruit.

Let cool and serve.

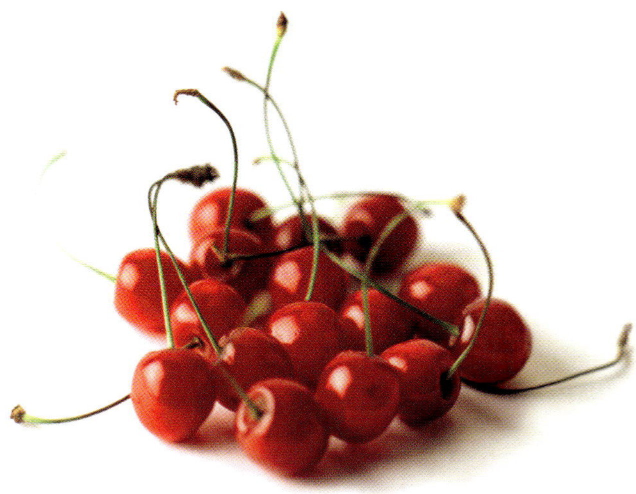

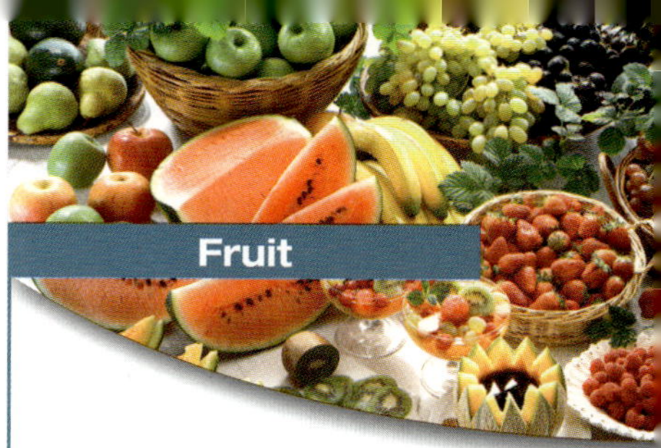

Strawberries, raspberries, and almonds

Ingredients and amounts for 4 people

✓ 14 oz (1¾ cups) large ripe strawberries
✓ 7 oz raspberries
✓ 20 almonds
✓ 3 tablespoons sugar

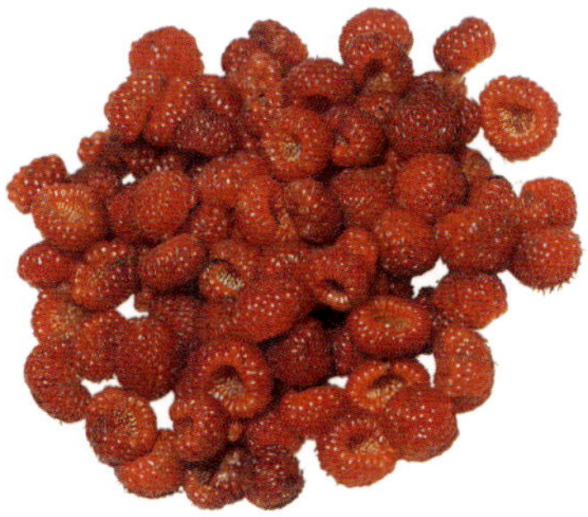

Preparation

Finely chop the almonds.
Wash, dry, and tail the strawberries; cut into pieces; and place in a bowl.
Wash the raspberries very gently and dry delicately with absorbent paper towels; place in a bowl, add the sugar and crush them, mixing with the sugar.
Pour the raspberry cream over the strawberries and then add the almonds.
Leave in the refrigerator for 30 to 40 minutes and then serve.

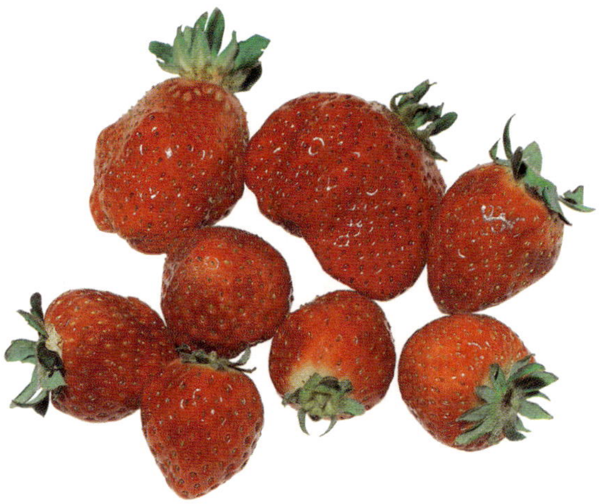

Bromatological evaluation per portion

Kcal	89
Protein (%)	7.2
Fats (%)	13.6
Carbohydrates (%)	79.2
Fiber (g)	5.4
Cholesterol (mg)	0

Valuable contents for the eye: ★★★

Strawberries are a good source of vitamin C and anthocyanosides.
Raspberries are rich in vitamin C and flavonoids.
Almonds are an excellent source of vitamin E; they also contain large quantities of magnesium in addition to zinc, calcium, and iron.
Sugar is a pure form of rapidly available energy.

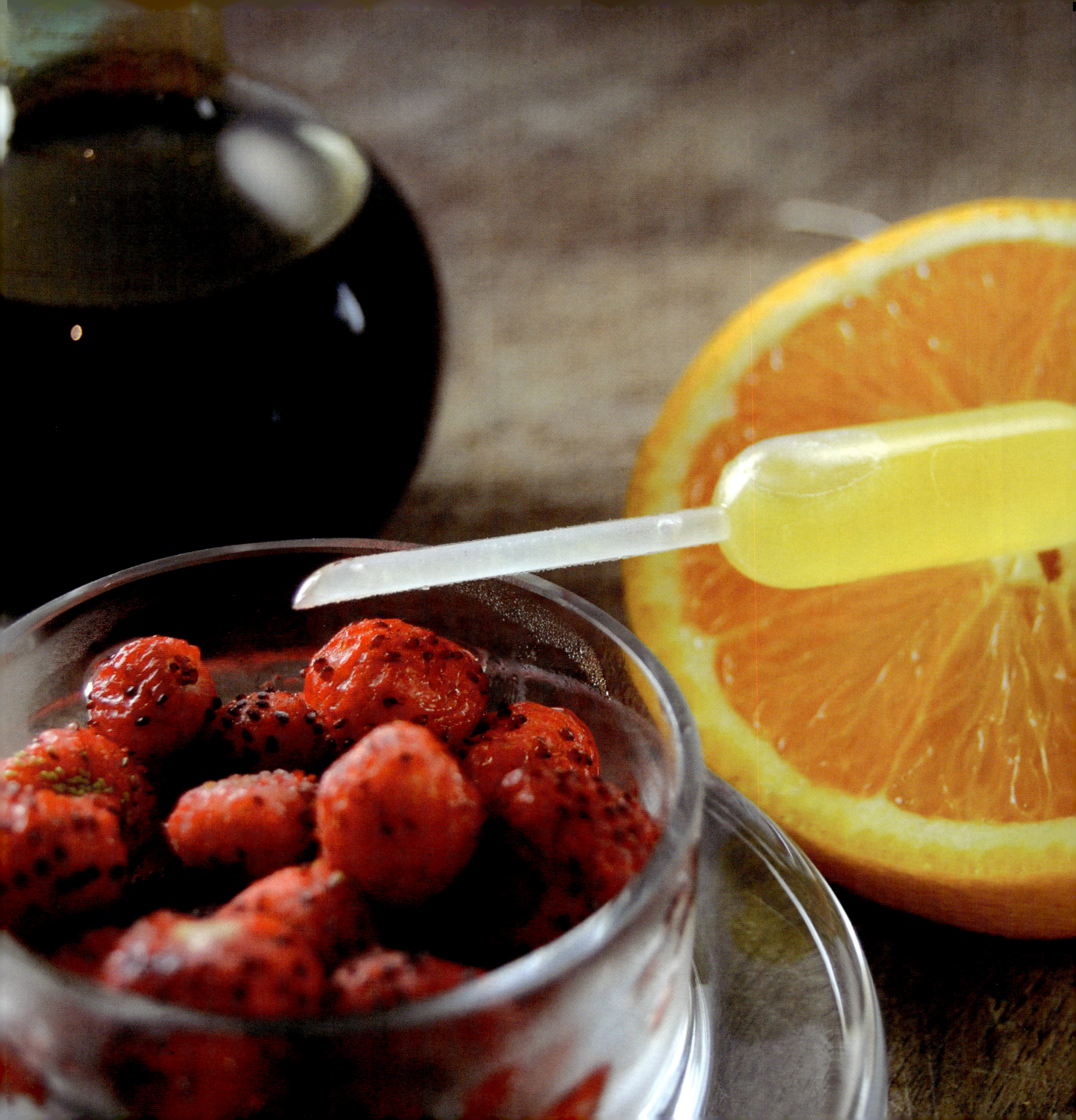

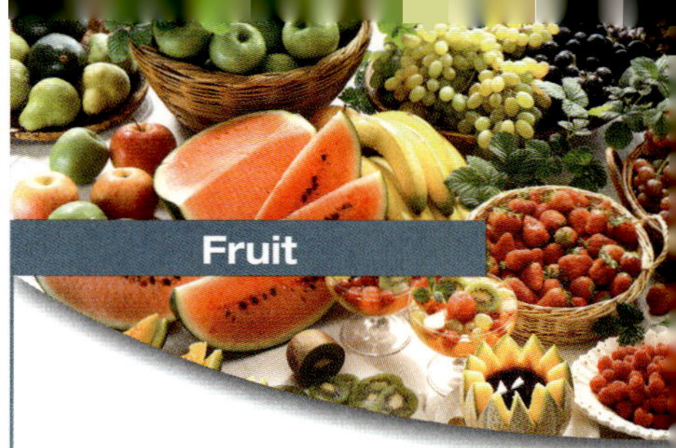

Wild strawberries with **balsamic vinegar**

Ingredients and amounts for 4 people

- ✓ 7 oz strawberries
- ✓ 4 teaspoons sugar
- ✓ 1 tablespoon balsamic vinegar
- ✓ juice of 1 orange

Preparation

Wash the strawberries. Place them in a bowl and add the orange juice, sugar, and balsamic vinegar.

Mix well.

Serve in small bowls; add a tablespoon of orange juice.

Bromatological evaluation per portion

Kcal	59
Protein (%)	3.7
Fats (%)	0
Carbohydrates (%)	96.3
Fiber (g)	0.7
Cholesterol (mg)	0

Valuable contents for the eye: ★★

Strawberries are a good source of vitamin C and anthocyanosides.

The **orange** is rich in sucrose and contains high quantities of vitamin C and β-carotene. It also contains flavonoids (particularly in the pith or albedo underneath the peel.)

Balsamic vinegar is low in calories but has a very intense flavor.

Sugar is a pure form of rapidly available energy.

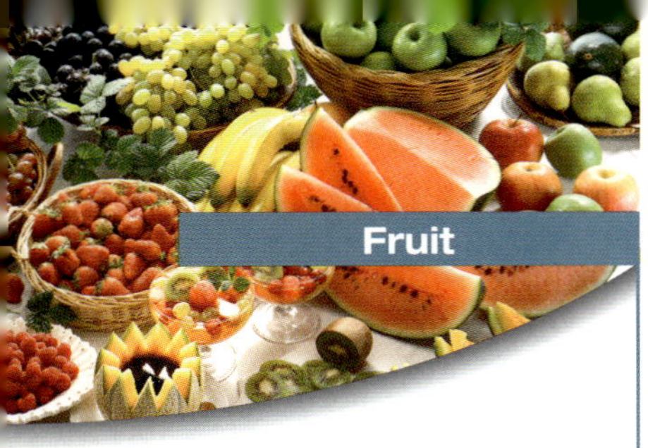

Strawberries in white wine

Bromatological evaluation per portion

Kcal	102
Protein (%)	3.4
Fats (%)	3.3
Carbohydrates (%)	93.3
Fiber (g)	1.5
Cholesterol (mg)	0

Valuable contents for the eye: ★ ★

Strawberries are a good source of vitamin C and anthocyanosides.

Sugar is a pure form of rapidly available energy.

Wine contains small quantities of flavonoids.

Ingredients and amounts for 4 people

✓ 14 oz (1¾ cups) large ripe strawberries

✓ 4 tablespoons sugar

✓ 6¾ tablespoons dry white wine

Preparation

Wash, dry, and tail the strawberries; cut them in half. Place in a bowl. Pour in the sugar and white wine. Store in the refrigerator for approximately 1 hour.

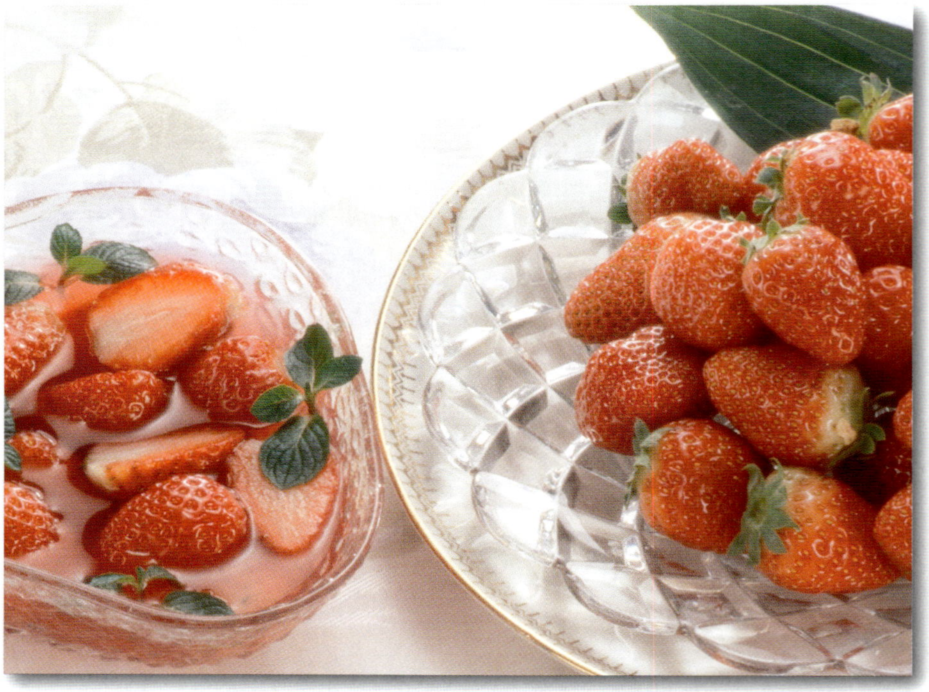

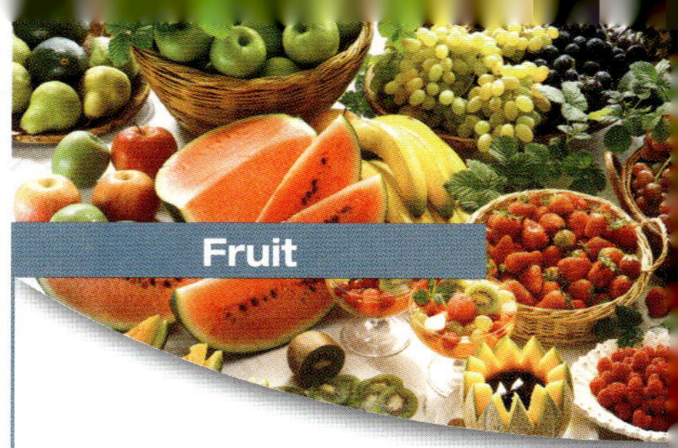

Mixed berries with yogurt

Ingredients and amounts for 4 people

- ✓ 1⅓ cups mixed berries (blueberries, raspberries, strawberries, blackberries)
- ✓ 10½ tablespoons plain yogurt
- ✓ 1 tablespoon honey (millefiori preferred)
- ✓ 4 tablespoons orange juice

Preparation

Wash and dry the fruit. Split into 4 portions with the same total quantity and an equal amount of each fruit.

Prepare the cream by adding the honey to the yogurt and mix well; then add the orange juice and mix.

Pour the cream over the fruit and place in the refrigerator for approximately 1 hour.

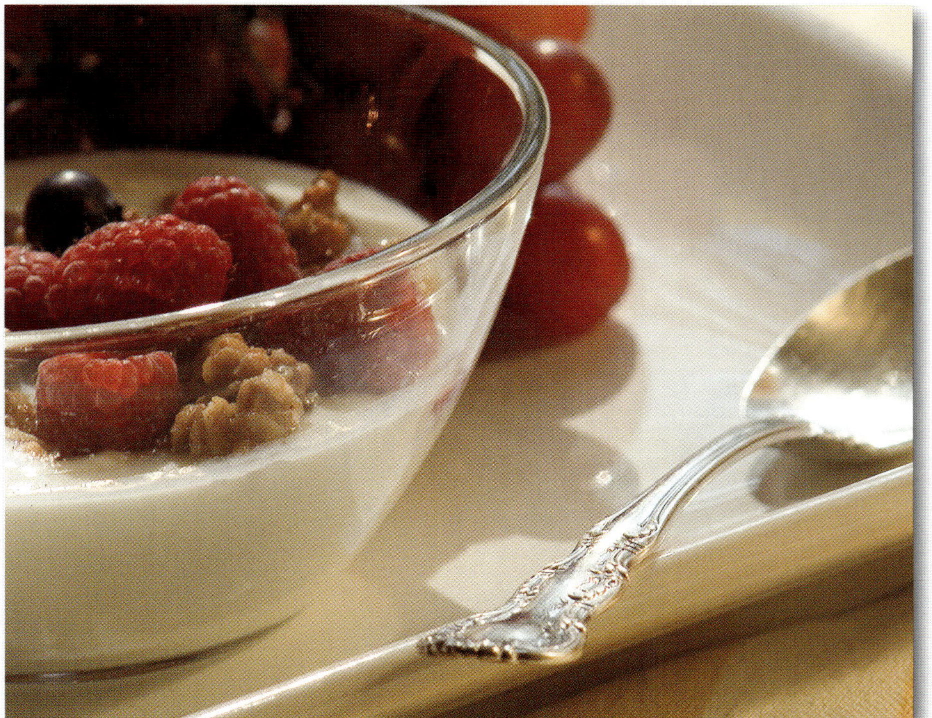

Bromatological evaluation per portion

Kcal	62
Protein (%)	16.7
Fats (%)	3
Carbohydrates (%)	80.3
Fiber (g)	5.4
Cholesterol (mg)	2.4

Valuable contents for the eye: ★ ★ ★

Blueberries are rich in vitamin C and anthocyanosides.

Raspberries are rich in vitamin C and flavonoids.

Strawberries are a good source of vitamin C and anthocyanosides.

The **orange** is rich in sucrose and contains high quantities of vitamin C and β-carotene. It also contains flavonoids.

Yogurt has a high repletion index; in addition to the live milk enzymes, it contains vitamins of the B group and folic acid.

Honey is rich in sugars (glucose and fructose).

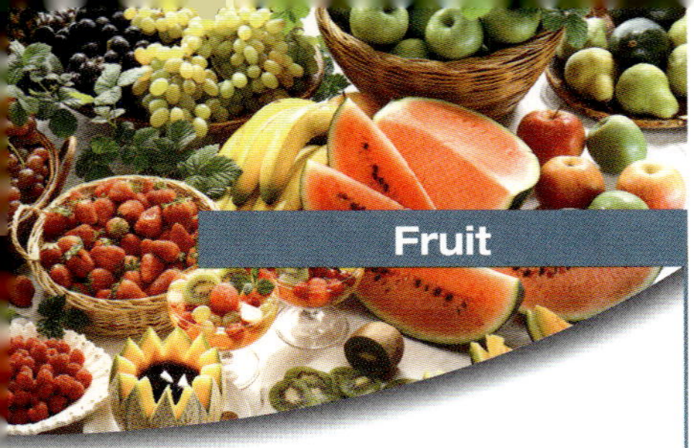

Mixed fruit with yogurt cream

Bromatological evaluation per portion

Kcal	111
Protein (%)	9.7
Fats (%)	0.9
Carbohydrates (%)	89.4
Fiber (g)	2.6
Cholesterol (mg)	0

Valuable contents for the eye: ★★★

Melon is rich in vitamin C and carotenoids.
The **orange** is rich in sucrose and contains high quantities of vitamin C and β-carotene. It also contains flavonoids.
The **banana** is rich in potassium and sugars; it contains vitamins C, A, and some of the B group.
Strawberries are a good source of vitamin C and anthocyanosides.
Grapes contain sugars, flavonoids, and melatonin (in the peel).
Yogurt has a high repletion index; in addition to the live milk enzymes, it contains vitamins of the B group and folic acid.
Honey is rich in sugars (glucose and fructose).

Ingredients and amounts for 4 people

- ✓ ½ melon
- ✓ 2 oranges
- ✓ 1 banana
- ✓ 3½ oz strawberries
- ✓ 3½ oz seedless grapes

For the cream

- ✓ 3½ oz (7 tablespoons) low fat yogurt
- ✓ 2⅓ tablespoons orange juice
- ✓ 1 tablespoon honey (acacia or millefiori preferred)
- ✓ 1 teaspoon grated orange zest
- ✓ 1 teaspoon chopped fresh mint

Preparation

Core and slice the fruit. Place on a large serving dish.
Prepare the cream by mixing the yogurt with the orange juice, honey, grated orange zest, and mint.
Pour over the fruit.

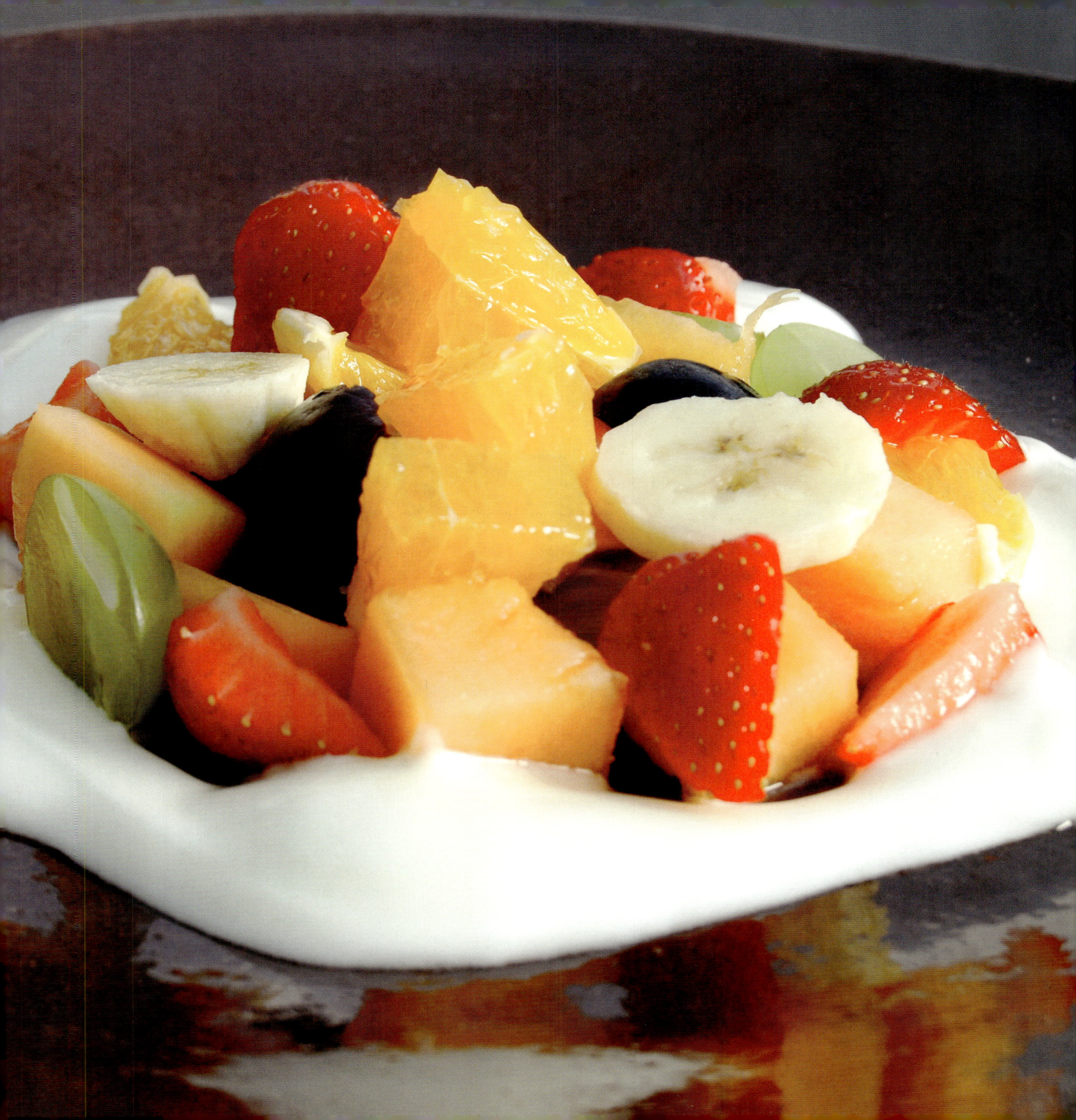

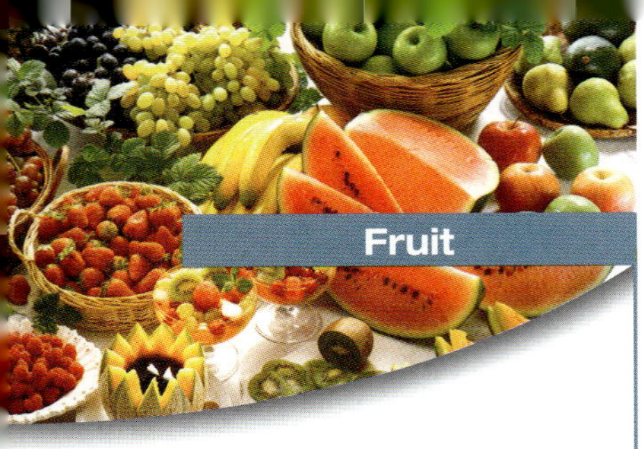

Fruit salad of apricot, kiwi, and banana

Bromatological evaluation per portion

Kcal	98
Protein (%)	3.6
Fats (%)	2.9
Carbohydrates (%)	93.5
Fiber (g)	1.8
Cholesterol (mg)	0

Valuable contents for the eye: ★ ★

Apricots are sweet and low in calories; they contain vitamin C and β-carotene.
Kiwis have a high content of vitamin C.
The **banana** is rich in potassium and sugars; it contains vitamins C, A, and some of the B group.
Lemon contains high quantities of vitamin C and β-carotene. It also contains flavonoids.

Ingredients and amounts for 4 people

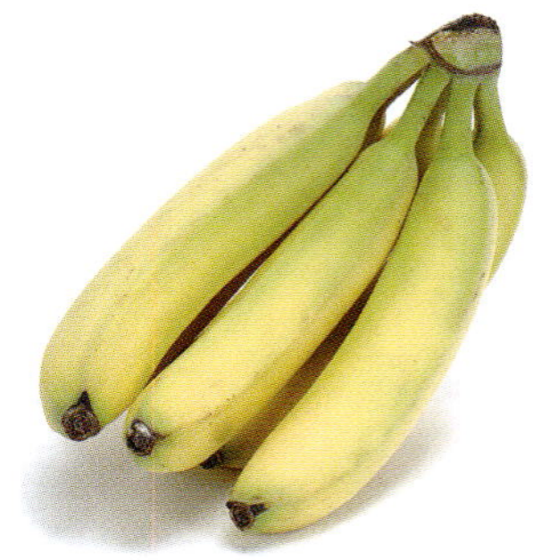

- ✓ 4 apricots
- ✓ 2 kiwi
- ✓ 1 banana
- ✓ juice of 1 lemon
- ✓ 4 tablespoon sugar
- ✓ 2 tablespoon dark rum

Preparation

Cut the apricots into segments; peel and dice the kiwi; slice the bananas; add the sugar, lemon juice, and rum.
Let sit for 20 to 30 minutes and then serve.
This fruit salad can be served with ice cream.

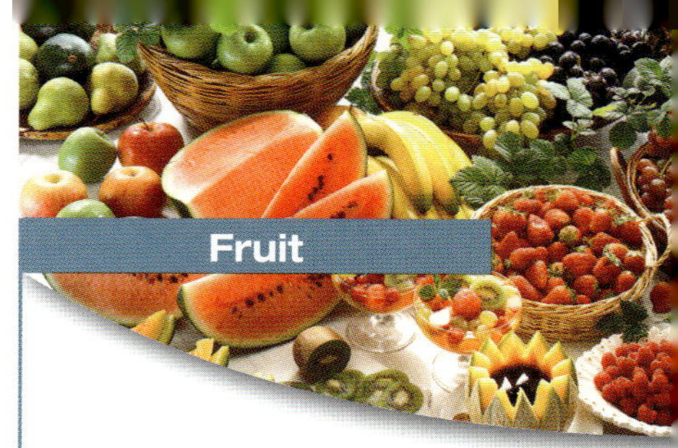

Fruit salad of watermelon, melon, and grapefruit

Ingredients and amounts for 4 people

- ✓ 1 watermelon
- ✓ 1 melon
- ✓ 1 grapefruit
- ✓ 1 glass of maraschino liqueur
- ✓ juice of 2 lemons
- ✓ 5 to 6 tablespoons sugar

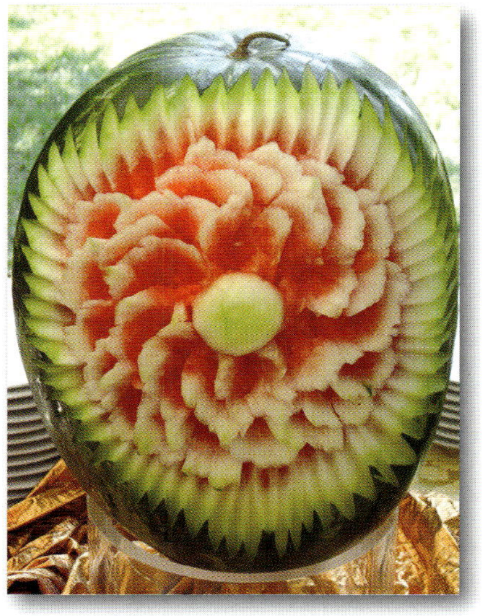

Preparation

Peel the melon and remove the seeds and the threads; dice the pulp.
Split the watermelon into two and dice the pulp, eliminating as many of the seeds as possible.
Peel the grapefruit; cut into slices. Dice the pulp.
Place the pieces of watermelon, melon, and grapefruit in a bowl; add the maraschino liqueur, lemon juice, and sugar. Mix and let sit for a few minutes in the refrigerator.
Instead of a bowl, an empty watermelon half can be used to serve the fruit.

Bromatological evaluation per portion

Kcal	182
Protein (%)	3.3
Fats (%)	0
Carbohydrates (%)	96.7
Fiber (g)	1.8
Cholesterol (mg)	0

Valuable contents for the eye: ★★

Watermelon is rich in water and fructose; it contains vitamins A and C and potassium. It also contains carotenoids, including lycopene.
Melon is rich in vitamin C and carotenoids.
Grapefruit is rich in vitamin C and flavonoids.
Lemon contains high quantities of vitamin C and β-carotene. It also contains flavonoids (particularly in the pith or albedo, underneath the peel).
Sugar is a pure form of rapidly available energy.

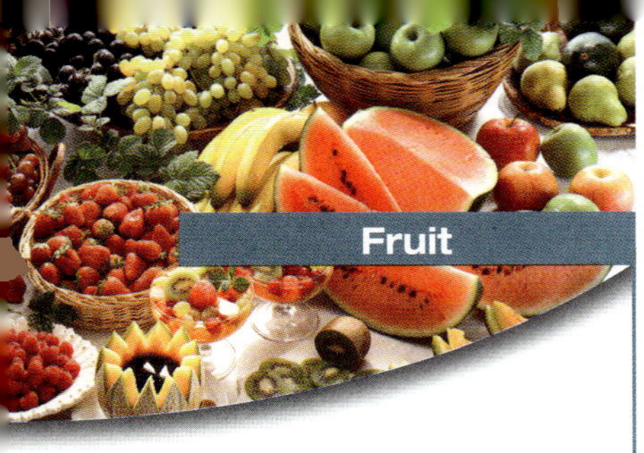

Fruit salad of grapefruit, strawberries, and grapes

Bromatological evaluation per portion

Kcal	180
Protein (%)	3.8
Fats (%)	1.8
Carbohydrates (%)	94.4
Fiber (g)	4.5
Cholesterol (mg)	0

Valuable contents for the eye: ★ ★

Grapefruit is rich in vitamin C and flavonoids.
Strawberries are a good source of vitamin C and anthocyanosides.
Grapes contain sugars, flavonoids, and melatonin (in the peel).
Lemon contains high quantities of vitamin C and β-carotene. It also contains flavonoids (particularly in the pith or albedo, underneath the peel).
Sugar is a pure form of rapidly available energy.

Ingredients and amounts for 4 people

✓ 1 grapefruit
✓ 12 strawberries
✓ 16 green grapes
✓ 16 black grapes
✓ juice of 1 lemon
✓ 2 tablespoons sugar

Preparation

Wash the grapes and remove the stems; cut them in half and remove the seeds.
Wash and dry the strawberries; remove the top and cut into quarters.
Peel and slice the grapefruit, removing the peel, the threads and the seeds; dice the pulp.
Mix the fruit in a bowl; add the sugar and the lemon juice.
Mix and leave for 20 to 30 minutes.
It can be served with low-fat yogurt.

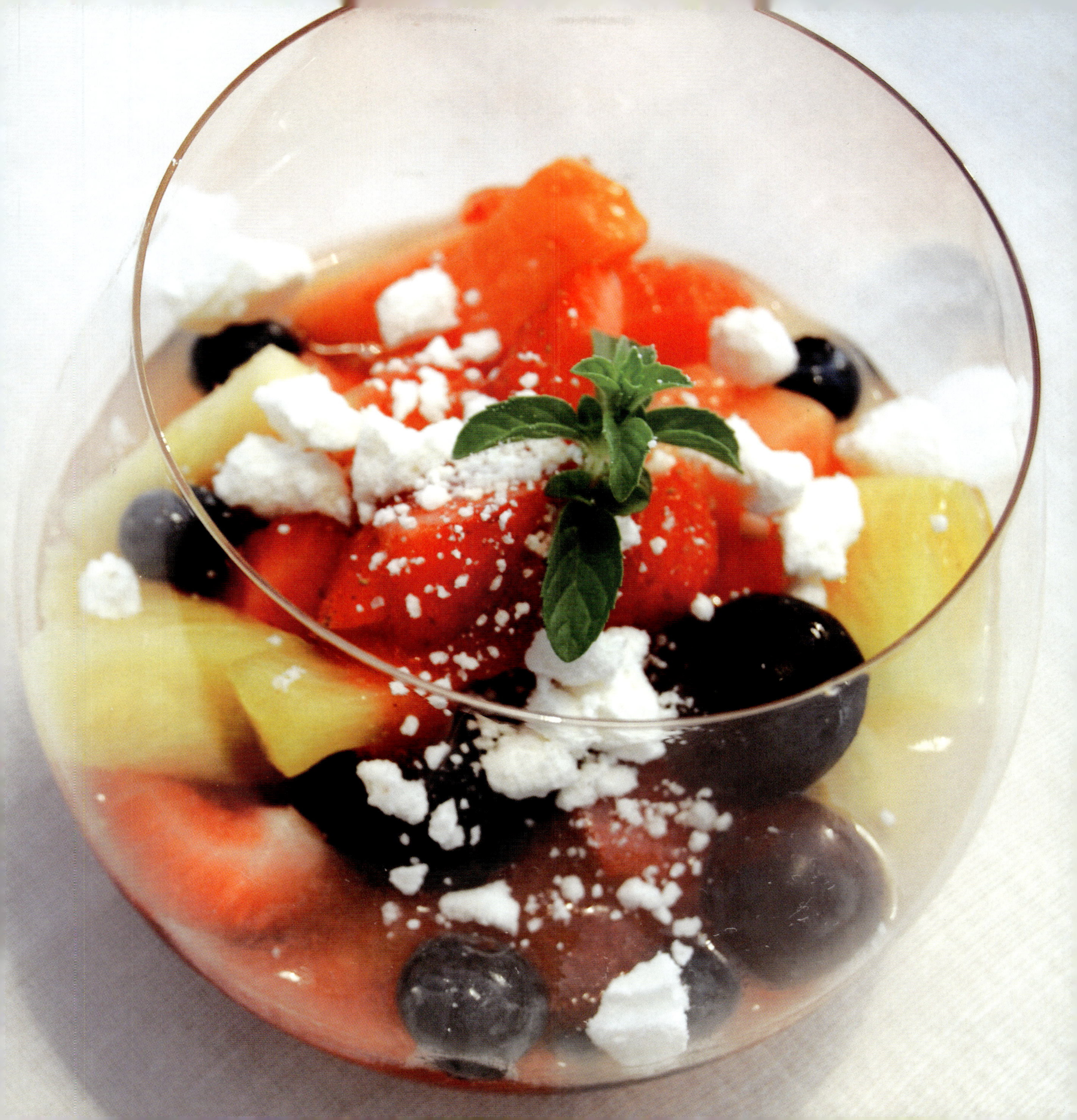

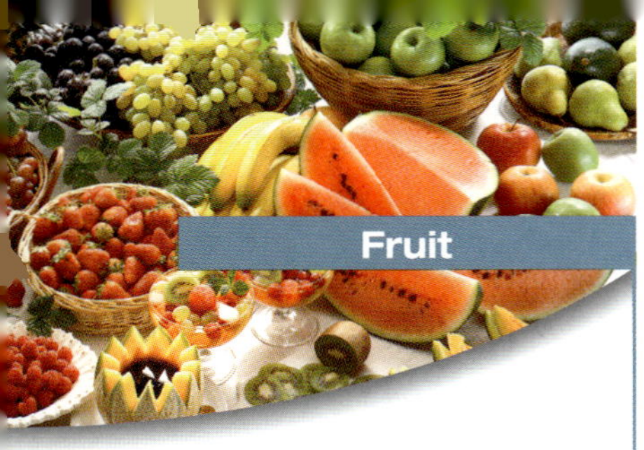

Fruit salad of apples, oranges, and walnuts

Bromatological evaluation per portion

Kcal	171
Protein (%)	6.4
Fats (%)	45.5
Carbohydrates (%)	48.1
Fiber (g)	3.8
Cholesterol (mg)	0

Valuable contents for the eye: ★★★

The **apple** is rich in fructose; it contains flavonoids (quercetin) and oligoelements such as zinc and selenium.

The **orange** is rich in sucrose and contains high quantities of vitamin C and β-carotene. It also contains flavonoids

Lime contains high quantities of vitamin C and β-carotene. It also contains flavonoids (particularly in the pith or albedo underneath the peel.)

Honey is rich in sugars (glucose and fructose).

Walnuts are high in calories and contain omega-3 fatty acids.

Ingredients and amounts for 4 people

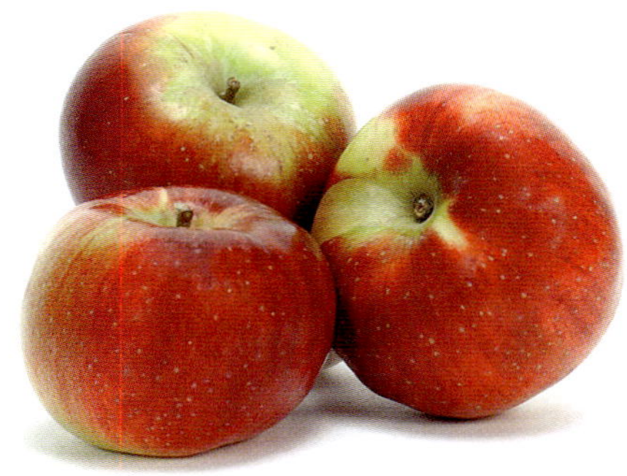

- ✓ 2 apples
- ✓ 2 oranges
- ✓ 1 lime
- ✓ 2 tablespoons honey (acacia or millefiori preferred)
- ✓ 6 walnuts

Preparation

Squeeze the lime.

Wash the oranges and cut them in half.

Squeeze one half of an orange.

Cut the other pieces of orange into thin slices, leaving the peel but removing the seeds.

Peel the apples and remove the core with a coring knife; slice the apples.

Alternate the slices of apple and orange on a serving plate, overlapping them slightly.

Mix the orange and lime juices, honey, and walnuts and pour over the fruit.

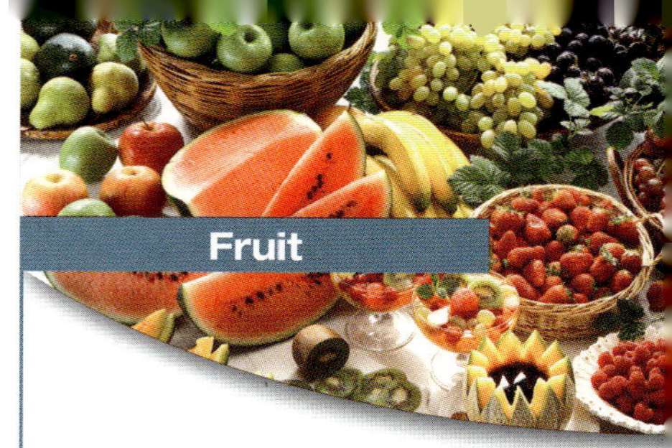

Blueberries and **peaches**

Ingredients and amounts for 4 people

- ✓ 5¼ oz blueberries
- ✓ 14 oz ripe yellow peaches
- ✓ 1 tablespoon sugar
- ✓ juice of 1 lemon
- ✓ 1 tablespoon water
- ✓ 1 teaspoon of grated lemon zest

Preparation

Dissolve the sugar by boiling in a pan with water for approximately 1 minute; let cool.

Wash, peel, and stone the peaches; cut into pieces and put in the blender.

Add the liquid sugar and the lemon juice to the blended fruit.

Add the blueberries and a pinch of the grated lemon zest; blend once again.

Alternately, the blueberries and lemon zest can be poured onto the blended peaches once they have been placed in the individual bowls for serving.

Bromatological evaluation per portion

Kcal	69
Protein (%)	8.9
Fats (%)	3.2
Carbohydrates (%)	87.9
Fiber (g)	3.9
Cholesterol (mg)	0

Valuable contents for the eye: ★ ★ ★

Blueberries are rich in vitamin C and anthocyanosides.

Peaches are rich in fiber, providing a high sense of fullness; they contain vitamin C, carotenoids, and flavonoids.

Lemon contains high quantities of vitamin C and β-carotene. It also contains flavonoids.

Sugar is a pure form of rapidly available energy.

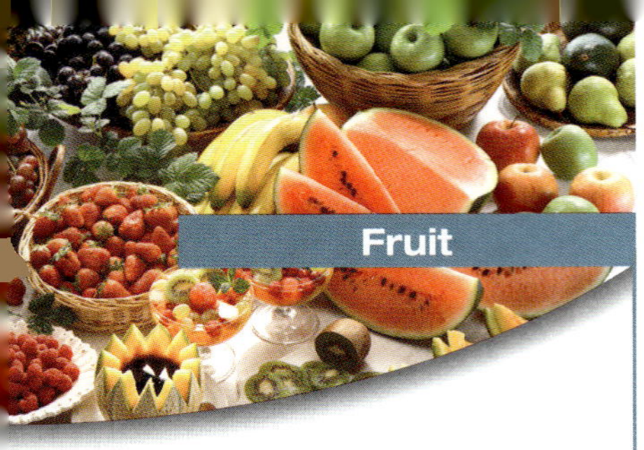

Fruit

Papaya and mango

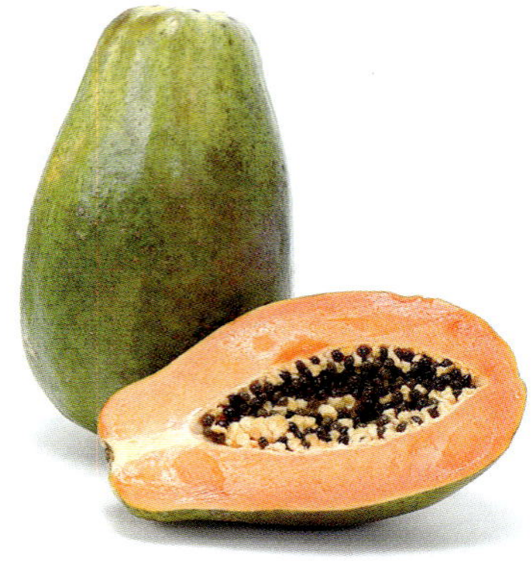

Ingredients and amounts for 4 people

- ✓ 2 very ripe mangoes
- ✓ 1 very ripe papaya
- ✓ juice of ½ lemon
- ✓ 4 tablespoons sugar

Preparation

Wash, peel, and dice the fruits, eliminating the inedible parts. Place the fruit in a bowl, and add the sugar and the lemon juice. Mix and leave for a few minutes before serving.

Bromatological evaluation per portion

Kcal	95
Protein (%)	4.2
Fats (%)	2
Carbohydrates (%)	93.8
Fiber (g)	2.2
Cholesterol (mg)	0

Valuable contents for the eye: ★★

Mango contains high quantities of vitamins A and C.

Papaya is rich in vitamin C, selenium, flavonoids, and carotenoids.

Lemon contains high quantities of vitamin C and β-carotene. It also contains flavonoids.

Sugar is a pure form of rapidly available energy.

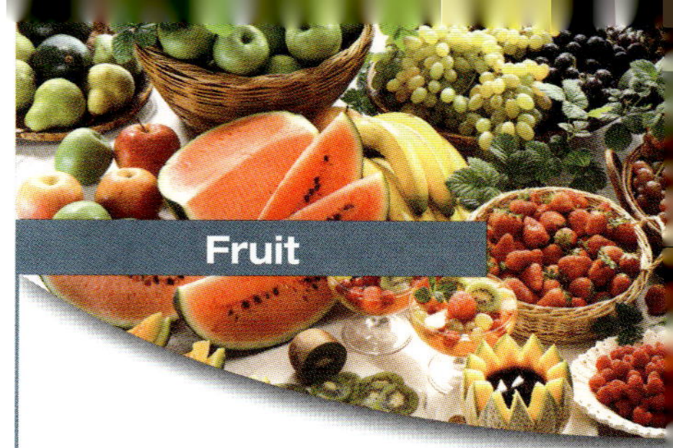

Pears with **blueberry** or **raspberry coulis**

Ingredients and amounts for 4 people

- ✓ 4 pears
- ✓ 10½ oz (1⅓ cups) blueberries or raspberries
- ✓ 8 tablespoons sugar
- ✓ 8 tablespoons dessert wine (Brachetto d'Aqui or Moscato d'Asti)
- ✓ juice of 2 lemons
- ✓ 2 glasses of water
- ✓ 3½ tablespoons icing sugar
- ✓ 1 piece of cinnamon

Preparation

Peel, core, and cut the pears; place in a casserole dish.

Add 2 glasses of water, the juice of 1 lemon, the cinnamon and half of the sugar; heat for approximately 10 minutes. Allow this mixture to cool.

Wash and dry the blueberries; place in a small casserole dish with the other half of the sugar, the remaining lemon juice, wine, and half a glass of water. Heat for 10 minutes and allow to thicken.

Place the blueberries in a blender; the cream obtained should be fairly dense.

Remove the pears from the syrup; place on a serving plate and cover with the blueberry coulis.

Bromatological evaluation per portion

Kcal	251
Protein (%)	2
Fats (%)	1.4
Carbohydrates (%)	96.6
Fiber (g)	5.6
Cholesterol (mg)	0

Valuable contents for the eye: ★★

Blueberries are rich in vitamin C and anthocyanosides.

Raspberries are rich in vitamin C and flavonoids.

Lemon contains high quantities of vitamin C and β-carotene. It also contains flavonoids.

Wine contains small amounts of flavonoids.

Cinnamon has a delicious aroma and is an aphrodisiac; it stimulates digestion, reduces the blood cholesterol and triglycerides, and stimulates the action of insulin.

Sugar is a pure form of rapidly available energy.

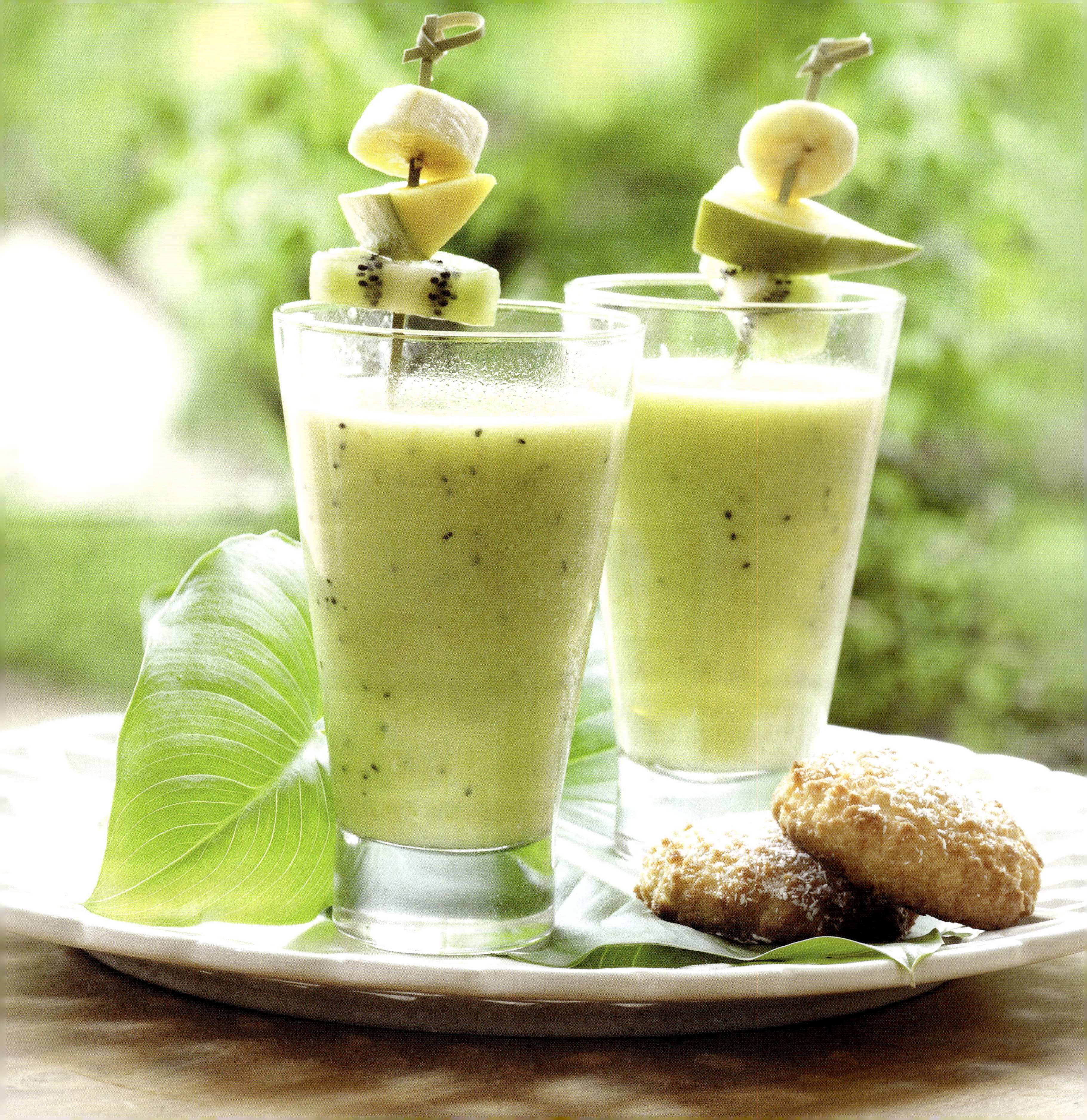

Juices, shakes, and smoothies

These drinks are obtained with an electrical appliance—the juicer—which separates the juice of fruit and vegetables from the pulp and the peel; it produces a concentrate of vitamins, minerals, sugars, starches, and enzymes without the fibrous parts. Ideally, these drinks should be consumed immediately, as soon as they have been made, to keep all the nutritional properties intact (they can be kept in the refrigerator but should be consumed within a couple of hours of preparation).
One of the major benefits of these drinks is that they can be digested very easily.
The most common juicer is the "citrus squeeze." Juicers (or separators) also exist for fruit and vegetables; these can be centrifugal or masticating juicers. The results are very similar as they all separate the juice from the pulp to produce the fruit drink.
Shakes contain fruit and crushed ice; they can also contain coffee, ice cream, and the like.
Smoothies are slightly different. These have the benefit of all the nutritional properties of fresh fruit, used in its entirety (including the skin if edible); therefore, they contain fibers, sugars, and vitamins.
Frequently, milk, cream, or yogurt is added to the blended fruit; this provides protein and fat and is, therefore, an extremely nutritious preparation. Sugar can be added in small quantities, but with caution as fruit already contains a considerable quantity of fructose.

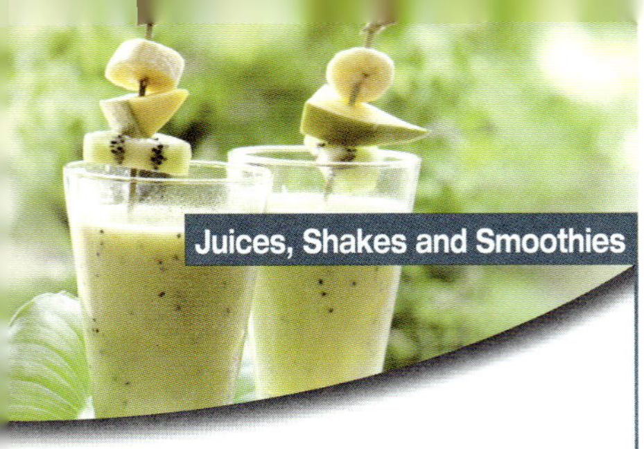

Apricots, peaches, strawberries, and kiwi

Bromatological evaluation per portion

Kcal	159
Protein (%)	11.6
Fats (%)	27.4
Carbohydrates (%)	61
Fiber (g)	3.1
Cholesterol (mg)	0

Valuable contents for the eye: ★★★

Apricots are sweet and low in calories; they contain vitamin C and β-carotene.
Peaches are rich in fiber, providing a great sense of fullness; they contain vitamin C, carotenoids, and flavonoids.
Strawberries are a good source of vitamin C and anthocyanosides.
Kiwis have a high content of vitamin C.
Milk (particularly whole milk) has a good balance of sugars, fats, and proteins; it contains high quantities of calcium and phosphorous, but particularly fat-soluble antioxidant vitamins and water-soluble vitamins.
Sugar is a pure form of rapidly available energy.

Ingredients and amounts for 4 people

- ✓ 4 ripe apricots
- ✓ 2 peaches or nectarines
- ✓ 7 oz ripe strawberries
- ✓ 1 kiwi
- ✓ 2 glasses of milk
- ✓ 2 tablespoons sugar

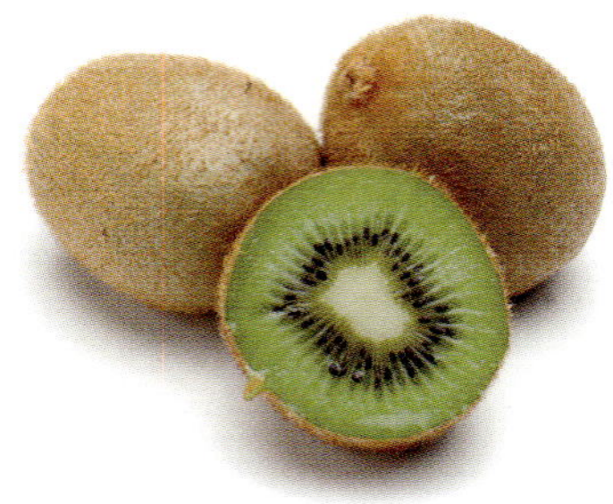

Preparation for blending

Wash and stone the peaches and the apricots.
Peel the kiwi.
Wash the strawberries and remove the stalks.
Cut the fruit into pieces and blend with the milk and sugar.

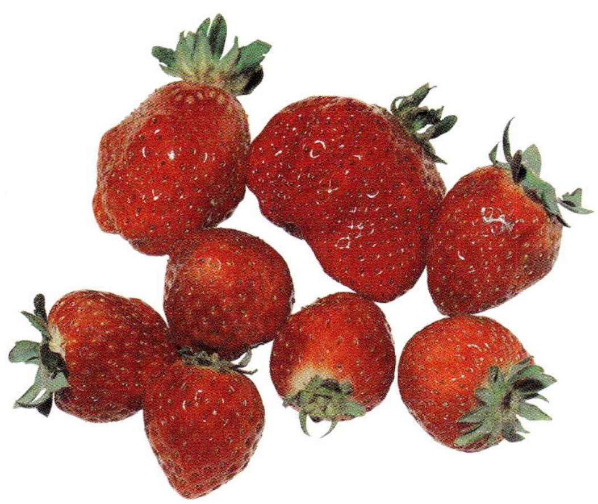

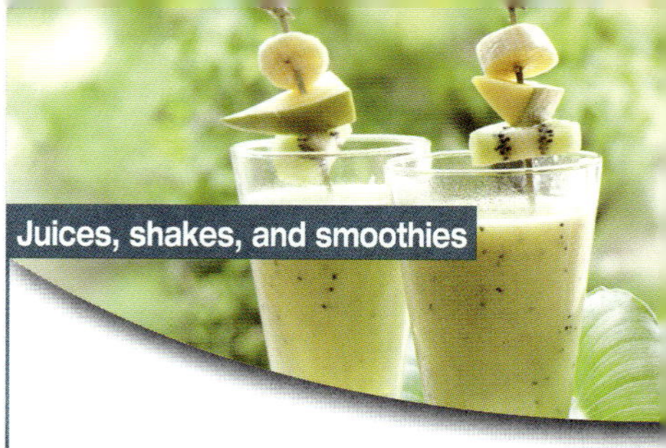

Oranges, banana, and strawberries

Bromatological evaluation per portion

Kcal	117
Protein (%)	8.9
Fats (%)	6.5
Carbohydrates (%)	84.6
Fiber (g)	4.8
Cholesterol (mg)	0

Ingredients and amounts for 4 people

- ✓ 2 oranges
- ✓ 2 bananas
- ✓ 10½ oz (1⅓ cups) strawberries

Preparation for squeezing and blending

Peel the oranges and divide into segments; remove the juice with a juicer or simply use a citrus squeezer.

Peel the banana and cut into pieces.

Wash the strawberries and remove the stalks.

Place all the fruit in the blender and blend until a creamy mixture is obtained.

Valuable contents for the eye: ★★★

The **orange** is rich in sucrose and contains high quantities of vitamin C and β-carotene. It also contains flavonoids (particularly in the pith or albedo underneath the peel).

The **banana** is rich in potassium and sugars; it contains vitamins C, A, and some of the B group.

Strawberries are a good source of vitamin C and anthocyanosides.

Oranges, carrots, and kiwi

Bromatological evaluation per portion

Kcal	101
Protein (%)	10.3
Fats (%)	7.4
Carbohydrates (%)	82.3
Fiber (g)	6.1
Cholesterol (mg)	0

Ingredients and amounts for 4 people

- ✓ 4 kiwis
- ✓ 4 carrots
- ✓ 4 navel oranges

Preparation for juicing

Wash, top, tail, and cut the carrots.

Peel the kiwi and the oranges.

Juice them all together.

Valuable contents for the eye: ★★★

Kiwis have a high content of vitamin C.

Carrots are an excellent source of β-carotene; they stimulate diuresis and intestinal motility.

The **orange** is rich in sucrose and contains high quantities of vitamin C and β-carotene. It also contains flavonoids (particularly in the pith or albedo underneath the peel).

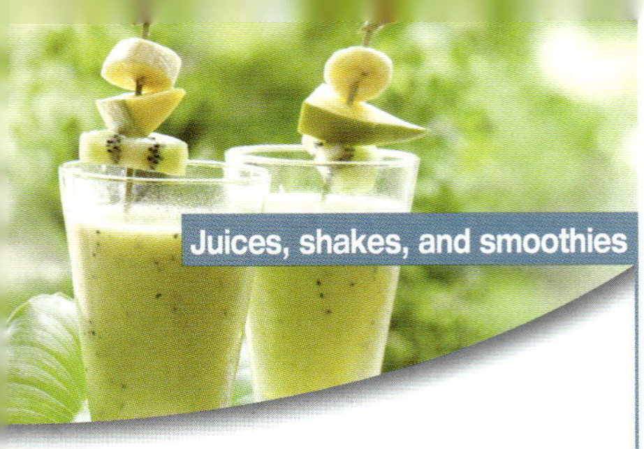

Oranges and **carrots**

Bromatological evaluation per portion

Kcal	71
Protein (%)	10
Fats (%)	5.2
Carbohydrates (%)	84.8
Fiber (g)	4.6
Cholesterol (mg)	0

Valuable contents for the eye: ★ ★ ★

Carrots are an excellent source of β-carotene; they stimulate diuresis and intestinal motility.

The **orange** is rich in sucrose and contains high quantities of vitamin C and β-carotene. It also contains flavonoids (particularly in the pith or albedo underneath the peel).

Ingredients and amounts for 4 people

✓ 6 carrots

✓ 2 oranges

Preparation for squeezing

Wash and peel the carrots and the oranges. Squeeze all together.

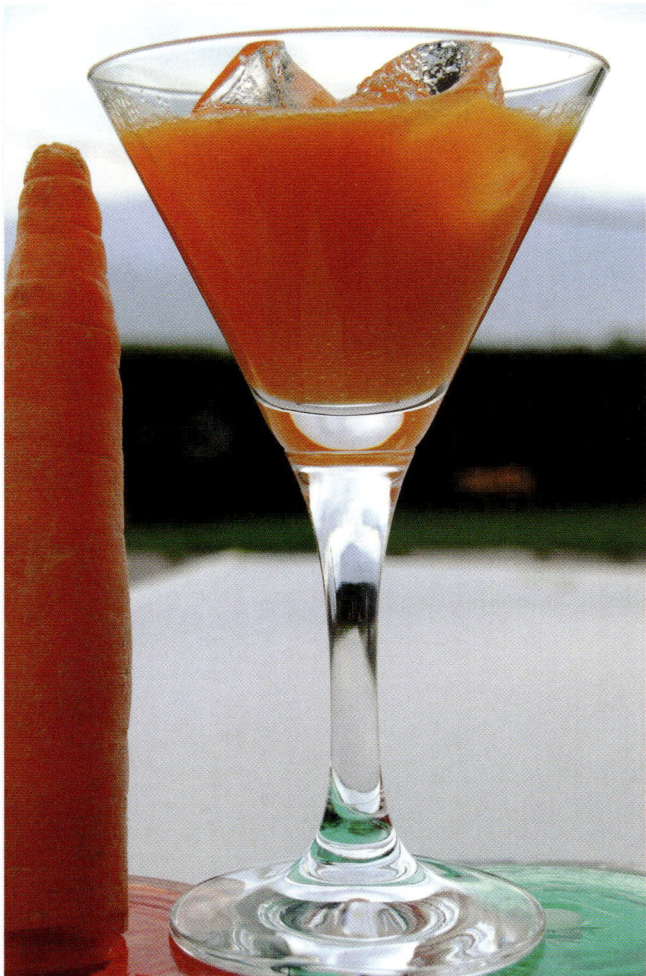

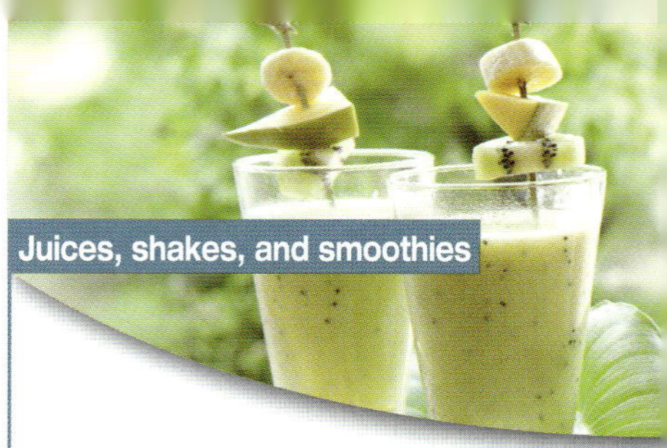

Banana, pineapple, apple, and pear

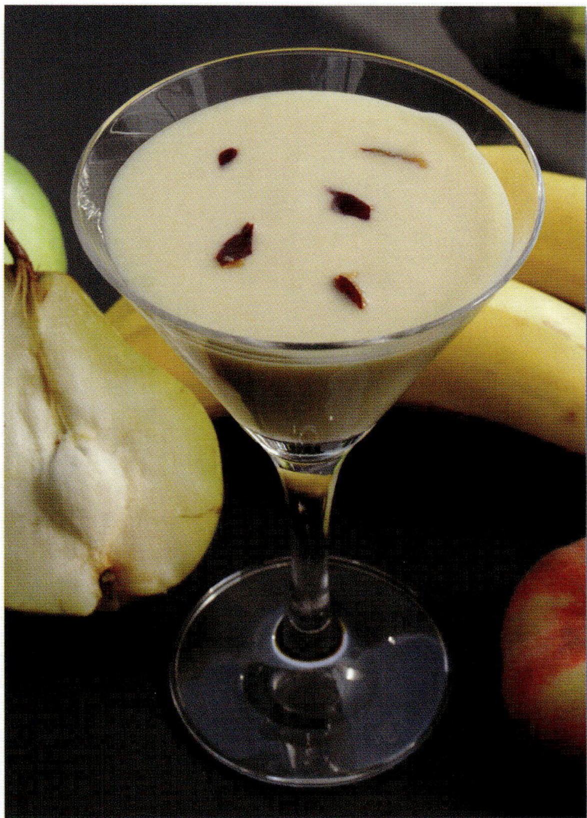

Ingredients and amounts for 4 people

- ✓ 1 banana
- ✓ ½ pineapple
- ✓ 1 apple
- ✓ 1 pear
- ✓ 2 tablespoons sugar
- ✓ 2 to 3 mint leaves of or 1 tablespoon mint syrup
- ✓ 2 glasses milk

Preparation for squeezing and blending

Peel the pineapple and eliminate the inedible parts; squeeze to extract the juice.
Wash and dry the apple and pear; remove the core and squeeze to extract the juice.
Peel the banana and cut into pieces.
Blend the banana with milk and sugar; add the pineapple, apple, and pear juices. Mix.
Decorate with a leaf of mint.

Bromatological evaluation per portion

Kcal	109
Protein (%)	5
Fats (%)	2.8
Carbohydrates (%)	92.2
Fiber (g)	3.2
Cholesterol (mg)	0

Valuable contents for the eye: ★ ★ ★

The **banana** is rich in potassium and sugars; it contains vitamins C, A, and some of the B group.
The **pineapple** is rich in potassium and β-carotene. It also contains bromeline, an anti-inflammatory.
The **apple** is rich in fructose; it contains flavonoids (quercetin) and oligoelements such as zinc and selenium.
The **pear** is rich in vitamins A and C and flavonoids.
Sugar is a pure form of rapidly available energy.
Milk (particularly whole milk) has a good balance of sugars, fats, and proteins; it contains high quantities of calcium and phosphorous, but particularly fat-soluble antioxidant vitamins and water-soluble vitamins.

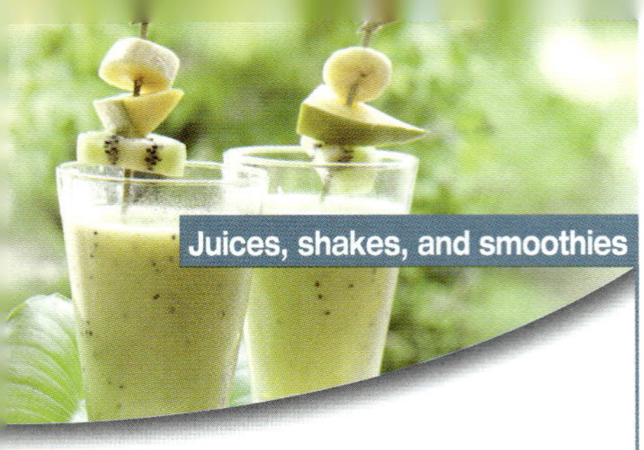

Carrots and apples

Bromatological evaluation per portion

Kcal	81
Protein (%)	5.9
Fats (%)	3.2
Carbohydrates (%)	90.9
Fiber (g)	4.5
Cholesterol (mg)	0

Valuable contents for the eye: ★★★

The **apple** is rich in fructose; it contains flavonoids (quercetin) and oligoelements such as zinc and selenium.

Carrots are an excellent source of β-carotene; they stimulate diuresis and intestinal motility.

Ingredients and amounts for 4 people

- ✓ 4 apples
- ✓ 3 large carrots

Preparation for juicing

Wash and scrub the carrots; top and tail.

Cut the apples.

Extract the juice separately from the carrots and then the apples and mix the juices in a glass.

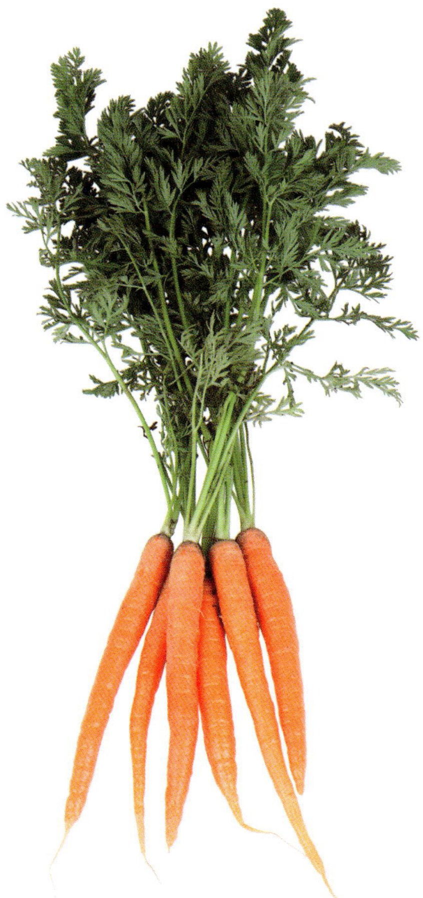

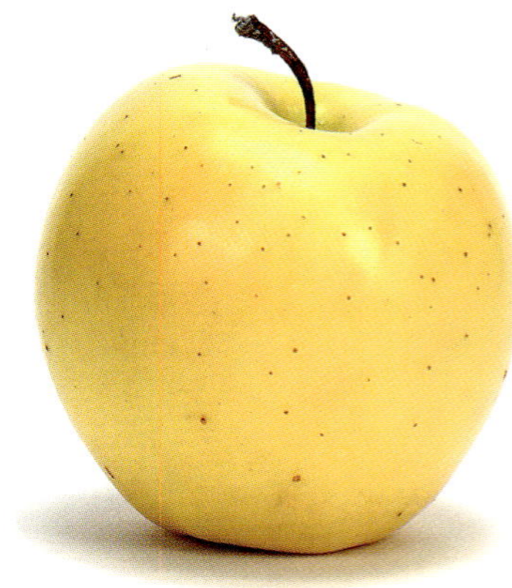

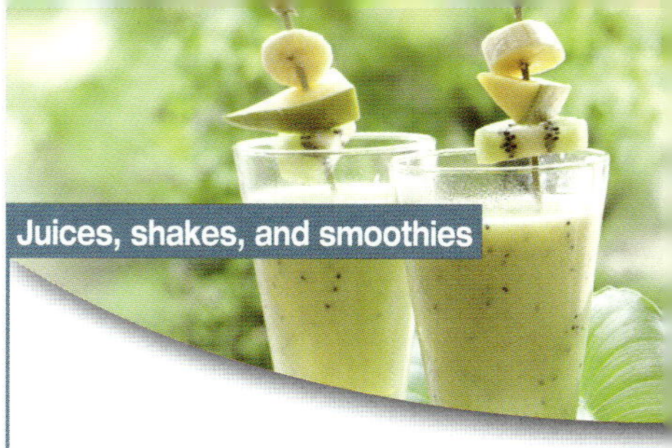

Strawberries or raspberries

Ingredients and amounts for 4 people

✓ 14 oz (1¾ cups) strawberries or raspberries
✓ 2 glasses of milk
✓ 2 tablespoons sugar

Preparation for blending

Wash and dry the strawberries and remove the stalks.
Cut into pieces.
Blend with sugar and milk.

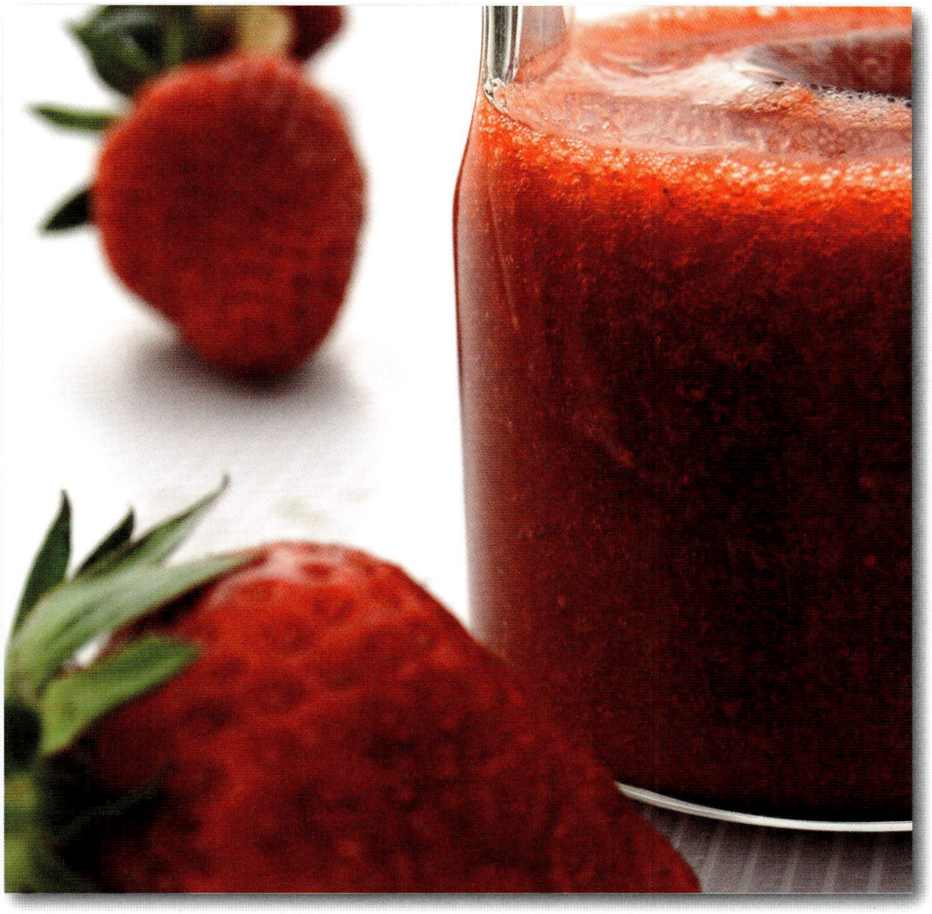

Bromatological evaluation per portion

Kcal	91
Protein (%)	14.2
Fats (%)	15.5
Carbohydrates (%)	70.3
Fiber (g)	1.5
Cholesterol (mg)	0

Valuable contents for the eye: ★★

Strawberries are a good source of vitamin C and anthocyanosides.
Raspberries are rich in vitamin C and flavonoids.
Milk (particularly whole milk) has a good balance of sugars, fats, and proteins; it contains high quantities of calcium and phosphorous, but particularly fat-soluble antioxidant vitamins and water-soluble vitamins.
Sugar is a pure form of rapidly available energy.

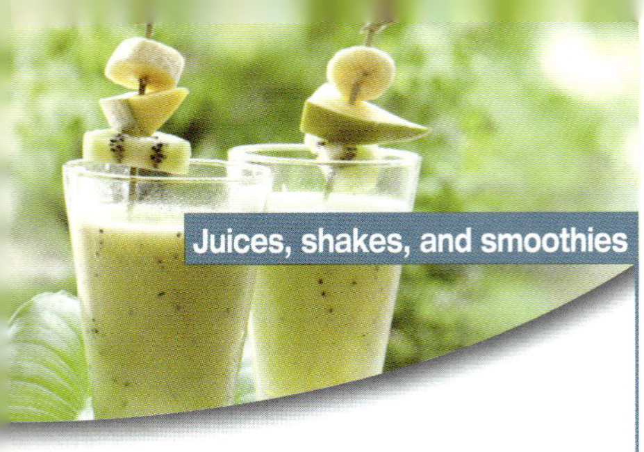

Strawberries, raspberries, and blueberries

Valuable contents for the eye: ★★

Strawberries are a good source of vitamin C and anthocyanosides.
Raspberries are rich in vitamin C and flavonoids.
Blueberries are rich in vitamin C and anthocyanosides.
Milk (particularly whole milk) has a good balance of sugars, fats, and proteins; it contains high quantities of calcium and phosphorous, but particularly fat-soluble antioxidant vitamins and water-soluble vitamins.
Sugar is a pure form of rapidly available energy.

Ingredients and amounts for 4 people

- ✓ 3½ oz raspberries
- ✓ 3½ oz strawberries
- ✓ 3½ oz blueberries
- ✓ 3 glasses of milk
- ✓ 3 tablespoons sugar

Bromatological evaluation per portion

Kcal	119
Protein (%)	13.5
Fats (%)	14.8
Carbohydrates (%)	71.7
Fiber (g)	3.6
Cholesterol (mg)	0

Preparation for blending

Wash the berries gently and dry on absorbent paper towels.
Remove the stalks from the strawberries.
Blend all the ingredients together.

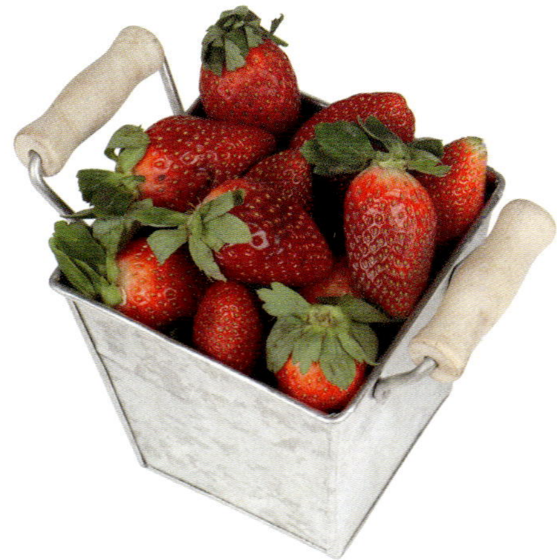

Strawberries and black currants

Valuable contents for the eye: ★★

Strawberries are a good source of vitamin C and anthocyanosides.
Black currants contain omega-6 and flavonoids.

Ingredients and amounts for 4 people

- ✓ 10½ oz strawberries
- ✓ 10½ oz black currants

Bromatological evaluation per portion

Kcal	47
Protein (%)	13.1
Fats (%)	0
Carbohydrates (%)	86.9
Fiber (g)	4.3
Cholesterol (mg)	0

Preparation for juicing or blending

Wash the strawberries and remove the stalks.
Wash the black currants and remove the fruit from the stalk.
Place each ingredient in the juicer and mix the juices in a glass. Alternately, blend the fruits.

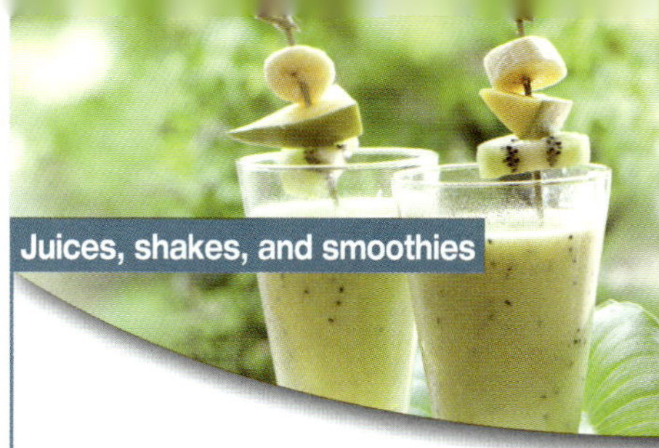

Kiwi

Ingredients and amounts for 4 people

✓ 4 kiwis

✓ 2 glasses of milk

✓ 2 tablespoons sugar

Preparation for blending

Peel the kiwi and cut into pieces. Remove the inedible parts. Blend with milk and sugar.

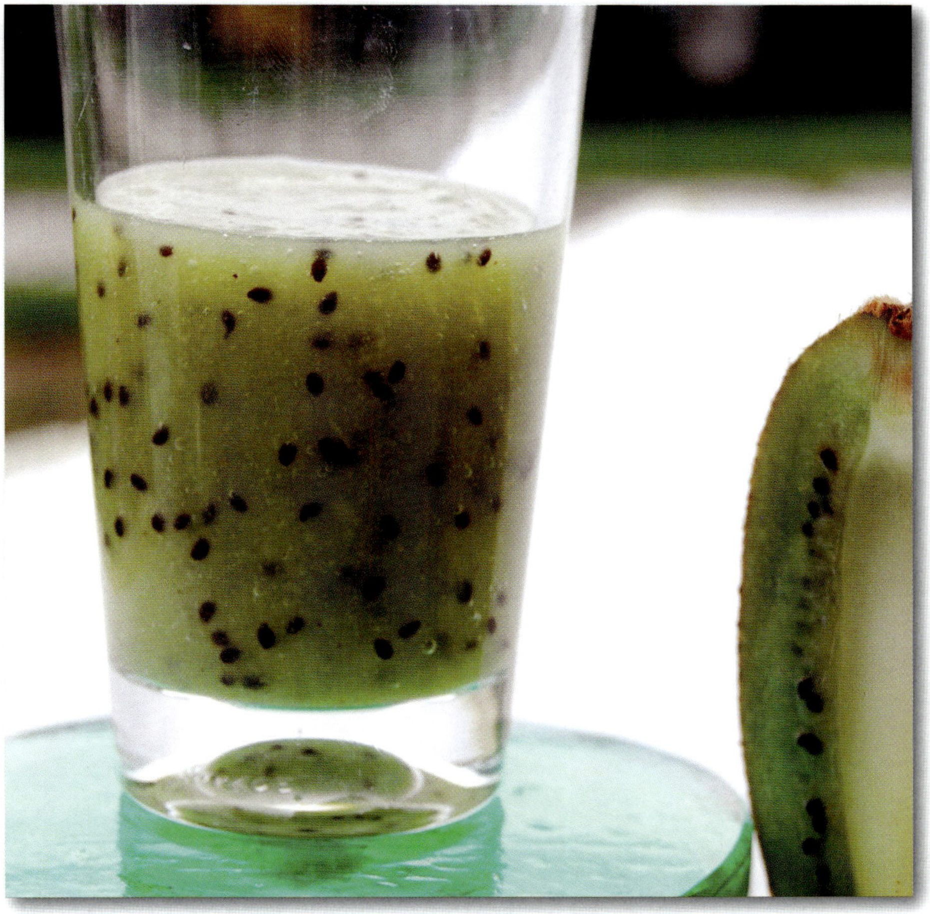

Bromatological evaluation per portion

Kcal	97
Protein (%)	13.4
Fats (%)	15
Carbohydrates (%)	71.6
Fiber (g)	1.5
Cholesterol (mg)	0

Valuable contents for the eye: ★ ★

Kiwis have a high content of vitamin C.

Milk (particularly whole milk) has a good balance of sugars, fats, and proteins; it contains high quantities of calcium and phosphorous, but particularly fat-soluble antioxidant vitamins and water-soluble vitamins.

Sugar is a pure form of rapidly available energy.

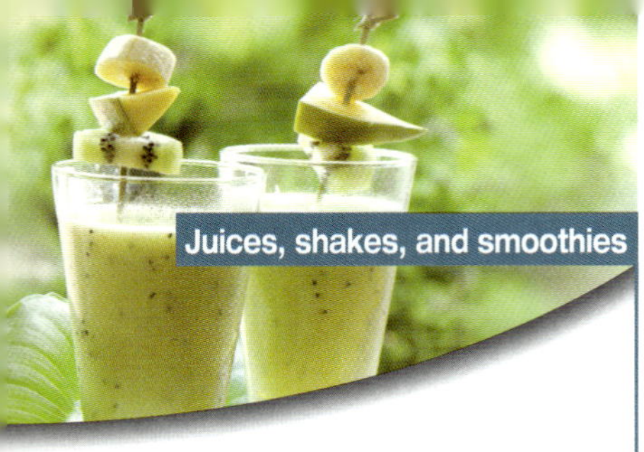

Raspberries and **blueberries**

Valuable contents for the eye: ★★

Raspberries are rich in vitamin C and flavonoids.
Blueberries are rich in vitamin C and anthocyanosides.

Ingredients and amounts for 4 people

✓ 14 oz raspberries

✓ 14 oz blueberries

Preparation for juicing

Wash the fruit and extract the juice.
Mix the juices in a glass and serve.

Bromatological evaluation per portion

Kcal	59
Protein (%)	13
Fats (%)	12.2
Carbohydrates (%)	74.8
Fiber (g)	10.5
Cholesterol (mg)	0

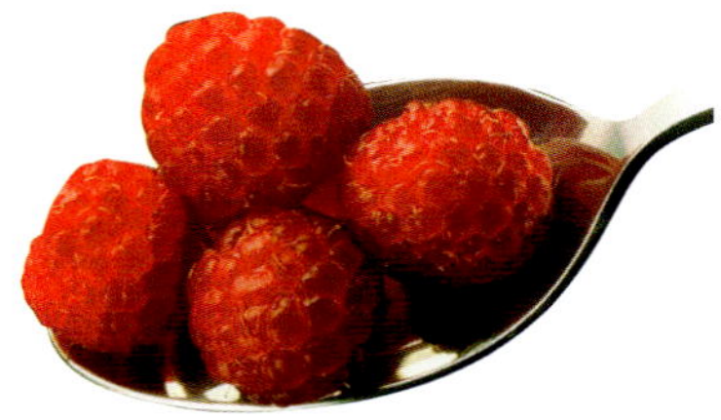

Raspberries and **peaches**

Valuable contents for the eye: ★★★

Raspberries are rich in vitamin C and flavonoids.
Peaches are rich in fiber, providing a great sense of fullness; they contain vitamin C, carotenoids, and flavonoids.

Ingredients and amounts for 4 people

✓ 10½ oz raspberries

✓ 6 peaches

Preparation for juicing

Wash the raspberries and extract the juice.
Cut the peaches into 4 parts and remove the pit; extract the juice.
Mix the peach and raspberry juices together in a glass.

Bromatological evaluation per portion

Kcal	75
Protein (%)	11.8
Fats (%)	7.6
Carbohydrates (%)	80.6
Fiber (g)	8.5
Cholesterol (mg)	0

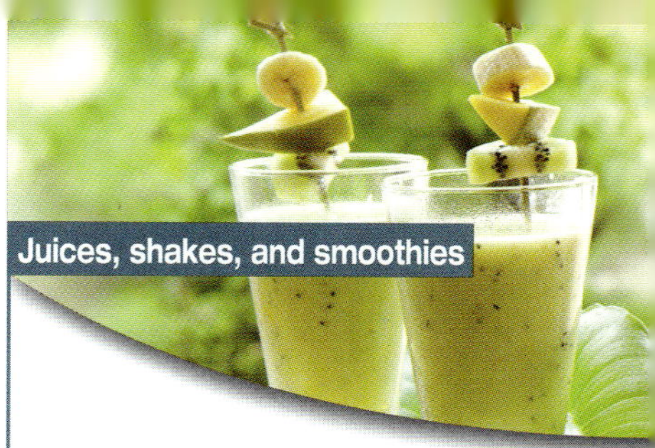

Apple and carrot

Bromatological evaluation per portion

Kcal	81
Protein (%)	6
Fats (%)	3.2
Carbohydrates (%)	90.8
Fiber (g)	4.5
Cholesterol (mg)	0

Ingredients and amounts for 4 people

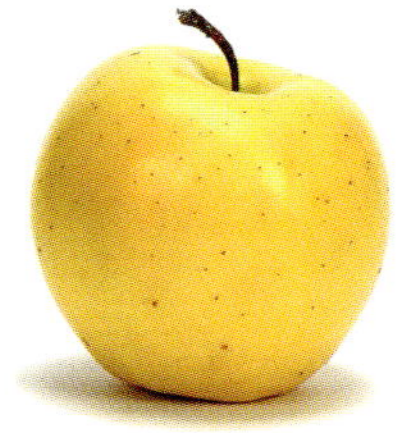

✓ 8 sprigs of mint
✓ 6 carrots
✓ 3 apples

Preparation for juicing

Wash and scrub the carrots. Top and tail.
Cut the apples into slices and remove the core.
Extract the juice from half of the sprigs of mint; repeat for the carrots and the apples. Mix the juices.
Decorate with a sprig of mint.

Valuable contents for the eye: ★★★

Carrots are an excellent source of β-carotene; they stimulate diuresis and intestinal motility.
The **apple** is rich in fructose; it contains flavonoids (quercetin) and oligo-elements such as zinc and selenium.
Mint contains flavonoids and essential oils, including menthol.

Apple, grapefruit, and black currants

Bromatological evaluation per portion

Kcal	89.2
Protein (%)	5.5
Fats (%)	0
Carbohydrates (%)	94.5
Fiber (g)	5
Cholesterol (mg)	0

Ingredients and amounts for 4 people

✓ 2 grapefruits
✓ 3 apples
✓ 5¼ oz black currants

Preparation for juicing

Peel the grapefruits and cut into pieces.
Wash the black currants and remove the fruit from the stalk.
Eliminate the core and cut the apple into slices.
Extract the juice separately from the black currants, grapefruit, and finally the apple.
Mix the juices in a glass.

Valuable contents for the eye: ★★★

Grapefruit contains vitamin C and flavonoids.
The **apple** is rich in fructose; it contains flavonoids (quercetin) and oligo-elements such as zinc and selenium.
Black currants contain omega-6 and flavonoids.

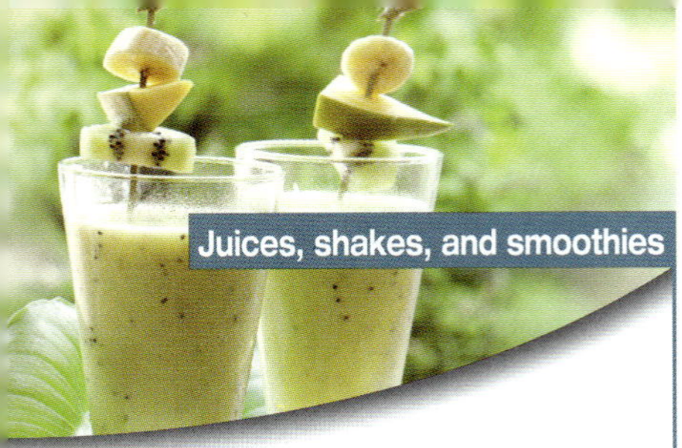

Melon, carrots, and oranges

Bromatological evaluation per portion

Kcal	102
Protein (%)	10
Fats (%)	5.3
Carbohydrates (%)	84.7
Fiber (g)	5.3
Cholesterol (mg)	0

Valuable contents for the eye: ★★★

Melon is rich in vitamin C and carotenoids.

Carrots are an excellent source of β-carotene; they stimulate diuresis and intestinal motility.

The **orange** is rich in sucrose and contains high quantities of vitamin C and β-carotene. It also contains flavonoids (particularly in the pith or albedo underneath the peel).

Ingredients and amounts for 4 people

- ✓ 1 melon
- ✓ 4 peeled carrots
- ✓ 2 oranges

Preparation for juicing

Peel the melon and remove the seeds.

Peel the oranges and divide into segments or cut into pieces.

Wash and scrub the carrots; top and tail.

Extract the juice separately from the 3 ingredients and then mix the juices.

Blueberries and yogurt

Ingredients and amounts for 4 people

✓ 10½ oz blueberries

✓ 10½ oz (1 ⅓ cups) yogurt

✓ 4 tablespoons honey (millefiori preferred)

✓ 2 tablespoons lemon juice

Preparation for blending

Wash the blueberries and dry on absorbent paper towels.
Place in the blender with the honey, the yogurt and the lemon juice. Blend.
Store in the refrigerator for 1 to 2 hours before drinking.

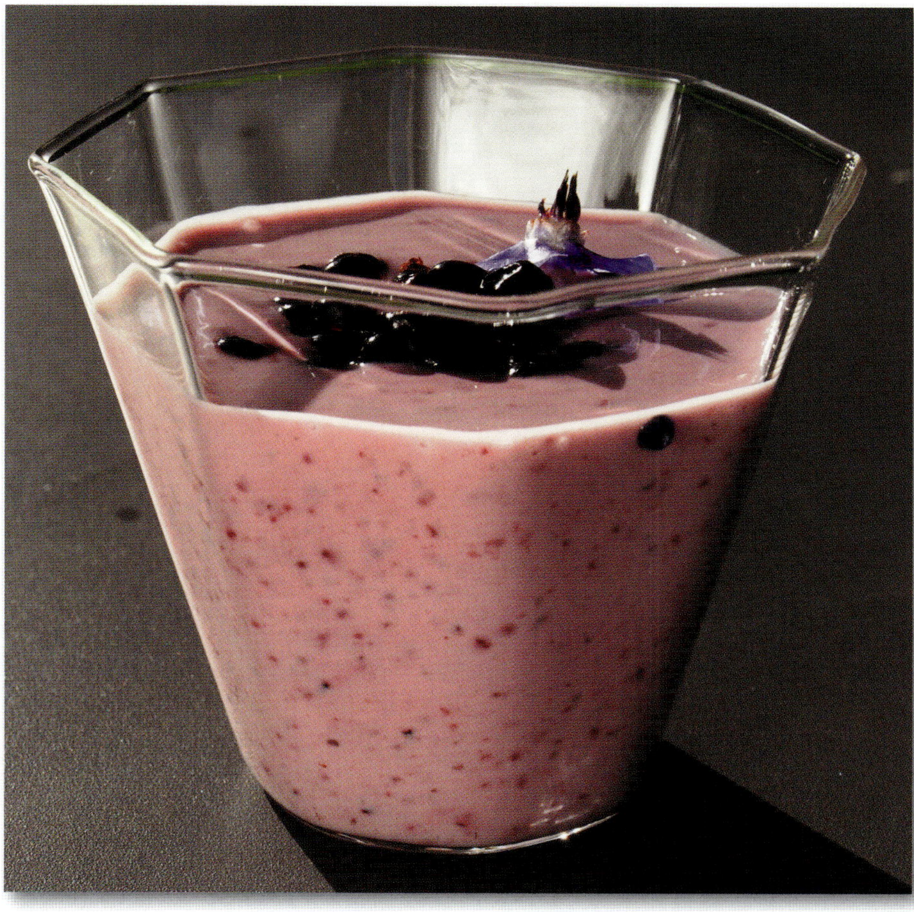

Bromatological evaluation per portion

Kcal	79
Protein (%)	17.3
Fats (%)	10
Carbohydrates (%)	72.7
Fiber (g)	2.4
Cholesterol (mg)	0

Valuable contents for the eye: ★★

Blueberries are rich in vitamin C and anthocyanosides.
Yogurt has a high repletion index and in addition to live milk enzymes, it contains vitamins of the B group and folic acid.
Honey is rich in sugars (glucose and fructose).

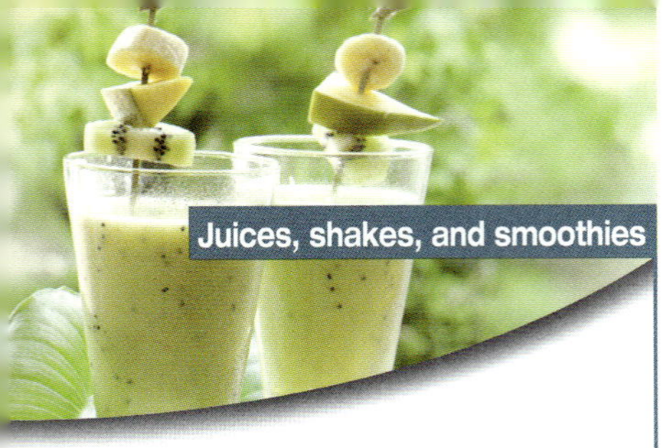

Tomato

Bromatological evaluation per portion

Kcal	64
Protein (%)	6.2
Fats (%)	73.1
Carbohydrates (%)	20.7
Fiber (g)	2
Cholesterol (mg)	0

Valuable contents for the eye: ★★

Tomatoes are rich in vitamins and oligominerals, but particularly they contain carotenoids and are the most important source of lycopene.

Olive oil is an excellent source of unsaturated fatty acids.

Oregano is rich in essential oils.

Ingredients and amounts for 4 people

✓ 6 ripe tomatoes

✓ ½ teaspoon oregano

✓ 1 tablespoon extra virgin olive oil

Preparation for blending

Wash the ripe tomatoes, cut into pieces, and place in the blender. Add the oregano and extra virgin olive oil and blend.

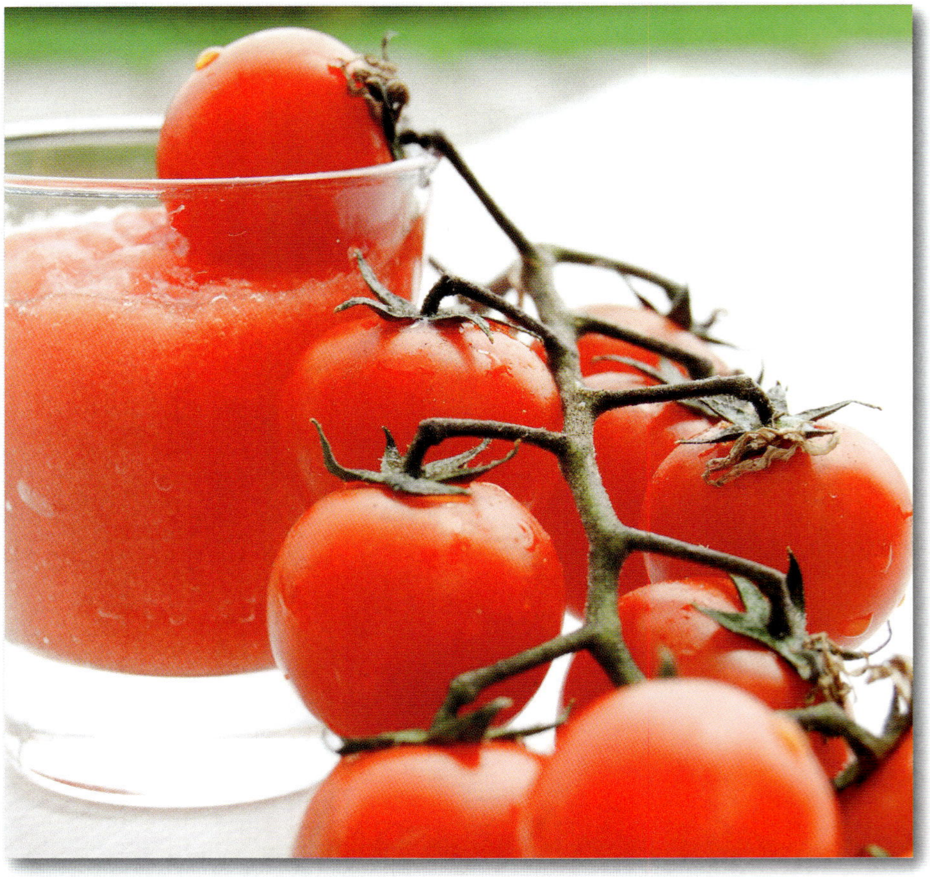

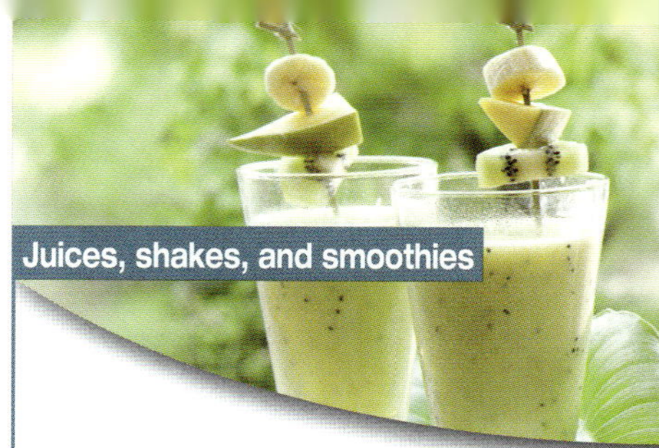

Tomatoes, basil, and parsley

Ingredients and amounts for 4 people

- ✓ 8 tomatoes
- ✓ 6 basil leaves
- ✓ 8 sprigs of fresh parsley

Preparation for juicing

Finely chop the basil and parsley.
Juice the tomatoes.
Mix all the ingredients together.

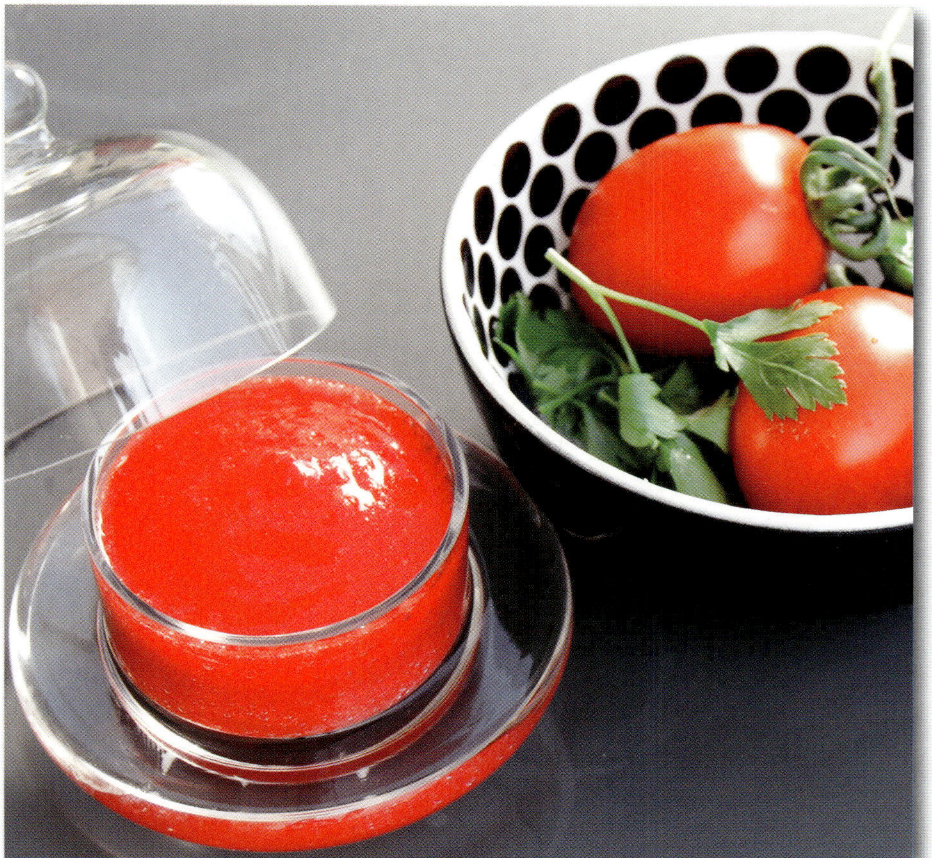

Bromatological evaluation per portion

Kcal	41
Protein (%)	23.4
Fats (%)	10.4
Carbohydrates (%)	66.2
Fiber (g)	4.4
Cholesterol (mg)	0

Valuable contents for the eye: ★★

Tomatoes are rich in vitamins and oligominerals, but particularly they contain carotenoids and are the most important source of lycopene.

Basil owes its aroma to the numerous essential oils it contains; these stimulate salivary and gastric secretions.

Parsley contains flavonoids and is also an apiol, an antispastic, and an antipyretic. It also stimulates uterine contractions.

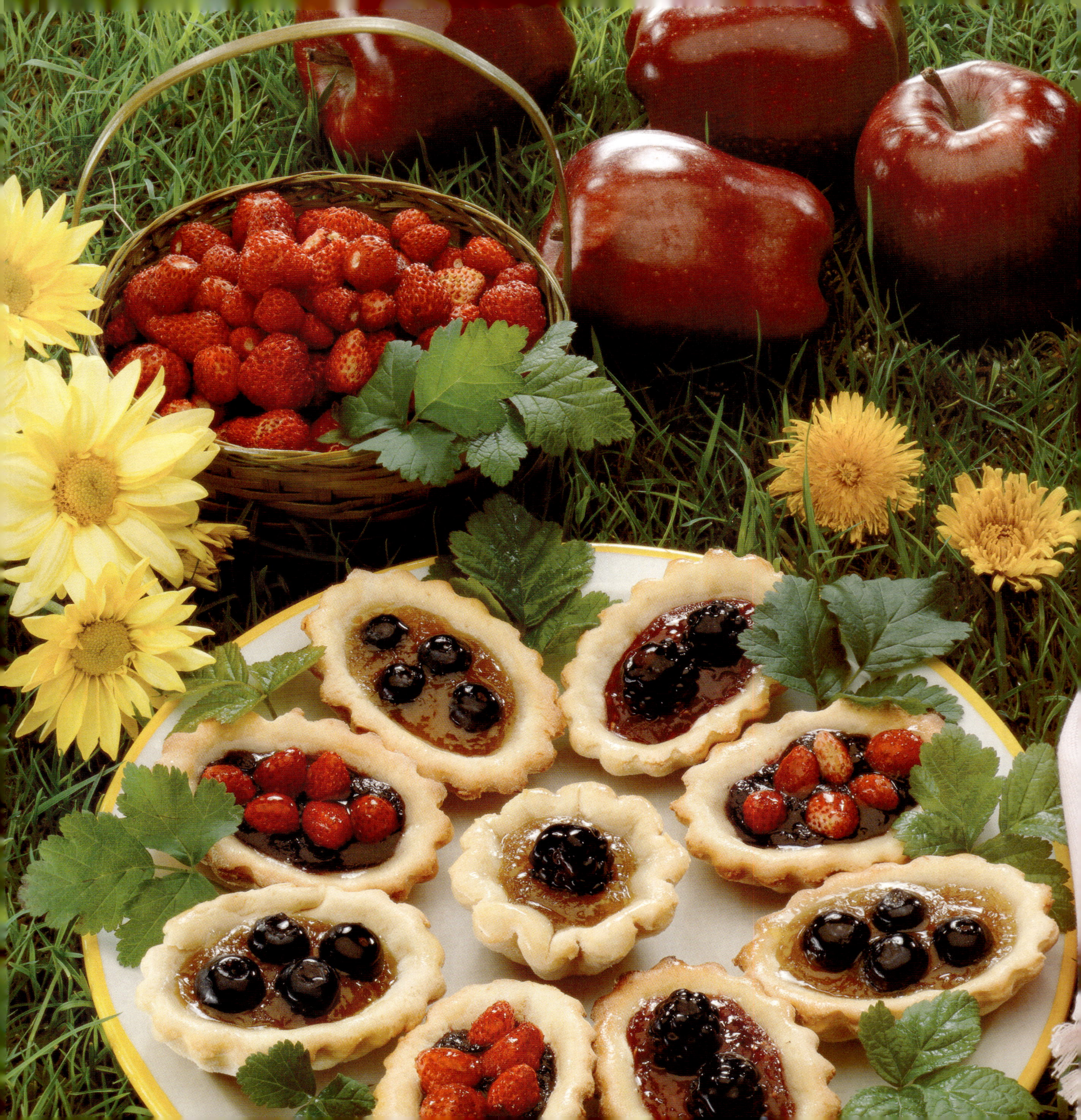

Desserts

Desserts are deeply rooted in history; in Ancient Greece, the common ingredient found in desserts was honey. The sacred fruit of the citronella was often accompanied by sesame seeds, walnuts, almonds, saffron (which has a powerful erotic association), raisins, and poppy seeds.
In modern times, the common ingredients of desserts are sugar and flour, produced by milling soft wheat flour; in nutritional terms, in addition to supplying essential nutrients, they are also extremely easy to digest.
Desserts are now synonymous with cakes: they are produced in the bakery, usually round in shape and frequently used to celebrate special occasions. Cakes can be hot or cold, baked or not.
Some traditional cakes are carrot cake, ricotta cheese cake, cakes with mascarpone (a type of clotted cream), jam, apple pies, cakes or crumbles, pine nut cakes, lemon sponges, Sacher cake, or the famous Italian tiramisu (literally meaning pick-me-up).
Chocolate is a frequent ingredient in desserts and cakes. From ancient times, this product has considerable nutritive properties. It has enlivening properties and, in some cases, is also classed as an aphrodisiac. It contains an alkaloid called theobromine, an analogue of teine and caffeine. Its properties are gently energetic and stimulating.
Another sweet that is often consumed at mealtimes is the cookie—a small sweet preparation common to many countries around the world.
Cookies are a baked preparation, a sweet confectionary, are small in size (usually 2 to 4 inches), and have a geometric shape with a variety of decorations. They are normally oven-baked to remove all traces of humidity.
There are records of cookies being prepared in ancient times. The 2 important characteristics that allow them to be stored for long periods of time are the presence of a sweetening agent (honey originally and sugar in more recent times) and the entire baking procedure in the oven.
Cookies are currently made from flour, eggs, butter, sugar, yeast, and a variety of flavors. The flour is predominantly wheat flour, although cookies are also produced using ground almonds (amaretti), ground hazel nuts from Piedmont (nocciolini di Chivasso) or corn flour (meliga pastry) typical of the Italian tradition. They are traditionally consumed in combination with a sweet dessert wine or at breakfast with tea, coffee, or milk.

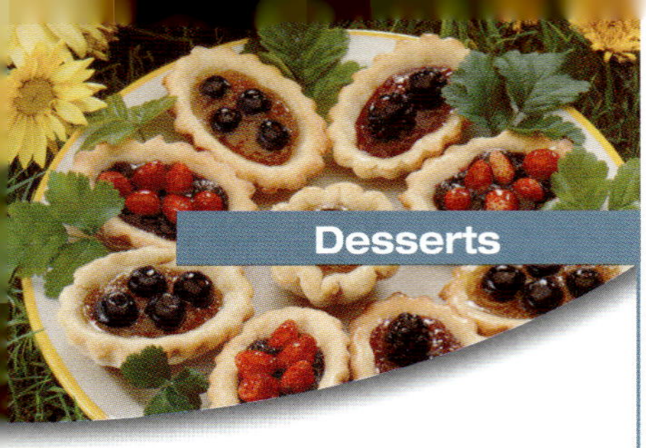

Confectioner's cream

Bromatological evaluation per portion

Kcal	283
Protein (%)	12.8
Fats (%)	40.4
Carbohydrates (%)	46.8
Fiber (g)	0.4
Cholesterol (mg)	401

Valuable contents for the eye: ★

Milk (particularly whole milk) has an excellent balance of sugars, fats, and proteins. It contains large quantities of calcium and phosphorous, fat-soluble anti-oxidant vitamins and water-soluble vitamins.

Eggs are rich in saturated fatty acids but also contain a good quantity of mono- and polyunsaturated fatty acids. Unfortunately, they contain cholesterol but they are also an important source of lutein.

The **sugar** is a pure form of rapidly available energy.

Ingredients and amounts for 4 people

- ✓ 2 cups milk
- ✓ 2 egg yolks
- ✓ 4 tablespoons sugar
- ✓ 2 tablespoons white flour
- ✓ grated zest of 1 lemon

Preparation

Heat the milk and the lemon zest in a saucepan.

Place the egg yolks and the sugar in a bowl and beat until yellow and smooth.

Gradually add the flour to the egg/sugar mixture and mix well.

Add this mixture to the milk; stir well to ensure that the cream does not stick to the saucepan or become lumpy.

When the mixture thickens, turn off the heat immediately.

This cream can be used in pies or other cakes and can also be eaten at breakfast.

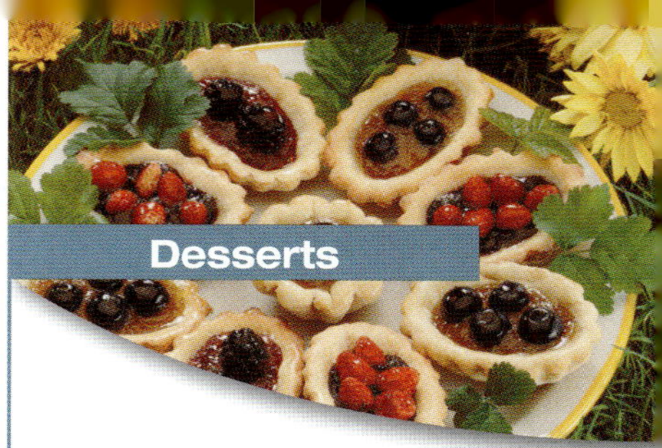

Blueberry cream

Ingredients and amounts for 4 people

✓ 10½ oz blueberries

✓ 5¼ oz rice malt

✓ 3 tablespoons corn flour

Preparation

Place ⅔ of the blueberries and the malt in a saucepan. Bring to a boil. Add the remaining blueberries and the corn flour and mix over low heat. Let cool.

This is an excellent cream for decorating cakes, spreading on fresh bread or toast, or mixing with plain white yogurt.

Bromatological evaluation per portion

Kcal	89.7
Protein (%)	9.9
Fats (%)	4.6
Carbohydrates (%)	85.5
Fiber (g)	2.6
Cholesterol (mg)	0

Valuable contents for the eye: ★★

Blueberries are rich in vitamin C and are anthocyanosidic.

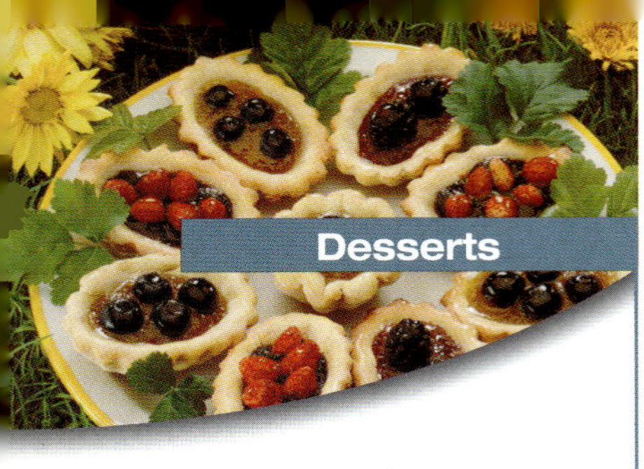

Bromatological evaluation per portion

Kcal	681
Protein (%)	7.1
Fats (%)	39.5
Carbohydrates (%)	53.4
Fiber (g)	3.0
Cholesterol (mg)	201

Valuable contents for the eye: ★★

Strawberries are a good source of vitamin C and are anthocyanosides.
Raspberries are rich in vitamin C and flavonoids.
Kiwis have a high vitamin C content.
Pears are rich in vitamin A, vitamin C, and flavonoids.
Apples are rich in fructose; they contain flavonoids (quercetin) and oligoelements such as zinc and selenium.
Milk (particularly whole milk) has an excellent balance of sugars, fats, and proteins; it contains large quantities of calcium, phosphorous, fat-soluble antioxidant vitamins and water-soluble vitamins.
Eggs are rich in saturated fatty acids but also contain a good quantity of mono- and polyunsaturated fatty acids. Unfortunately, they contain cholesterol but they are also an important source of lutein.

Strawberry, raspberry, black currant, kiwi fruit, pear, apple, or banana tart

Ingredients and amounts for 4 people

- ✓ 1 packet of puff pastry
- ✓ 14 to 17½ oz fresh fruit
- ✓ 2 sheets of gelatin
- ✓ parchment paper
- ✓ 17½ oz dried beans or rice
- ✓ confectioner's cream

Preparation

Grease a cake pan (of diameter 8½ to 9½ in) and dust with flour.
Soak the sheets of gelatin in water for a few minutes; remove and squeeze to remove some of the water. Melt in a saucepan.
Roll the pastry into a sheet of thickness ¼ in; cut a circle just slightly larger than the cake pan. Place the pastry disk in the pan and prick it all over with a fork.
Place a circle of parchment paper on top of the pastry and place the beans or rice on top.
Heat the oven to 350°F and bake the pastry base for approximately 20 minutes.
When the pastry base is baked, remove from the oven; remove the beans and the paper. Let cool and place on a serving dish.
When cool, add the confectioner's cream prepared previously and smooth.
Decorate the tart with the chosen fruit in the desired quantity and brush with gelatin to preserve the color of the fruit.

Preparation of the fruit

The fruit is used to decorate the cake; the pieces must be washed, dried, peeled, topped, and tailed.
Wash and dry the strawberries, raspberries, blackberries, or the black currants.
Slice the bananas, apples, pears, and kiwi and sprinkle them with lemon juice so that they do not oxidize.

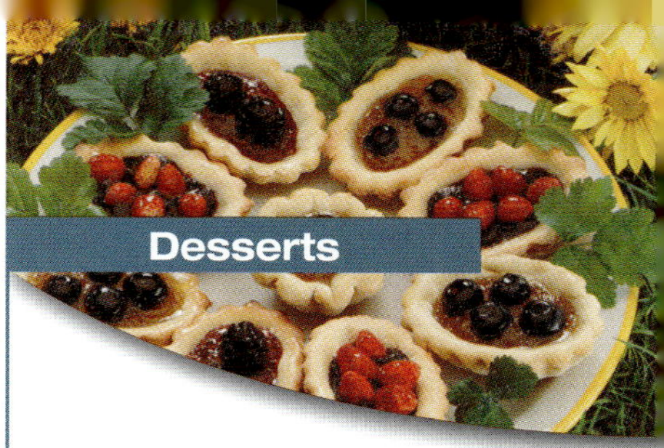

Blueberry fool

Ingredients and amounts for 4 people

- ✓ 10½ oz blueberries
- ✓ 10½ oz fresh ricotta (sheeps' milk)
- ✓ 2 tablespoons sugar
- ✓ 1 teaspoon orange-flower extract
- ✓ ¾ cup water
- ✓ ½ vanilla bean

Preparation

Drain the ricotta well. Place in a mixer with the sugar, water, vanilla bean, the orange-flower extract, and half of the blueberries; mix to produce a smooth cream.
Add the remainder of the blueberries and pour into a mold.
Leave in the refrigerator for a couple of hours.

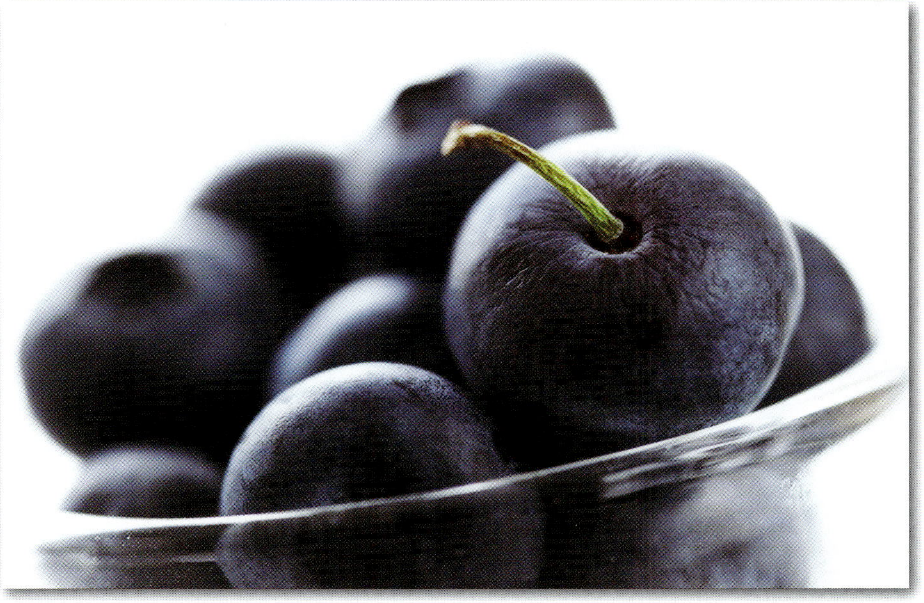

Bromatological evaluation per portion

Kcal	165
Protein (%)	20.2
Fats (%)	51
Carbohydrates (%)	28.8
Fiber (g)	2.5
Cholesterol (mg)	33.6

Valuable contents for the eye: ★★

Blueberries are rich in vitamin C and anthocyanosides.
Ricotta is a tasty light milk-based product that contains a high quantity of calcium and a small quantity of vitamins.

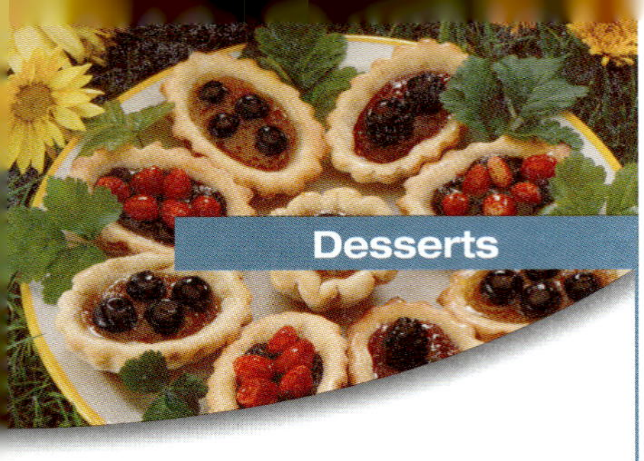

Bromatological evaluation per portion

Kcal	237
Protein (%)	9.1
Fats (%)	64
Carbohydrates (%)	26.9
Fiber (g)	1.48
Cholesterol (mg)	0

Valuable contents for the eye: ★

Blueberries are rich in vitamin C and anthocyanosides.

Eggs are rich in saturated fatty acids but also contain a good quantity of mono- and polyunsaturated fatty acids. Unfortunately, they contain cholesterol but they are also an important source of lutein.

Cream has a high fat content but it is also very delicious.

Blueberry mousse

Ingredients and amounts for 4 people

✓ 8¾ cups blueberries

✓ 3 sheets of gelatin

✓ 2 egg whites

✓ ¾ cup whipping cream

✓ 3 tablespoons sugar

Preparation

Wash and dry the blueberries; liquidize them and pour the liquid into a bowl.

Whip the cream and add to the liquidized blueberries.

Beat the egg whites with a pinch of salt and when stiff, add to the blueberry mixture.

Soak the gelatin in cold water; dissolve it by heating in a small saucepan and then add to the blueberry mixture.

Mix all the ingredients together and leave in the refrigerator for at least 3 hours. Then serve.

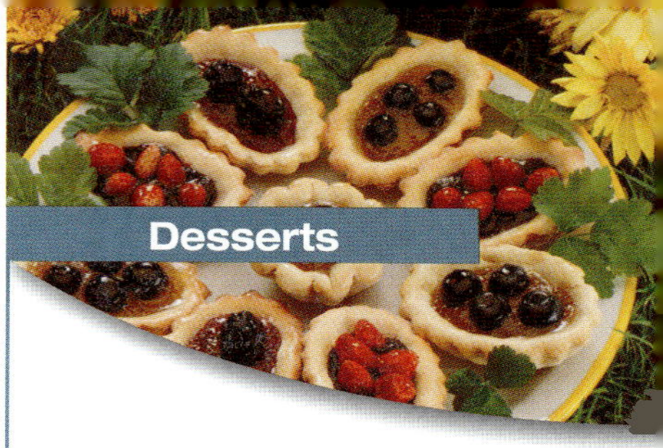

Mother's recipe for stuffed peaches

Ingredients and amounts for 4 people

- ✓ 8 peaches
- ✓ 8 amaretti cookies
- ✓ 1½ oz almonds
- ✓ 1 whole egg
- ✓ 2 tablespoons butter
- ✓ 1 glass of white wine
- ✓ 7 tablespoons sugar

Preparation

Select high-quality peaches because the stone will be easier to remove. Wash the peaches and cut them in half. Remove some of the flesh from the center; place the half-peaches in an oven dish.
Crush the amaretti cookies and the almonds, but not too finely.
Mix the peach flesh with the amaretti cookie/almond mixture;
add melted butter and the egg.
Fill the cavity in the half-peaches with this mixture.
Sprinkle with sugar (about 2 tablespoons depending on taste), white wine, and pats of butter and place the peaches in the oven. Toast gently for a few minutes until the surface has browned.
Excellent when served warm, possibly accompanied by bread.

Bromatological evaluation per portion

Kcal	439
Protein (%)	7.2
Fats (%)	34.7
Carbohydrates (%)	58.1
Fiber (g)	6.3
Cholesterol (mg)	89.5

Valuable contents for the eye: ★

Peaches are rich in fiber; this fruit produces a high degree of repletion. It contains vitamin C, carotenoids, and flavonoids.
The **almond** is an excellent source of vitamin E; it contains a lot of magnesium and quantities of zinc, calcium, and iron.

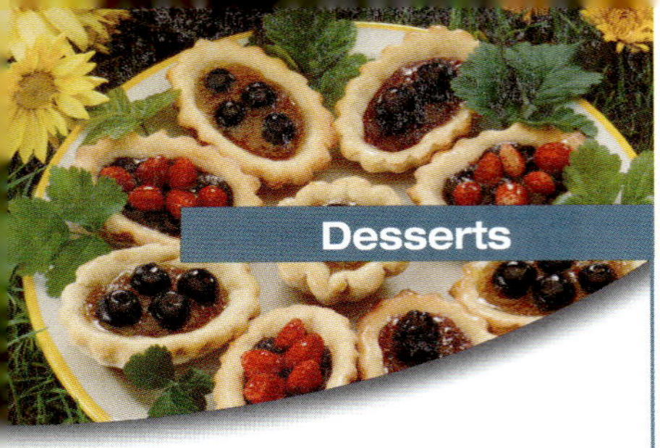

Carrot cake (1)

Bromatological evaluation per portion

Kcal	725
Protein (%)	6.3
Fats (%)	35.4
Carbohydrates (%)	58.3
Fiber (g)	2.9
Cholesterol (mg)	129

Valuable contents for the eye: ★

Carrots are an excellent source of β-carotene; they also stimulate diuresis and intestinal motility.

Olive oil is an excellent source of unsaturated fatty acids.

Eggs are rich in saturated fatty acids but also contain a good quantity of mono- and polyunsaturated fatty acids. Unfortunately, they contain cholesterol but they are also an important source of lutein.

Once the skin has been washed well, the external part of the **lemon** skin, the flavedo, contains essential oils and carotenoids.

Lemon juice is rich in vitamin C and β-carotene.

Ingredients and amounts for 4 people

- ✓ 7 oz carrot
- ✓ 7 tablespoons extra virgin olive oil
- ✓ 1 cup flour
- ✓ 1 cup sugar
- ✓ 3 eggs
- ✓ zest of ½ lemon
- ✓ juice of ½ lemon
- ✓ 1 packet of yeast

Preparation

Wash the carrots; top and tail them and peel.

Cut them into pieces and place in a blender with the oil; blend for a few minutes. Add the sugar, flour, eggs, yeast, lemon juice, and zest; blend for a few more minutes to mix well.

Grease a baking pan with flour and dust all the surfaces with flour.

Bake for 35 minutes at 350°F.

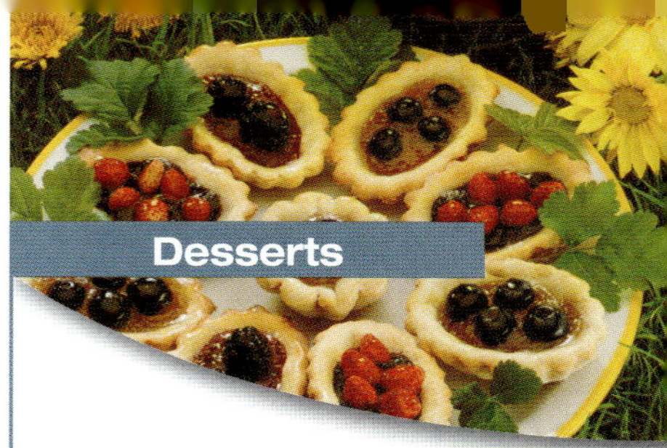

Carrot cake (2)

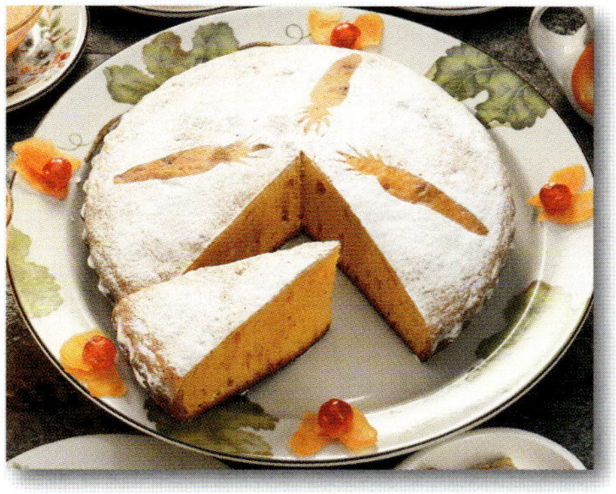

Ingredients and amounts for 4 people

- ✓ 10½ oz carrots
- ✓ 10½ oz almonds or walnuts
- ✓ 3 eggs
- ✓ 7 tablespoons sugar
- ✓ 2 tablespoons flour
- ✓ 1 measure of rum
- ✓ zest of 1 grated lemon
- ✓ 1 sachet of rising agent for cakes
- ✓ pinch of salt

Preparation

Put the eggs in the blender. Add the flour, salt, sugar, lemon zest, and rising agent. Blend well.

Add the rum and blend again until a homogeneous mixture is obtained. Pour the mixture into a bowl and add the chopped almonds or walnuts and the finely grated carrots.

Mix well; grease a cake pan with butter and dust all the surfaces with flour. Pour in the mixture.

Heat the oven and bake at 390°F for 30 to 35 minutes.

Bromatological evaluation per portion

Kcal	305
Protein (%)	13.1
Fats (%)	40.8
Carbohydrates (%)	46.1
Fiber (g)	5.1
Cholesterol (mg)	129

Valuable contents for the eye: ★

Carrots are an excellent source of β-carotene; they also stimulate diuresis and intestinal motility. **Almonds** are an excellent source of vitamin E; they contain a lot of magnesium and considerable quantities of zinc, calcium, and iron. **Walnuts** are extremely high in calories and contain omega-3 fatty acids.

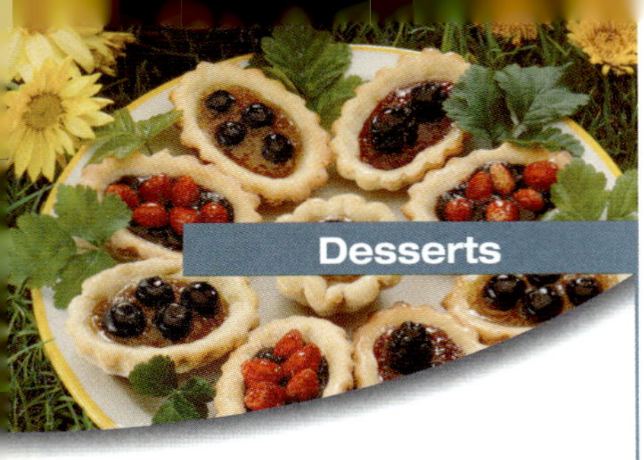

Mango fruit au gratin

Bromatological evaluation per portion

Kcal	256
Protein (%)	1.6
Fats (%)	59.1
Carbohydrates (%)	39.3
Fiber (g)	1.4
Cholesterol (mg)	50

Valuable contents for the eye: ★

Mango fruit contains high levels of vitamin A and vitamin C.

Butter is made from milk and contains high quantities of saturated fatty acids.

Ingredients and amounts for 4 people

✓ 4 ripe mangos

✓ 5 tablespoons butter

✓ 6 tablespoons sugar

✓ 1 tablespoon dark rum

Preparation

Peel the mangos, cut them in half, and remove the stone.

Melt the butter in a casserole dish, add the sugar, and stir until melted. Add the mangos to the dissolved sugar and pour the remaining butter over the top. Place in the oven heated to 350°F for a few minutes and then under the broiler to brown.

When cooked, heat the rum, pour over the mangos, and set afire.

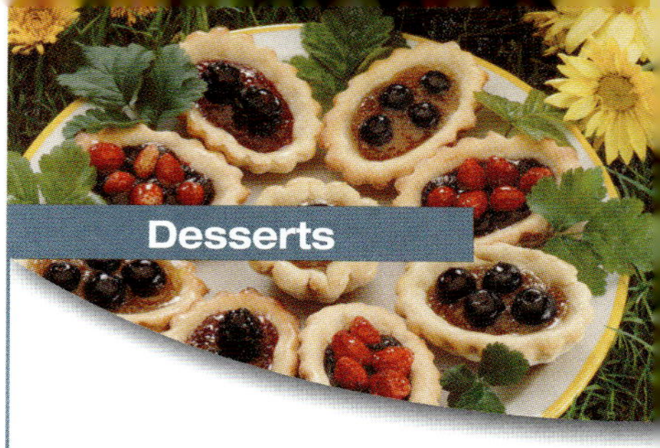

Hot crêpes with mixed berries

Ingredients and amounts for 4 people

- ✓ 1 cup flour
- ✓ 4 tablespoons sugar
- ✓ 1½ cups milk
- ✓ 3 eggs (beaten)
- ✓ 2¾ tablespoons butter
- ✓ 1 tablespoon of orange or mandarin liqueur (optional)
- ✓ 3½ oz raspberries
- ✓ 3½ oz wild strawberries
- ✓ 3½ oz blackberries
- ✓ 3½ oz blueberries
- ✓ 7 oz zabaglione
- ✓ 2¾ tablespoons icing sugar
- ✓ 6¾ oz red port
- ✓ pinch of salt

Preparation of the mixed berries: Wash the mixed berries, dry them gently, and soak them for an hour in the port.

Preparation of the batter: Mix the flour, sugar, and a pinch of salt; dilute with warm milk, add the beaten eggs and mix all the ingredients together. Flavor with the orange or mandarin liqueur (optional); leave the batter in the refrigerator for approximately 1 hour. Add the butter that has been melted over gentle heat.

Preparation for the crêpes: Coat a nonstick pan with butter, heat, and add a ladleful of the batter; cook the first crêpe, turning it to cook on both sides, keep warm. Continue in this way until all the batter has been used; coat the pan with butter between the preparation of one crepe and the next.

Filling: Fill the freshly made warm crêpes with the mixed berries and the warm zabaglione (see separate recipe on p. 375), sprinkle with icing sugar, and serve immediately.
For a lighter recipe, exclude the zabaglione even though it would be a great pity not to include it.

Bromatological evaluation per portion

Kcal	996
Protein (%)	10.2
Fats (%)	21.3
Carbohydrates (%)	68.5
Fiber (g)	4
Cholesterol (mg)	611

Valuable contents for the eye: ★★★

Raspberries are rich in vitamin C and flavonoids.
Strawberries are a good source of vitamin C and anthocyanosides.
Blackberries contain iron, vitamin C, and a good quantity of flavonoids.
Blueberries are rich in vitamin C and anthocyanosides.
Red port contains resveratrol and flavonoids.
Milk (particularly whole milk) has a good balance of sugars, fats, and proteins; it contains high quantities of calcium and phosphorous, but particularly fat-soluble anti-oxidant vitamins and water-soluble vitamins.
Sugar is pure rapidly available energy.

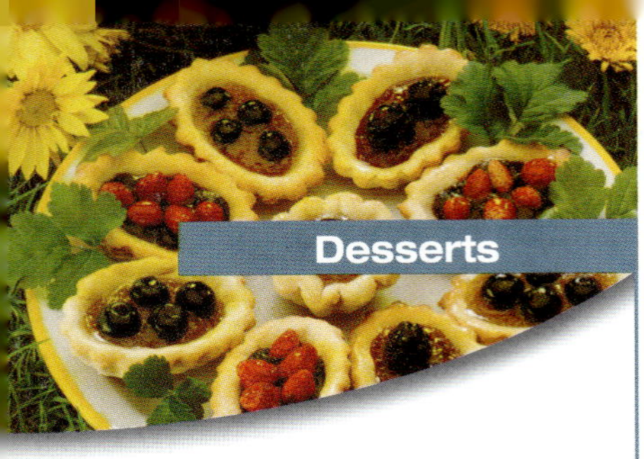

Bromatological evaluation per portion

Kcal	231
Protein (%)	1.2
Fats (%)	5.7
Carbohydrates (%)	93.1
Fiber (g)	0.2
Cholesterol (mg)	0

Valuable contents for the eye: ★★★

Raspberries are rich in vitamin C and flavonoids.
Strawberries are a good source of vitamin C and anthocyanosides.
Blackberries contain iron, vitamin C, and good quantities of flavonoids.
Blueberries are rich in vitamin C and anthocyanosides.
Sugar is pure, rapidly available energy.
Lemon contains high quantities of vitamin C and β-carotene. It also contains flavonoids (particularly in the pith or albedo) underneath the peel.

Mixed berry sorbet

(this recipe requires an ice cream machine)

Ingredients and amounts for 4 people

✓ 14 oz mixed berries (raspberries, wild strawberries, blackberries, blueberries)
✓ 10½ tablespoons sugar
✓ juice of 1 lemon
✓ 2 tablespoons of grenadine syrup

Preparation

Pour the lemon juice over the mixed berries that have been cut into pieces; add the sugar and the syrup, stir, and pour the mixture into the drum of the ice cream making machine.
Activate the machine for approximately 25 to 30 minutes.

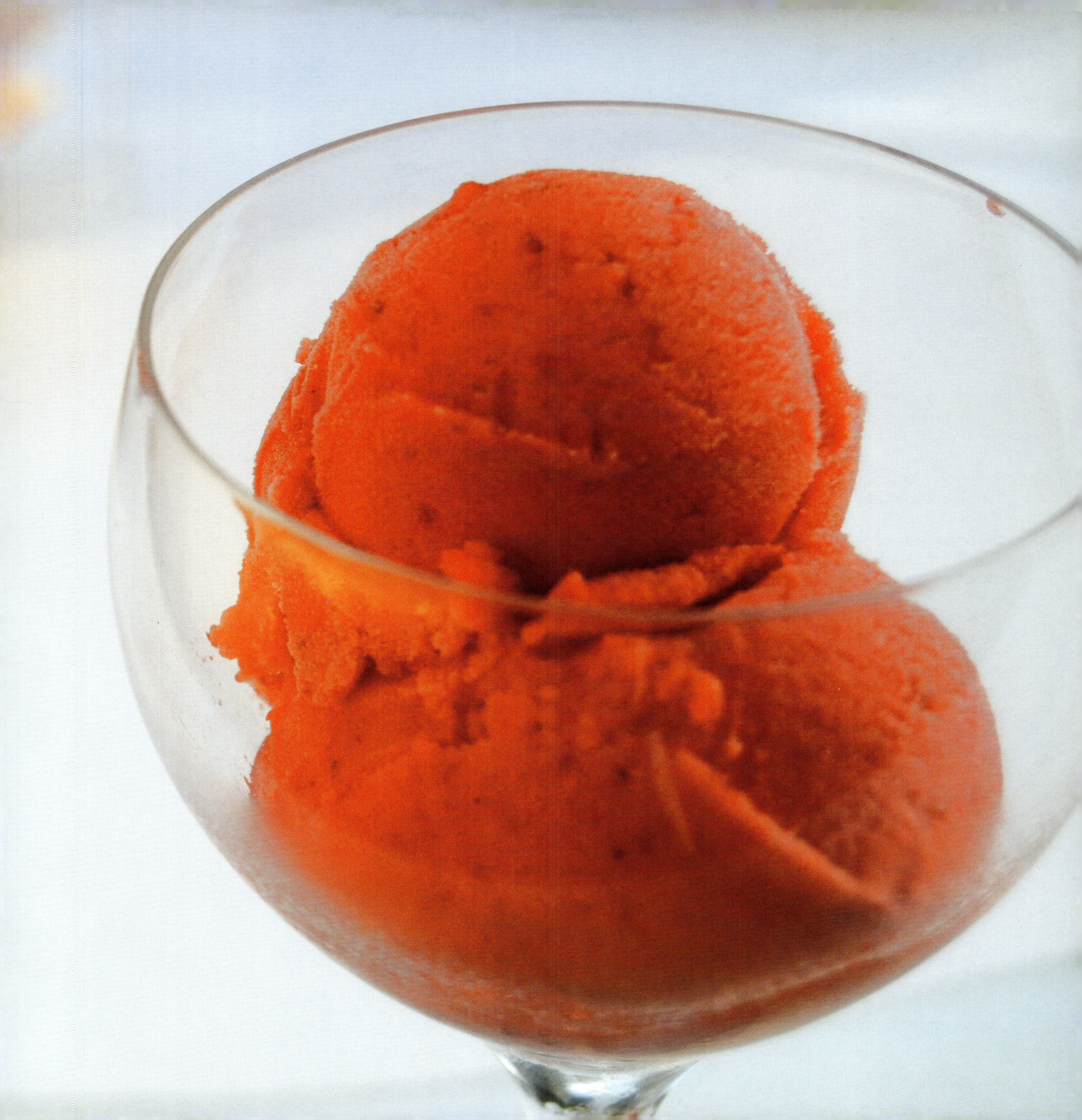